Body Contouring Surgery

Springer Nature More Media App

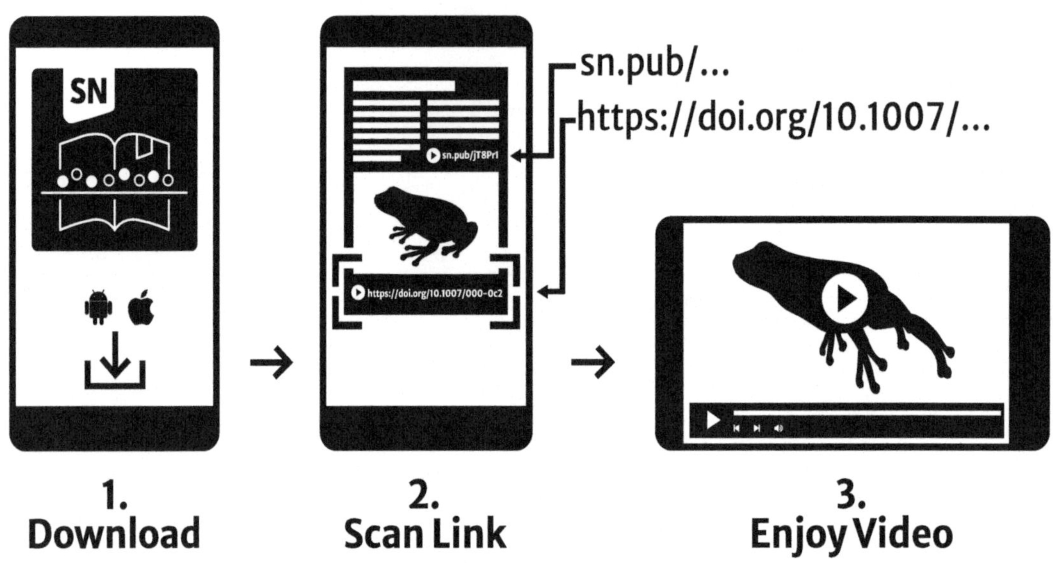

Support: customerservice@springernature.com

Evgeni Sharkov

Body Contouring Surgery

The Role of Non-Invasive, Minimal-Invasive and Surgical Technologies

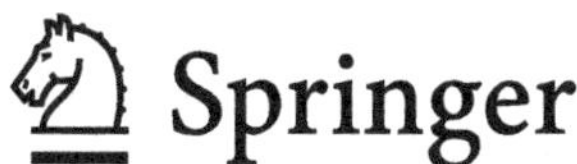

Evgeni Sharkov
Private Aesthetic Clinic VDERM
Sofia, Bulgaria

This work contains media enhancements, which are displayed with a "play" icon. Material in the print book can be viewed on a mobile device by downloading the Springer Nature "More Media" app available in the major app stores. The media enhancements in the online version of the work can be accessed directly by authorized users.

ISBN 978-3-031-33352-1 ISBN 978-3-031-33350-7 (eBook)
https://doi.org/10.1007/978-3-031-33350-7

This Springer imprint is published by the registered company Springer Nature Switzerland AG
The registered company address is: Gewerbestrasse 11, 6330 Cham, Switzerland

I would like to dedicate this book to my wife Irina Sharkova, MD, to our daughter Ivana Sharkova, and to my parents.

Preface

In my practice as a specialist in Plastic, Reconstructive and Aesthetic Surgery during the last years, I have seen a growth in the percentage of patients looking to improve their appearance through procedures which are characterized with minimal or no recovery period, minimal or no risk of side effects and of course to achieve the best results.

After a long period of careful research and exchange of experience with specialists in different fields of aesthetic medicine from all around the world, I was able to select and offer different types of non-invasive and minimally invasive technologies to our patients together with Dr. Irina Sharkova who is a Dermatology Specialist and a leading specialist in her field in Bulgaria.

Many of my patients ask for my professional opinion about body contouring in case of obesity or massive weight loss. Nowadays, the patients I take for consultations are very well informed about different types of technologies which have a positive effect on their aesthetic problem. The hardest part is to provide an accurate information to the patient about the extent to which a particular technology could help solve the aesthetic problem in question.

The surgeon's assessment about whether the particular aesthetic problem is solvable with a non-invasive technology, minimally invasive technology, operative technology, or a combination of these technologies is of a big essence. Depending on the chosen method and the specific preoperative status, we need to explain to the patients to what extent will their condition improve:

- **Obesity**—in this case, the method needs to be in accordance with the extent of obesity and depending on this the patient needs to be redirected to a specialist on bariatric surgery and needs additional guidelines for weight loss through physical and/or diet plan. The patient may need to improve his/her condition through non-invasive interventions such as Evolve X™ or minimally invasive techniques such as BodyTite™, FaceTite™, AccuTite™, Morpheus8™, Morpheus8 Body™ radio frequency procedures, vibrational type of lipoaspiration, and VASERlipo®. A combination of surgical excision procedure and one or more of the abovementioned minimally invasive techniques in the treated area and/or other nearby body areas together with the non-invasive additional treatment during the postoperative period—Evolve X™, Ultherapy®, truSculpt® flex.
- **massive weight loss**—in these cases, I do not make compromises in my practice and the only option for this particular patient to be treated by me

is through surgical excisional procedures and all of the technologies can be applied in nearby body areas and/or during the postoperative period which aims to optimize the final result. In my practice, I have started to frequently apply FaceTite™ which is a radiofrequency procedure that aims to tighten the skin in the neck area, and it gives positive results for me and the patient in regard to the final result. My observations are that although there is a massive weight loss and a decrease in the collagen potential the radio frequent energy contributes extremely for the tightening of the skin even in such cases. In the light of this, in my practice I treat 90% of these patients through this type of minimally invasive procedure as opposed to the facelift surgical intervention.

- **young patients with normal body weight** who are searching for a slight improvement in a particular body area—improvement of the condition through non-invasive interventions like Evolve X™, truSculpt® flex, Ultherapy®, or minimally invasive techniques like BodyTite™, FaceTite™, AccuTite™, Morpheus8™, Morpheus8 Body™ radiofrequency procedures, vibrational type of lipoaspiration, and VASERlipo®.
- **fit patients who want their muscle groups sculpted and defined**—improvement in the condition through non-invasive interventions like Evolve X™, truSculpt®flex. Muscle definition through VASERlipo® ultrasound intervention combined with vibrational type of lipoaspiration with or without radiofrequency procedures—all of this in one intervention.
- in my practice, I frequently use operative interventions as a solution for patients who have a normal **body weight with excessive skin after weight loss, but not massive weight loss**. In cases where patients request a definition, my approach is a combination of excisional procedure with VASERlipo® ultrasound intervention combined with vibrational type of lipoaspiration with or without radiofrequency procedures. We add the non-invasive techniques during the postoperative period so that we can optimize the recovery period and the final results.

The plan is in accordance with the patient's choice whether they want to undergo a surgical procedure. Patients who do not consent to a surgical procedure have to be acquainted with the possible alternatives. Whereas patients who are willing to undergo a surgical procedure should not be urged to use an alternative solution to the problem through other methods. The alternative approach is an option after which the patients can assess the situation again and make a decision whether the achieved results are sufficient, or they would like an additional improvement through a surgical intervention. I can state that my collaboration with Dr. Irina Sharkova as a leading specialist in dermatology has always led to the successful and complex managing of my patients. With reference to this, we can list various injection and laser procedures performed by Dr. Irina Sharkova and her team of dermatologists in our clinics, and we aim to always optimize the final result.

The influence in my practice, the approach towards my patients and guiding them through their preoperative and postoperative period is a result from my practice in Aleksandrovska University Hospital, Sofia, Bulgaria, where I had the opportunity to study under the guidance of Assoc. Prof. Roman

Romanski MD. The decision to believe in the radiofrequency procedures and their effectiveness I owe to Dr. Pier Paolo Rovatti who educates internationally for many years in radiofrequency technologies. The thing that changed everything in regard to my abilities to precisely contour the bodies of my patients is the practice which was led under the guidance of the doyenne of body contouring procedures Dr. Alfredo Hoyos in Bogota, Colombia. I can bravely state that for me Dr. Alfredo Hoyos is not only a surgeon and a doctor, but a brilliant creator and visionary in the field of plastic surgery. During the years, I have had the opportunity to meet people like Al Ali, MD, and Prof. Denis Hurwitz. The techniques they use and implement are in the core of my practice. I would like to express my gratitude to Dr. Francois Petit for sharing his techniques in buttock augmentation.

My everyday work and the success of our practice could not be possible without the dedication and the professionalism of our team—including our team of surgeons, dermatologists, and anaesthesiologists as well as the treatment and care of patients from the team of nurses in our clinics. Through this book, I would like to present how I apply combinations of different kinds of technologies and surgical interventions in my practice. My aim is to optimize the final results in body contouring. Based on the information that I gathered when performing the interventions during the last couple of years I will attempt to systemize when, how, and which technologies to combine—the combination of technologies and the combination of technologies with surgical excision techniques. In this book, I have presented combined approaches, pure excision procedures as well as pure non-invasive and pure minimally invasive procedures and the results from them.

Sofia, Bulgaria Evgeni Sharkov

Disclosure

International trainer for INMODE radiofrequency devices—BodyTite™, FaceTite™, AccuTite™, Morpheus8™, Morpheus8 Body™, EVOLVE X™.

Contents

Introduction

Obesity and Overweight

Obesity is a health problem that itself poses an immediate health risk. Globally, there has been a threefold increase in the number of people suffering from overweight and obesity since 1975. Statistics show that in 2016, more than 1.9 trillion people over 18 years of age were overweight, of which 650 million were obese. In 2016, 41 million children under the age of 5 were overweight or obese, and in the age group between 5 and 19 years, the figure was 340 million. The majority of the world's population lives in countries where overweight and obesity prevail over malnutrition as a cause of death [1].

Characteristics

Obesity is a chronic pathological condition characterized by the accumulation of an excessive amount of adipose tissue in the human body. Obesity is the result of a disturbed energy balance—the ratio between the energy value of food and the energy consumption of a person. Depending on the degree of accumulation of adipose tissue, the condition is defined as overweight or obesity [1–3]. *The overweight factor leads to a potential increase in the risk of cardiovascular and cerebrovascular diseases, type 2 diabetes, joint and respiratory diseases, and malignant neoplasms. The excessive accumulation of adipose tissue is a risk factor for the development of osteoarthritis, sleep apnoea, gastro-oesophageal reflux, arterial hypertension, diabetes mellitus, heart failure, pulmonary asthma, postmenopausal breast cancer, and carcinoma of the endometrium, colon, prostate, gall bladder and biliary tract* [2, 3].

Risk Factors

1. *Genetic factors*: If one of the parents is obese, the probability for the child to develop obesity is 40%; if both parents are obese, the probability is 80%. Without family burden, the percentage is 10 [1, 4, 5].
2. *Environmental factors*: In many cases, the living environment is not conducive to a healthy lifestyle [1, 4, 5]. Examples of this are the lack of accessible sporting facilities, parks and bike lanes; the large portion sizes; the composition of food, etc.
3. *Physiological factors* [1, 4, 5]: This group of factors involves disorders in the exchange of adipose tissue, hormonal changes, etc.
4. *Psychological factors* [1, 4, 5]: In some people, the emotional state affects nutrition. This group of factors includes eating disorders.
5. *Conditions and diseases* such as insulin resistance, hypothyroidism and Cushing's syndrome [1, 4, 5].
6. *Medications*: Taking some medications is associated with an increase in body mass: antidepressants, anticonvulsants, some medications used in the treatment of diabetes, some hormonal preparations, corticosteroids, etc. [1, 4, 5].

E. Sharkov, *Body Contouring Surgery*, https://doi.org/10.1007/978-3-031-33350-7_1

Types of Obesity

Depending on the distribution of the subcutaneous adipose tissue, there are three types of obesity [1, 6]:

1. Generalized—the thickness of the subcutaneous adipose tissue increases throughout the body.
2. Female type (gynoid) or peripheral—the deposition of fats is mainly in the lower part of the body (hip); the body becomes pear-shaped.
3. Male type (android) or central—the largest amount of adipose tissue is deposited on the abdomen and chest; the body becomes apple-shaped.

Body Mass Index (BMI)

Body mass index (BMI) is a measure used to assess obesity. It is calculated by dividing the weight in kilograms by the height in square meters: BMI = kg/m^2. It is usually assumed that people with BMI ≥ 30 kg/m^2 have excessive accumulation of adipose tissue, but BMI is not an indicator to distinguish between muscle and adipose tissue [7–10].

Degrees of obesity according to body mass index (BMI) and risk of comorbidities

Classification	BMI (kg/m^2)	Risk of obesity-related complications
Normal weight	18.5–24.9	Not high
Overweight	25.0–29.9	High
Obesity I degree	30.0–34.9	Moderately high
Obesity II degree	35.0–39.9	Very high
Obesity III degree	40	Extremely high

Waist Circumference and Waist-Hip Ratio

Waist circumference measurement is another metric used to assess obesity. Increased waist circumference is associated with a significantly higher risk of cardiovascular disease through increased systolic and diastolic blood pressure values [11].

The waist-hip ratio (WHR) can be used to assess the redistribution of adipose tissue in the body and determine the type of obesity. A normal waist-hip ratio should be less than 1.0 for men and 0.85 for women [12]. The incidence of cardiovascular and cerebrovascular accidents has been shown to increase with increasing waist-hip ratio in both sexes.

Risk of developing obesity-related complications

	Waist circumference in centimetres	
Risk of complications	Men	Women
Increased	≥94	≥80
Significantly increased	≥102	≥88

Massive Weight Loss

Massive weight loss is defined as losing more than 45 kg or more than 100% of the ideal weight for the individual. Epidemiological and clinical studies indicate a positive influence of comorbidity in patients with obesity after significant weight reduction [13]. Patients with II–III degree obesity are more often resistant to significant weight reduction through conventional methods such as diet, physical and behavioural regimen, as well as various pharmaceuticals. Obesity leads to psychogenic, hormonal, metabolic and anatomical changes, which in themselves lead to further obesity [1, 13]. On the psychogenic side, a distress syndrome develops, which stimulates the production of hormones and neuropeptides that increase the accumulation of adipose tissue and lead to deviations in the diet. Hormonal changes include increased production of insulin and cortisol, decreased levels of dehydroepiandrosterone, decreased production of growth factors, increased levels of oestrogen relative to testosterone in males, increased levels of progesterone and increased levels of androgen hormones in females. The listed hormonal changes lead to both an increased accumulation of fat in the fat depots and the inhibition of lipolysis processes.

Statistically, this type of patients, after stopping the nutritional and/or physical regimen, not only regain the lost kilograms, but often even gain extra body weight.

Bariatric Surgery

The idea of surgical treatment of obesity arose from the fact that patients who underwent gastric and small intestinal resections experienced weight loss. The jejunoileal bypass (JIB) performed by Kremen et al. in 1954, consisting of anastomosing the 40th cm of the jejunum with the ileum, but 10 cm from the ileocecal valve, was accepted as the beginning of bariatric surgery. Despite the initial efforts to improve this technique, it was rejected due to serious side effects associated with bacterial overgrowth, diarrhoea, dehydration and liver damage [1, 14]. In the 1970s, Mason introduced vertical banded gastroplasty with a ring (VBG), which is based on the restriction of the size of the stomach and the additional placement of a reinforcing ring. In recent years, however, it has also been denied due to frequent complications such as vomiting, reflux and, above all, repeated weight gain [14, 15]. Again, Mason also introduced the Roux-en-Y gastric bypass, in which part of the stomach is bypassed by creating an anastomosis between it and the jejunum. This operation remains one of the most popular even today [15, 16]. The first operation with the idea of malabsorption as a weight loss mechanism was performed by Scopinaro in 1972. In it, after horizontal resection of the stomach and reduction of its capacity to absorb food, biliopancreatic diversion (BPD) is performed—bypass of biliopancreatic juices or shortening of the length of the small intestine through which resorption of nutrients is possible, by separating them from the biliopancreatic juices [17, 18]. This leads to certain malabsorption. Similar is also Marceau's operation—duodenal switch (DS), in which, however, the passage of food through the pylorus is preserved by interrupting the duodenum below it and anastomosing it with the distal ileum [19]. This also leads to a lot of weight loss, even in patients who are unable to fully comply with a dietary regimen, reducing the incidence of side effects such as diarrhoea and malabsorption of important nutrients.

With maturation of laparoscopic gastrointestinal surgery in the 1990s, minimally invasive techniques were applied to bariatric surgery. As Wittgrove performed the first laparoscopic gastric bypass, he is considered the father of laparoscopic bariatric surgery [20]. Laparoscopic operations are quickly becoming the 'gold standard'. Later, after the work of various teams from Italy, Belgium, Sweden and the USA, new, typical laparoscopic operations were also introduced, such as placing an adjustable gastric banding (AGB) and the most modern operation that is gaining more and more popularity in recent times—sleeve gastrectomy (SG) [21].

Indications

According to the recommendations of the U.S. National Institutes of Health Consensus Conference in 1991, bariatric surgery should be done considering the following patient characteristics and other factors [22]:

- BMI >40 kg/m^2
- BMI >35 kg/m^2 with proven one of the following accompanying diseases that can be influenced by the operation—type 2 diabetes, arterial hypertension, sleep apnoea and dyslipidaemia
- Age between 18 and 60 years
- Long-term history of obesity with unsuccessful conservative treatment for at least 6 months
- Absence of an endocrine disease that is the cause of obesity
- Mentally stable patient, without alcohol and drug addiction
- Well-motivated patients, understanding the principle and risks of the operation, capable of long-term post-operative follow-up
- Acceptable operational risk
- Centres specialized in performing these operations with well-trained and experienced surgical team and medical staff

An increasing number of studies have accumulated on bariatric surgery in patients with BMI >30 kg/m^2 and <35 kg/m^2 and the presence of type 2 diabetes mellitus, which demonstrate an advantage of operative treatment over conservative treatment in terms of weight loss and control of type 2 diabetes mellitus [23].

In recent years, much has been speculated about the application of bariatric surgery in the treatment of severe obesity in patients under 18 years of age. There are opposing opinions on this issue, which has a moral, ethical and legal side. The results show a significant and lasting reduction in the body weight, with the surgery preventing the emotional and physical consequences of obesity in the growing population [13, 24]. However, further research and society tuning are needed for bariatric surgery to be accepted as a method for treatment of severe obesity in patients under 18 years of age. A strict selection and case-by-case assessment are currently recommended in this group of patients.

References

1. Grozdev K. Multidisciplinary approach in bariatric/metabolic surgery. 2021;9–30.
2. Bray G, Bouchard C. Handbook of obesity. CRC Press Taylor & Francis Group; 2014.
3. Bray GA, Kim KK, Wilding JPH, World Obesity Federation. Obesity: a chronic relapsing progressive disease process. A position statement of the World Obesity Federation. Obes Rev. 2017;18:715–23.
4. Keith SW, Redden DT, Katzmarzyk PT, Boggiano MM, Hanlon EC, Benca RM, et al. Putative contributors to the secular increase in obesity: exploring the roads less traveled. Int J Obes. 2006;30:1585–94.
5. Janesick AS, Shioda T, Blumberg B. Transgenerational inheritance of prenatal obesogen exposure. Mol Cell Endocrinol. 2014;398:31–5.
6. Vague J. The degree of masculine differentiation of obesities: a factor determining predisposition to diabetes, atherosclerosis, gout, and uric calculous disease. 1956. Obes Res. 1996;4:204–12.
7. WHO. Obesity: preventing and managing the global epidemic: report of a WHO Consultation on Obesity, Geneva, 3–5 June 1997. Epidemic Opamtg. Geneva: World Health Organization; 1998.
8. Webster JD, Hesp R, Garrow JS. The composition of excess weight in obese women estimated by body density, total body water and total body potassium. Hum Nutr Clin Nutr. 1984;38:299–306.
9. Willett WC, Dietz WH, Colditz GA. Guidelines for healthy weight. N Engl J Med. 1999;341:427–34.
10. Staiano AE, Bouchard C, Katzmarzyk PT. BMI-specific waist circumference thresholds to discriminate elevated cardiometabolic risk in White and African American adults. Obes Facts. 2013;6:317–24.
11. Romero-Corral A, Lopez-Jimenez F, Sierra-Johnson J, Somers VK. Differentiating between body fat and lean mass-how should we measure obesity? Nat Clin Pract Endocrinol Metab. 2008;4:322–3.
12. Bjorntorp P, Bengtsson C, Blohme G, Jonsson A, Sjostrom L, Tibblin E, et al. Adipose tissue fat cell size and number in relation to metabolism in randomly selected middle-aged men and women. Metabolism. 1971;20:927–35.
13. Inge TH, Courcoulas AP, Jenkins TM, Michalsky MP, Helmrath MA, Brandt ML, et al. Weight loss and health status 3 years after bariatric surgery in adolescents. N Engl J Med. 2016;374(2):113–23.
14. Baker MT. The history and evolution of bariatric surgical procedures. Surg Clin North Am. 2011;91:1181–201.
15. Mason EE, Ito C. Gastric bypass in obesity. Surg Clin North Am. 1967;47:1345–51.
16. Mason EE, Printen KJ, Hartford CE, Boyd WC. Optimizing results of gastric bypass. Ann Surg. 1975;182:405–14.
17. Scopinaro N, Gianetta E, Civalleri D, Bonalumi U, Bachi V. Bilio-pancreatic bypass for obesity: II. Initial experience in man. Br J Surg. 1979;66:618–20.
18. Scopinaro N. Biliopancreatic diversion: mechanisms of action and long-term results. Obes Surg. 2006;16:683–9.
19. Marceau P, Biron S, Bourque RA, Potvin M, Hould FS, Simard S. Biliopancreatic diversion with a new type of gastrectomy. Obes Surg. 1993;3:29–35.
20. Wittgrove AC, Clark GW, Tremblay LJ. Laparoscopic gastric bypass, Roux-en-Y: preliminary report of five cases. Obes Surg. 1994;4:353–7.
21. Sánchez-Pernaute A, Herrera MA, Pérez-Aguirre ME, Talavera P, Cabrerizo L, Matía P, et al. Single anastomosis duodeno-ileal bypass with sleeve gastrectomy (SADI-S). One to three-year follow-up. Obes Surg. 2010;20:1720–6.
22. NIH conference Consensus Development Conference Panel. Gastrointestinal surgery for severe obesity. Ann Intern Med. 1991;115:956–61.
23. Serrot FJ, Dorman RB, Miller CJ, Slusarek B, Sampson B, Sick BT, et al. Comparative effectiveness of bariatric surgery and nonsurgical therapy in adults with type 2 diabetes mellitus and body mass index <35 kg/m^2. Surgery. 2011;150(4):684–91.
24. Hazzan D, Chin EH, Steinhagen E, et al. Laparoscopic bariatric surgery can be safe for treatment of morbid obesity in patients older than 60 years. Surg Obes Relat Dis. 2006;2(6):613–6.

Part I

Non-invasive Techniques

Non-invasive Radiofrequency and Myostimulation-Based Procedures

Non-invasive Radiofrequency-Based Procedures

EVOLVE X™ is a radiofrequency device based on the principle of bipolar radiofrequency, which allows, through accommodation in the parameters, to achieve an improvement in skin tone through collagen stimulation, reduction in fat deposits and stimulation of muscle tone [1–3]. Performed as an independent procedure, the improvement is 20–30% of the optimal expectations (Table 1), and for this purpose a physical and nutritional regimen is also recommendable (Figs. 1, 2) .

Non-invasive Myostimulation Procedures

This type of non-invasive procedures, independently applied without previous surgical intervention, would also have a satisfactory result, if a nutritional and physical regimen is observed and no accompanying metabolic disorders are present [4–8]. **truSculpt® flex** is one of the devices that rely on electric muscle stimulation. It has three modes of operation and allows toning and tightening of the muscles in up to eight areas at the same time (Fig. 3a, b; Table 2).

E. Sharkov, *Body Contouring Surgery*, https://doi.org/10.1007/978-3-031-33350-7_2

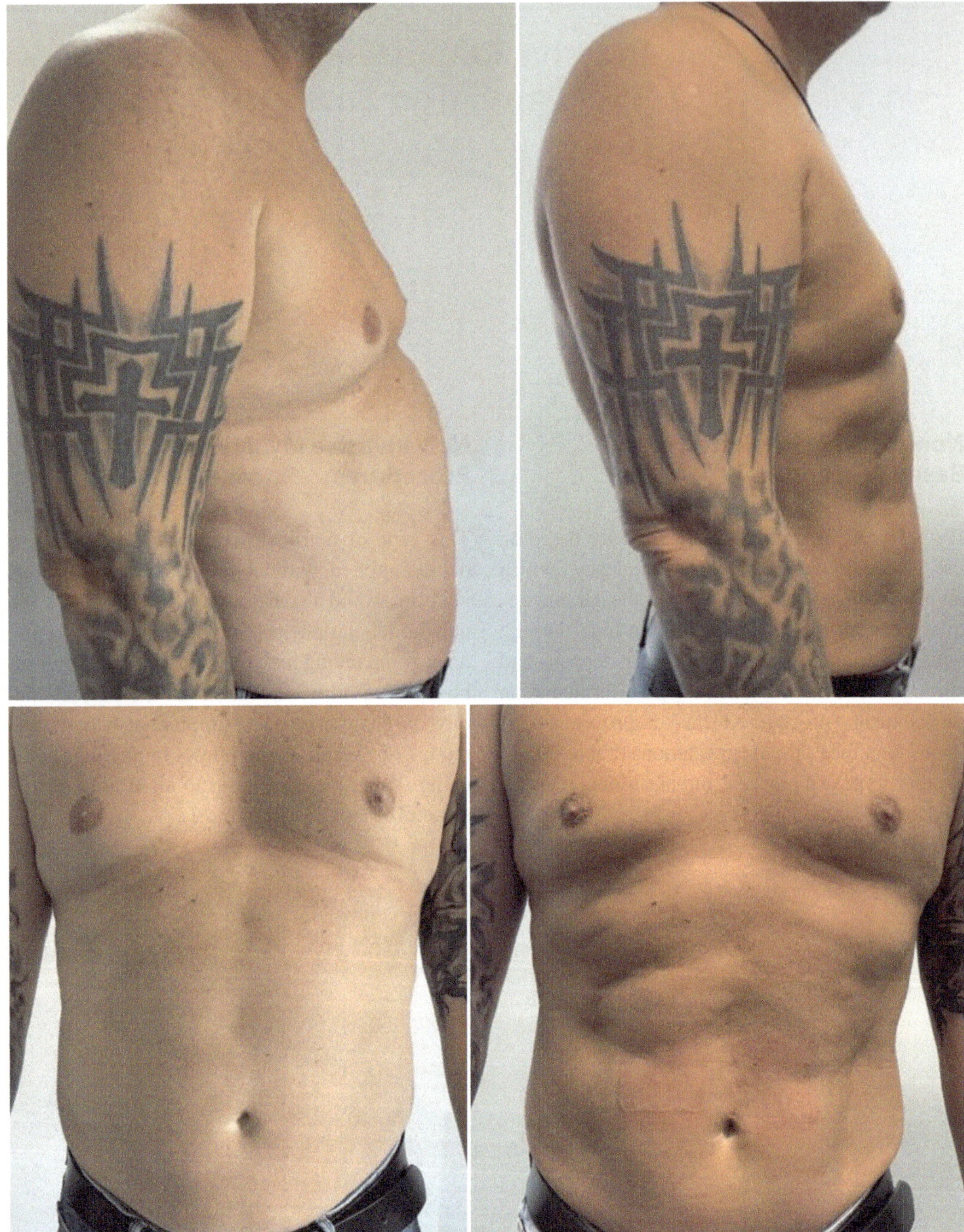

Fig. 1 Patient before and after 4 sessions with EVOLVE X™

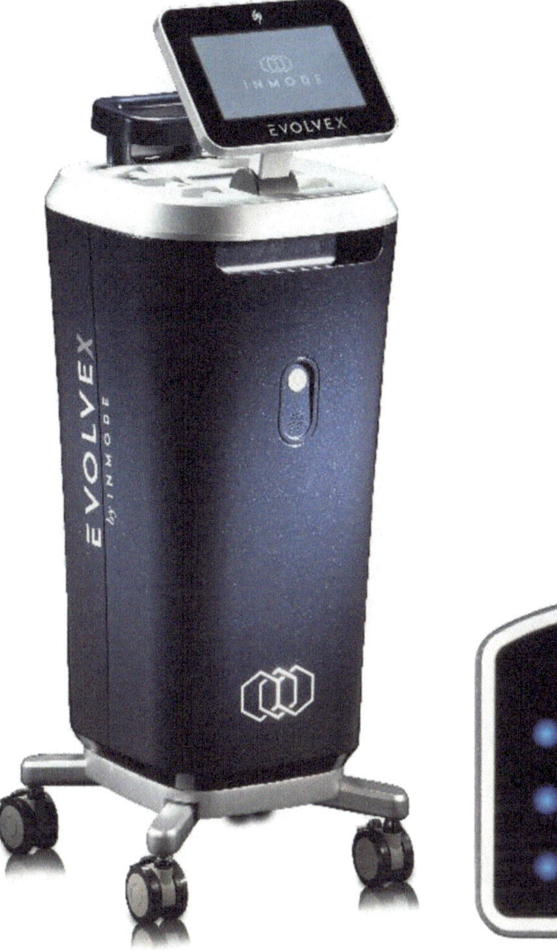

Fig. 2 EVOLVE X™ with 'TRANSFORM' applicators that can simultaneously together "Tite", "Tone" and "Trim" in a single session, meaning tightening the skin, stimulate the muscle contraction and melt the subcutaneous fat

Table 1 EVOLVE X™: treatment protocol used by the author

Effect	Tightens skin, lipolysis, muscle stimulation
Number of procedures	6–8, once a week
Areas	Legs, arms, abdomen, flank area
RF level	Starting from 20 J and gradually increasing to 30 J
Temperature	Starting from 40° and gradually increasing during the procedure
EMS (electromyostimulation)	Starting at level 5 and gradually increasing according to the patient's tolerance
Final result	6 weeks after the last procedure

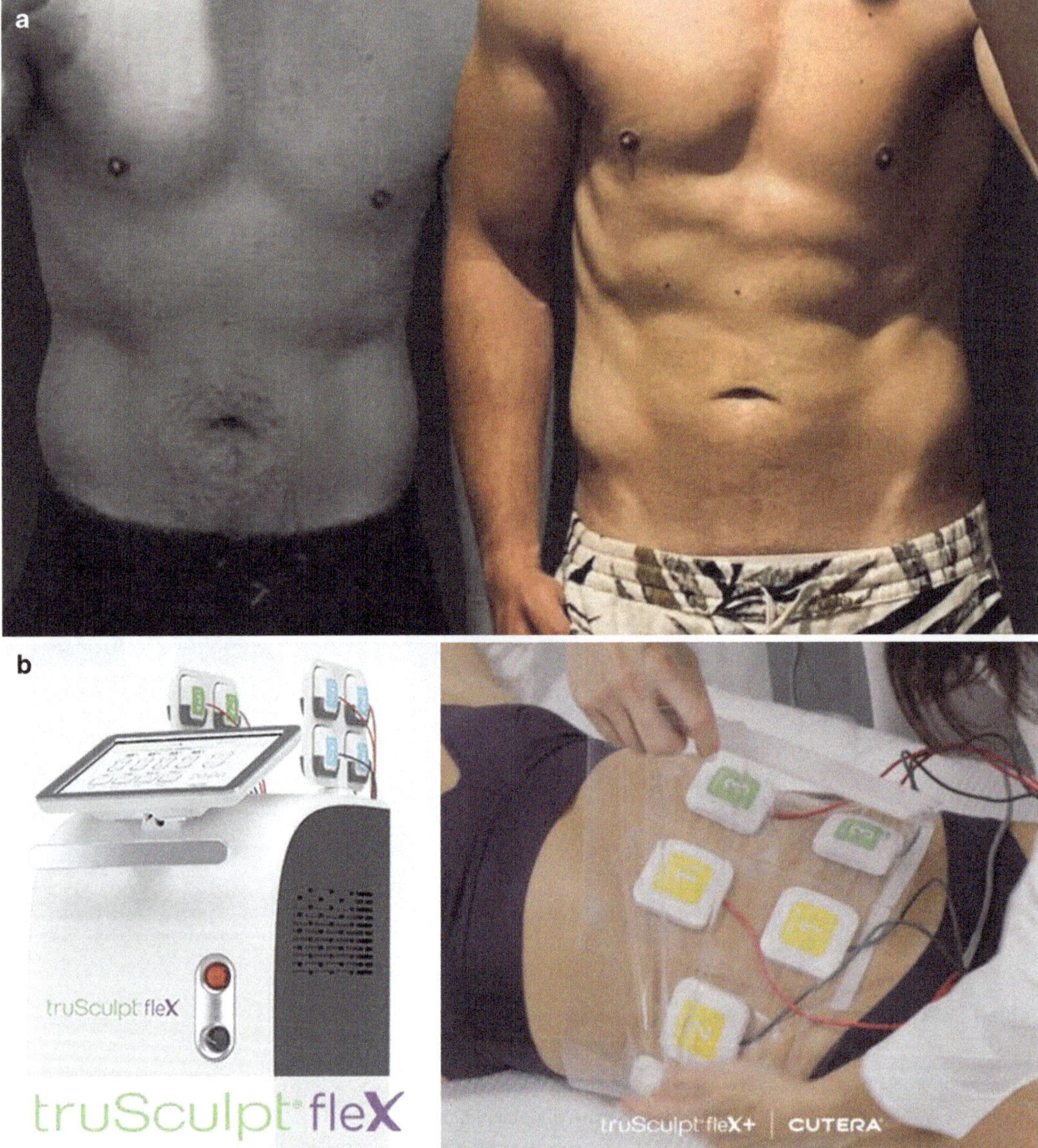

Fig. 3 (**a**) Before and after 4 sessions truSculpt® flex done by Irina Sharkova MD, following the protocol described in Table 2. (**b**) truSculpt® flex with the applicators for myostimulation

- Stimulates twisting movements and smooth stretching that mimic a warm-up workout with gradually increasing muscle stimulation.
- Stimulates retention and relaxation similar to strength training such as squats, and leads to increased muscle endurance.
- Fast, deep, successive contractions that cause the muscle to increase in volume, i.e. to grow.

Table 2 **trusculpt® flex**—treatment protocol used by the author

Effect	Myostimulation (causes 52–55 thousand muscle contractions in 45 min
Number of procedures	Overall 4–6 / 1–2 times a week
EMS (electromyostimulation)	Starting from 20% and gradually increasing according to the patient's tolerance
A peep mode	Patients who do not sport and do not have an active lifestyle/ the first two procedures to prepare for the next mode
B tone mode	– Sporting and active people Or – After 2 procedures peep mode
C sculpt mode	After several A or B procedures, the specific being that it maintains the muscles in a state of isometric contraction for a period of 30 min

References

1. Mulholland RS. The bodytite book, vol. 261. 2nd ed. Rijeka: IntechOpen; 2021. p. 734–50.
2. Mulholland RS. Radiofrequency energy for non-invasive and minimally invasive skin tightening. Clin Plast Surg. 2011;38:437–48.
3. Hernandez Zendejas G, Reavie DW, Azabache R, et al. Lipoplasty combined with percutaneous radio-frequency Dermaplasty: a new strategy for body contouring. Aesth Plast Surg. 2020;44:455–63.
4. Babault N, Cometti G, Bernardin M, Pousson M, Chatard J-C. Effects of electromyostimulation training on muscle strength and power of elite rugby players. J Strength Cond Res. 2007;21(2):431–7.
5. Billot M, Martin A, Paizis C, Cometti C, Babault N. Effects of an electrostimulation training program on strength, jumping, and kicking capacities in soccer players. J Strength Cond Res. 2010;24(5):1407–13.
6. Watson T, Nussbaum EL, editors. Electrophysical agents: evidence-based practice. Edinburgh: Elsevier; 2021.
7. Watson T. The role of electrotherapy in contemporary physiotherapy practice. Man Ther. 2000;5(3):132–41.
8. Demidas A. Electrical stimulation: then and now. Applications and limitations. Physiother quart. 2021;29(4):81–6.

Non-invasive Ultrasound Based Procedures

Ultrasound Procedures

Ultrasound procedures as a stand-alone intervention are mainly used to tighten and lift the skin by collagen stimulation [1–3]. This type of procedure can be used both as a self-supporting technique and as maintaining the durability of surgically performed interventions such as facelift [4–6]. Ultherapy® is a non-invasive ultrasound device that focuses ultrasound energy at a temperature between 65 and 70 °C in the deep dermal layers and thus stimulates neocollagenogenesis (Fig. 1a, b).

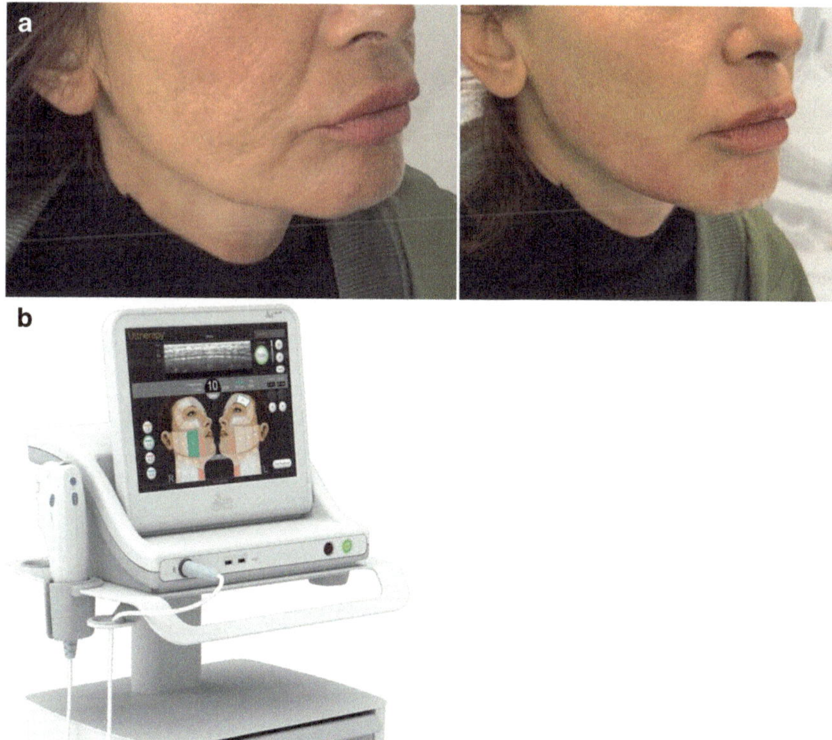

Fig. 1 (**a**) Before and after one procedure with Ultherapy®. Patient of Irina Sharkova MD, who was done following the protocol described in Table 1. (**b**) Ultherapy® device

E. Sharkov, *Body Contouring Surgery*, https://doi.org/10.1007/978-3-031-33350-7_3

Table 1 Ultherapy® treatment protocol

Effect	Tightening skin on neck (necklift)
Number of procedures	2–3 procedures per year. The interval in between the procedure could be 3 or 6 or 9 months, depending on the morphotype
Initial treatment depending on the BMI and the level of the SMAS determined by ultrasound visualization	4 mm depth/0,4–1,2 J mm²/ 4–10 MHz/approximately 75 pulses per area with tip no. 4,5 (DS 4,5) 3 mm depth/ 0,4–1,2 J mm²/ 4–10 MHz/ approximately 75 pulses per area with tip no. 3 (DS 3) 1 mm depth /0,4–1,2 J mm²/ 4–10 MHz/ approximately 75 pulses per area with tip no. 1,5 (DS 1,5)
Following procedures	The amount of pulses is overall half of the initial treatment

References

1. Sklar LR, El Tal AK, Kerwin LY. Use of transcutaneous ultrasound for lipolysis and skin tightening: a review. Aesthet Plast Surg. 2014;38:429–41.
2. Hwang JH, Crum LA. Current status of clinical high-intensity focused ultrasound. Annu Int Conf Proc IEEE Eng Med Biol Soc. 2009;2009:130–3.
3. Chan NP, Shek SY, Yu CS, Ho SG, Yeung CK, Chan HH. Safety study of transcutaneous focused ultrasound for noninvasive skin tightening in Asians. Lasers Surg Med. 2011;43:366–75.
4. Kennedy JE, Ter Haar GR, Cranston D. High-intensity focused ultrasound: surgery of the future? Br J Radiol. 2003;76:590–9.
5. Capla JM, Rubin JP. Discussion: randomized sham-controlled trial to evaluate the safety and effectiveness of a high-intensity focused ultrasound device for noninvasive body sculpting. Plast Reconstr Surg. 2011;128:263–4.
6. Jewell ML, Solish NJ, Desilets CS. Noninvasive body sculpting technologies with an emphasis on high-intensity focused ultrasound. Aesthet Plast Surg. 2011;35:901–12.

Part II

Minimally Invasive Techniques

Minimally Invasive Radiofrequency-Based Procedures: Morpheus8™, Morpheus8 Body™, BodyTite™, FaceTite™, AccuTite™

Introduction

Morpheus8 is a minimally invasive bipolar radiofrequency microneedling procedure. The device uses 2 mm diameter ejecting needles to deliver energy deep into the skin, creating micro-injuries that trigger the body's natural response and encourage the production of new collagen and elastin to tighten the skin [1, 2]. It can be used anywhere on the body, including the abdomen or buttocks, although it is most popular on the face, jawline and neck (Fig. 1a–c). Due to the 40 needle plate with penetration up to 7–8 mm, Morpheus8 Body™ allows non-operative skin tightening and fat destruction to be performed on larger areas of the body as abdomen, thighs and buttocks [3–5] (Fig. 2).

The protocols recommended by the author are as follows:

Face and Neck

Thin Skin

4 mm/35–40 energy/3 stacks per place/50% overlapping/wherever the skin is thicker/cycle mode/1 pps/don't go on fillers

+

3 mm/30–35 energy/2 stacks per place/30–40% overlapping/everywhere except the forehead and upper eyelid area/cycle mode/1 pps/

+

1 or 2 mm/12–25 energy/1 stacks per place/no overlapping/everywhere, including the forehead and periorbital area/Cycle mode/1pps/

Those are applied for the neck, having the same pattern

Face and Neck

Thicker Skin and Submental Fat, also Acne Scaring Tissue

4 mm/35–40 energy/3 stacks per place/50% overlapping/wherever the skin is thicker/fixed mode/1 pps/don't go on fillers

+

3 mm/30–35 energy/2 stacks per place/30–40% overlapping/everywhere except the forehead and upper eyelid area/fixed mode/1pps/

+

2 mm/12–25 energy/1 stacks per place/no overlapping/everywhere, including the forehead and periorbital area/Cycle MODE/1ppp/

those are applied for the neck, having the same pattern

Supplementary Information The online version contains supplementary material available at https://doi.org/10.1007/978-3-031-33350-7_4. The videos can be accessed individually by clicking the DOI link in the accompanying figure caption or by scanning this link with the SN More Media App.

E. Sharkov, *Body Contouring Surgery*, https://doi.org/10.1007/978-3-031-33350-7_4

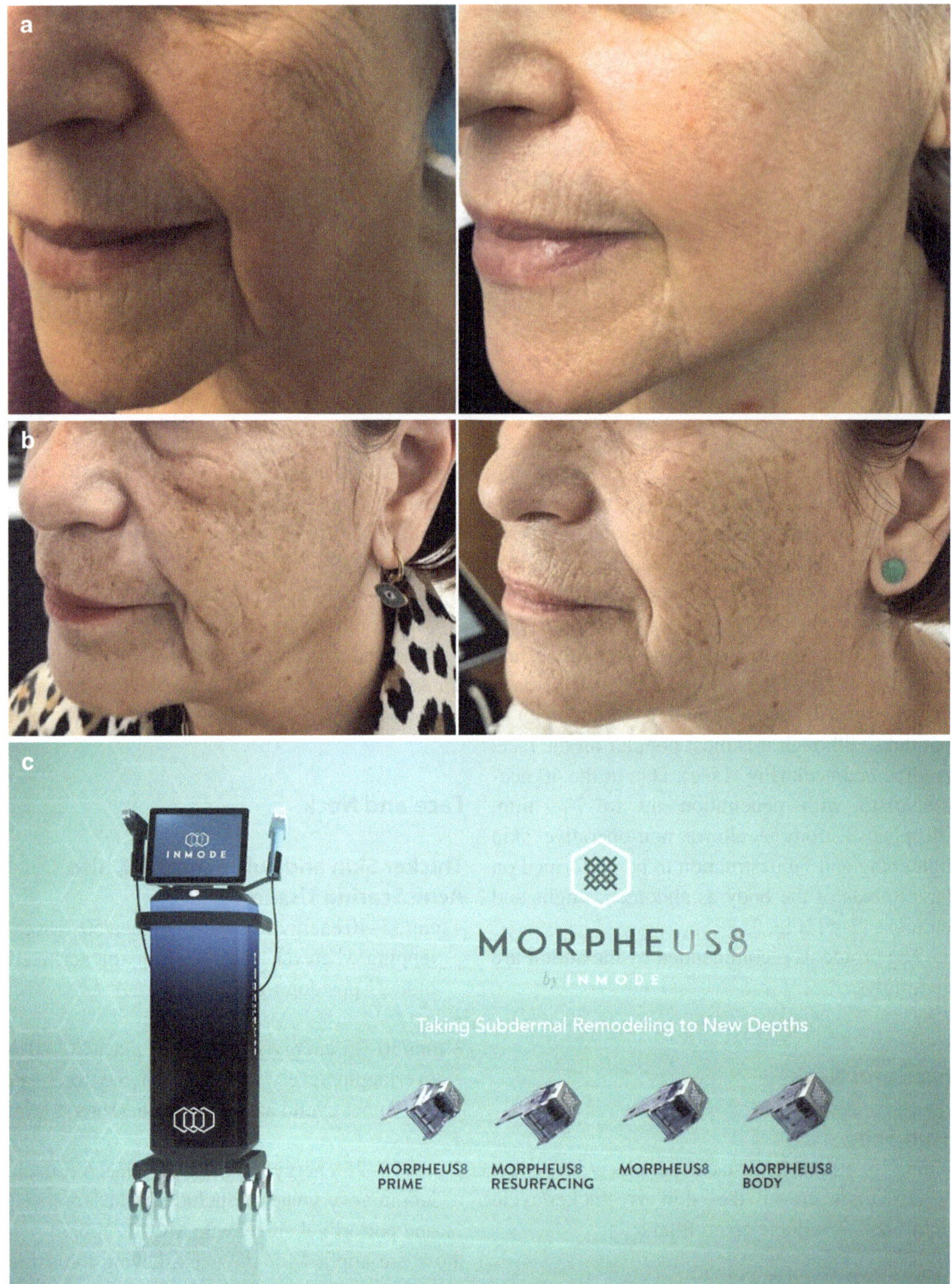

Fig. 1 (**a**) Before and 45 days after one session Morpheus8™. (**b**) Before and 45 days after two session Morpheus8™. (**c**) Morpheus8™ with the different types of tips—Morpheus8 Prime™, Morpheus8 Resurfacing™, Morpheus8, Morpheus8 Body. Morpheus8™ delivers the deepest fractional treatments available. Morpheus8 Body with 3D Smart Frame and Burst technology provides up to 8 mm subdermal adipose tissue remodelling (thermal profile of 7 mm + an additional heat profile of 1 mm)

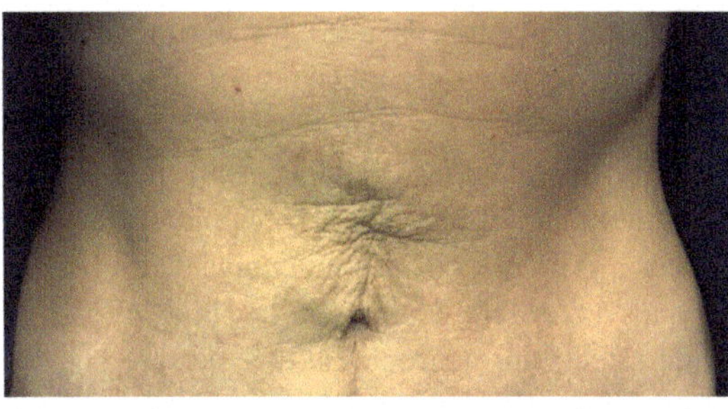

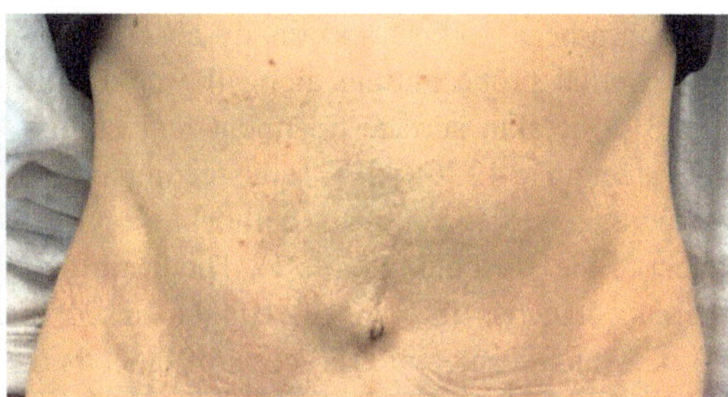

Fig. 2 Before and after Morpheus8 body™ in combination with BodyTite™. BodyTite™—20 kJ were done on the skin above the umbilicus with parameters as follows—40 energy; 40 °C external cut off. Tightening the skin from just one entry point just below the xyphoid. Morpheus8 body—**Burst mode—7-5-3 mm/30 energy/ 3 stacks per place/ 25–30% of overlapping**

Periorbital Rejuvenation: 8 Pin Handpiece-Morpheus8 Prime™

3 mm/ 30–35 energy/2 stacks per place/30–40% overlapping/except upper eyelid area/fixed mode/1pps/to tighten the skin and melt fat in the lower eyelid

+

1 or 2 mm/12–25 energy/1 stacks per place/20% overlapping/everywhere, including the forehead and periorbital area

Morpheus8 body™ allows non-operative skin tightening and fat destruction to be performed on larger areas of the body as abdomen, thighs and buttocks (Fig. 2).

Protocols recommended by the author are as follows:

Morpheus8 Body

To Tighten Skin: Elbows, Neck, Arms, Knees, etc.

4 mm/35–40 energy/3 stacks per place/50% overlapping/wherever the skin is thicker/fixed mode/1pps/

+

3 mm/30–35 energy/2 stacks per place/30–40% overlapping fixed mode/1pps/

+

2 mm/12–25 energy/1 stack per place/cycle

No overlapping

Morpheus8 Body

To Tighten Skin, Melt Superficial Fat and Cellulite—Abdomen, Flanks, Arms, Thighs, Knees, etc./Also for Stretch Marks

1. 7–8 mm/35–40 energy/3 stacks per place/50% overlapping/wherever the skin is thicker/fixed mode/1pps

   +

2. 4–6 mm/30–35 energy/2 stacks per place/30–40% overlapping/fixed mode/1pps/

   +

3. 2 mm/ 12–25 energy/1 stacks per at place/ cycle

   No overlapping

Possible—Burst mode—7-5-3 mm/30 energy/3 punches per place/25–30% of overlapping instead of the above points 1; 2; 3. Advantages—faster procedure as for the patients, as for the doctor.

FaceTite™—a bipolar radiofrequency handpiece. The internal probe emits radiofrequency energy which traverses the intervening soft tissue causing a heat gradient and finally absorbed by the external probe gliding along the epidermis [1–13]. The skin surface treatment temperature can be set up to 42 °C (40 °C is the recommended temperature settlement by the author) for optimal effect of the procedure (Table 1). The heating of the subcutaneous fat deposits can be raised to 70 °C, which results in destruction of fat cells in the treated area. The radiofrequency energy between the two probes stimulates the collagen in the vertical and oblique septa of the subcutaneous adipose, resulting in skin tightening and lifting. The procedure can be performed under local anaesthesia. There is a short recovery period of mild to moderate swelling. The desired effect is observed within a day, with an upward projection towards the final result gradually appearing over the next 6 months. Results persist for a minimum of 6 years. FaceTite is applied in the face and neck, and in smaller areas of the body such as 'banana roll', knees, elbows and armpits. FaceTite can also be used for optimization of results from previous open surgery procedures—an insufficiently satisfactory result of an operative facelift; contour irregularities from previous liposuctions; lifting and tightening of residual excess skin in previous operative lifting techniques in different areas of the body. Possible side effects are neuropraxia that subsides within days or weeks, thermal injury in the area of the entrance holes or on the tip of the internal electrode in case of incorrect handling of the probe; hematomas, fibrous nodules that are successfully treated by corticosteroid application in the area (Figures 1, 2, 3, 4, 5, 6 and 7 video of preoperative markings and the procedure).

AccuTite™—in essence, it is a procedure identical to FaceTite™, the difference being in the physical parameters of the probe, which is designed to treat smaller areas of the face. AccuTite™ can treat the neck and jaw areas for lifting the skin and destroying fatty deposits;

Table 1 FaceTite™ treatment protocols used by the author

Area	Energy	Temperature parameters	Technique
Neck	5–12 kJ	40° ext. t 70° int. t	Tightening and melting fat
Lower 1/3 of face	1–2 kJ per side	-ll-	-ll-
Small areas of the body: – Knees – Armpits – Banana roll – Contour deformities after previous liposuction	8–10 kJ per 10 sq.cm of treated area	-ll-	-ll-

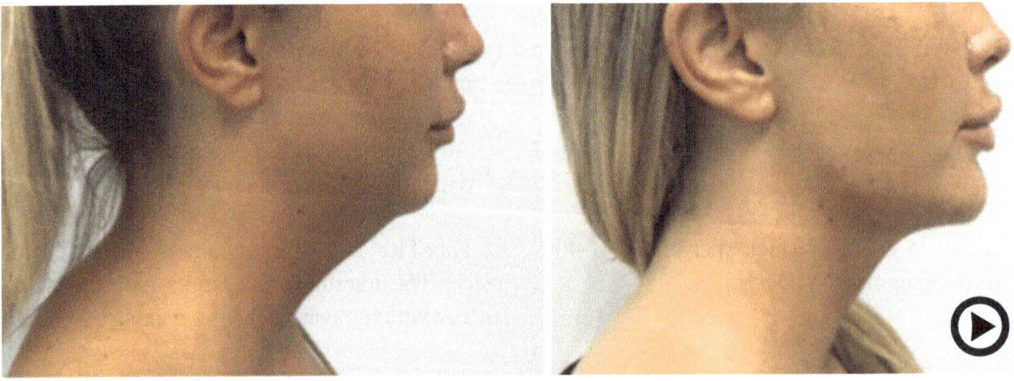

Fig. 3 Before and 6 months after FaceTite™ in a 33-year-old female patient. FaceTite™ of the submental area with liposuction and Morpheus8 in one procedure (▶ https://doi.org/10.1007/000-b0c)

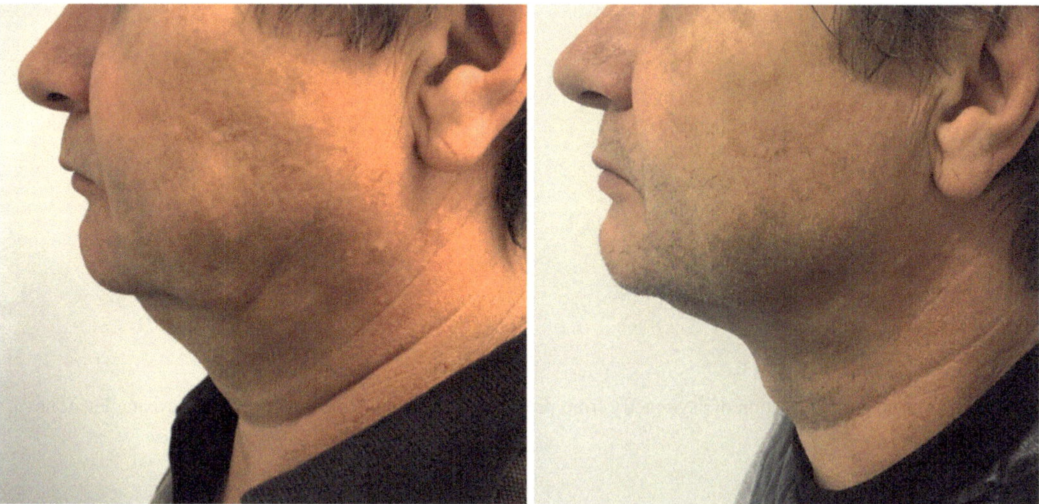

Fig. 4 A 44-year-old male patient. Before and 6 months after FaceTite™

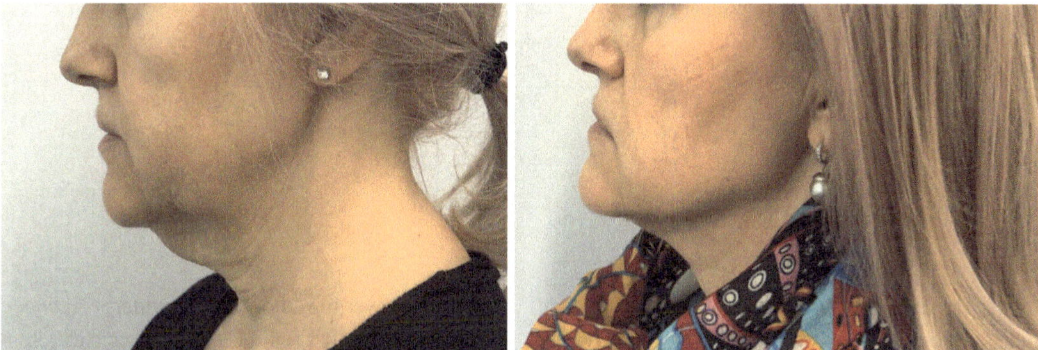

Fig. 5 A 50-year-old female patient. Before and 6 months after FaceTite™

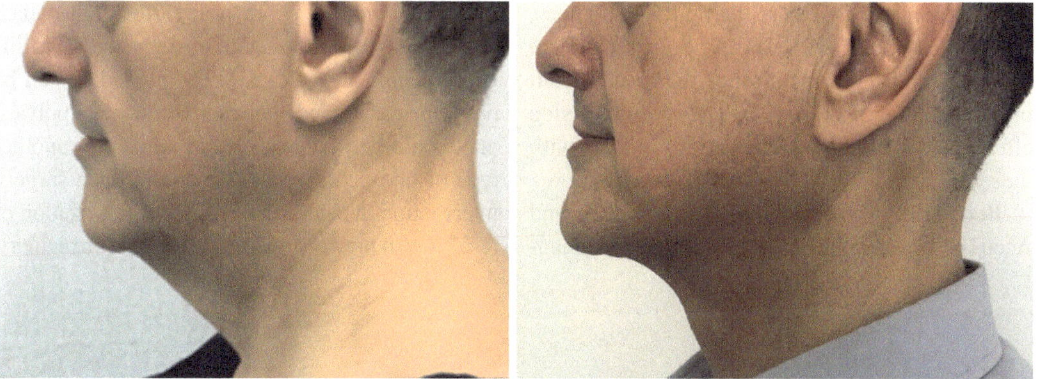

Fig. 6 A 52-year-old male patient after massive weight loss. Before and 1 year after FaceTite™

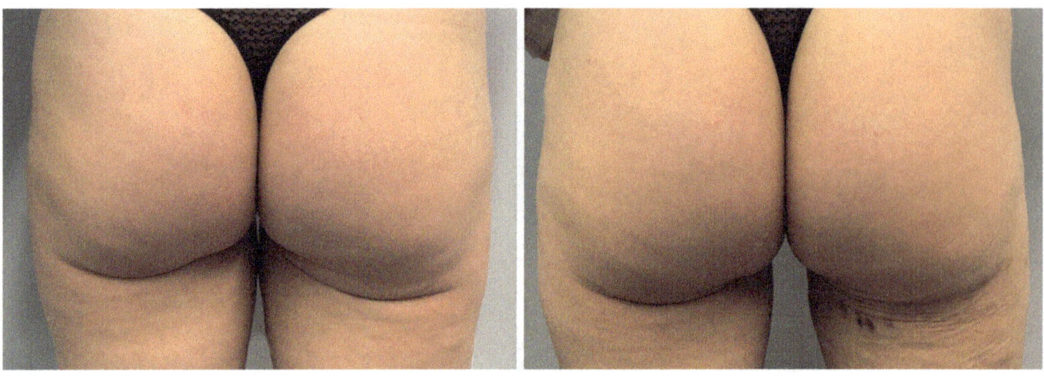

Fig. 7 Before and after correction of asymmetry from previous liposuction in the banana roll area, using FaceTite™

Table 2 AccuTite™ treatment protocols used by the author

Area	Energy	Temperature parameters	Technique
Neck	5–8 kJ	40° ext. t/ 70° int. t	Tightening/melting
Lower 1/3 of the face	1–2 kJ per side	-ll-	-ll-
NLF	0.3–0.5 kJ per side	-ll-	Melting
Malar fat pad	0.2–0.4 kJ per side	-ll-	Melting
Lower eyelids	0.2–0.4 kJ per side	39° ext. t/ 69° int. t	Tightening
Upper eyelids	0.2–0.3 kJ per side	37–38° ext. t/ 67–68° int. t	Tightening
Brow lift	0.4–0.6 kJ per side	40° ext. t/ 70° int. t	-ll-
Small areas of the body	5–8 kJ	-ll-	Tightening and melting

lower facial third for correction in the area of marionette wrinkles; contouring of the jawline; malar fat pad reduction; nasolabial fold reduction; brow lift; upper & lower eyelids for skin tightening. In certain cases, the probe can also be used to treat small areas of the body—the knees, elbows, labia (Table 2). The procedure can also be used for the optimization of the results from previous surgeries [1–19]. The possible side effects and methods of correction overlap with those of FaceTite (Figs. 8, 9 and 10).

BodyTite™—procedure similar to FaceTit and AccuTite with a probe of significantly larger dimensions and power of radiofrequency energy between 20 and 40 W. BodyTite finds application in different parts of the body with the aim of destruction of fat deposits and at the same time tightening of the skin (Table 3). The probe is equipped with an option to adjust the working depth from 1 to 6 cm, which makes it possible to treat the subcutaneous fat at different depths [1–6, 20–23]. The procedure can be performed as a standalone radiofrequency lipolysis, or it could be performed as an adjunct to another type of liposuction technique and/or open surgery intervention. It can be used also for optimization of results from previous surgeries—contour irregulari-

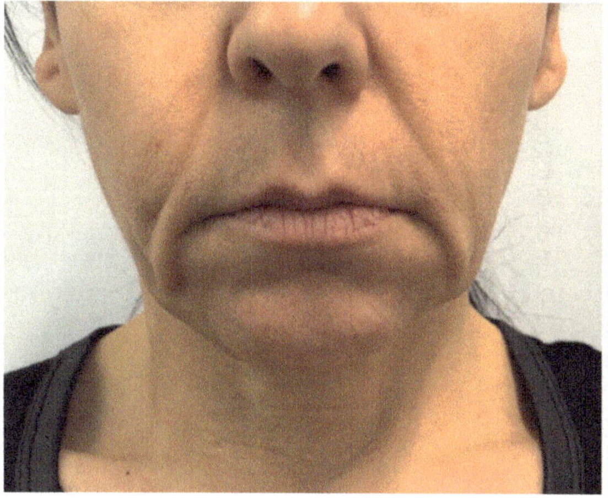
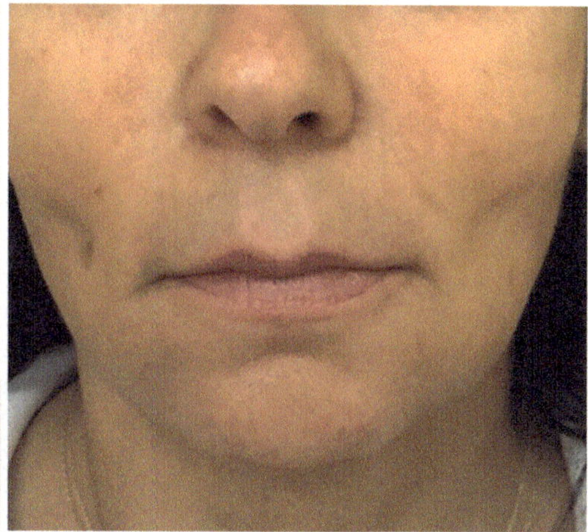

Fig. 8 Before and after lifting in the lower third of the face using AccuTite™. Two sessions in between 6 months. The final result is 1 year after the first and 6 months after the second procedure. AccuTite™ probe. /40 ext. & 70 int. cut off/1Kj per side per procedure

Fig. 9 Before and after correction of nasolabial folds using AccuTite™. One session with AccuTite™ probe—0.4 kJ per side/40 ext & 70 int cut off/energy was applied to melt the fat laterally of the nasolabial fold. The final result is 6 months after the procedure

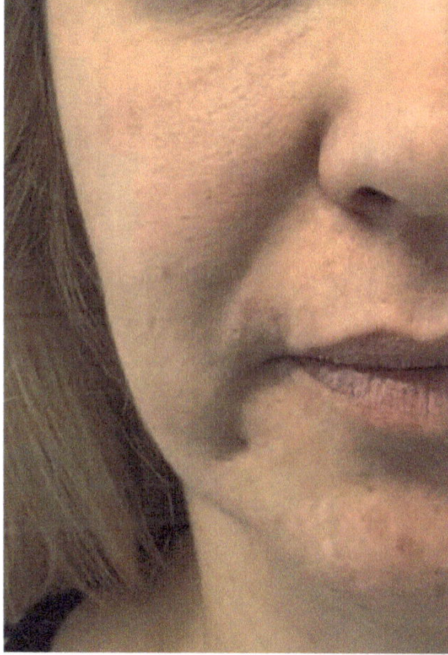
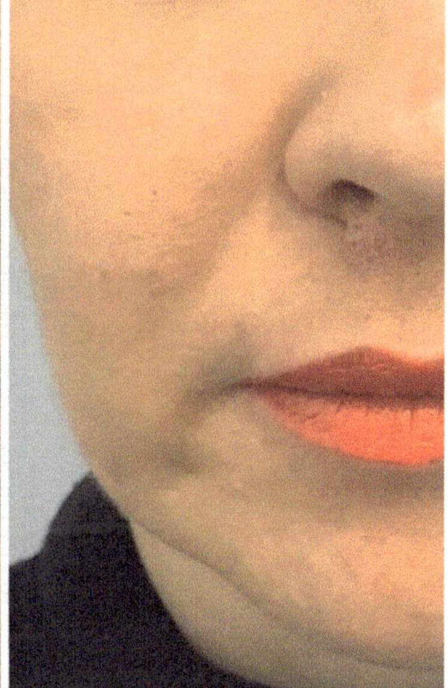

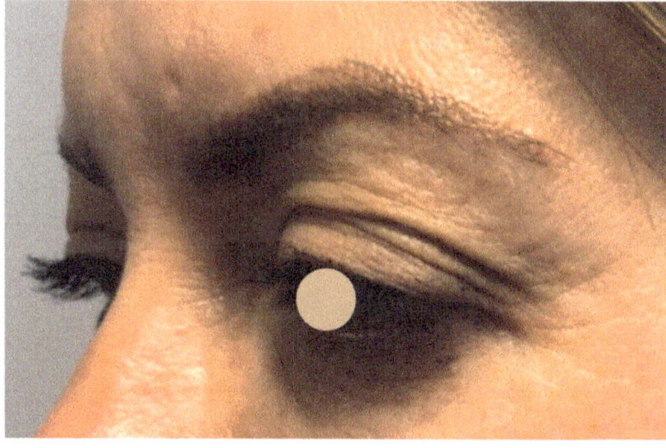
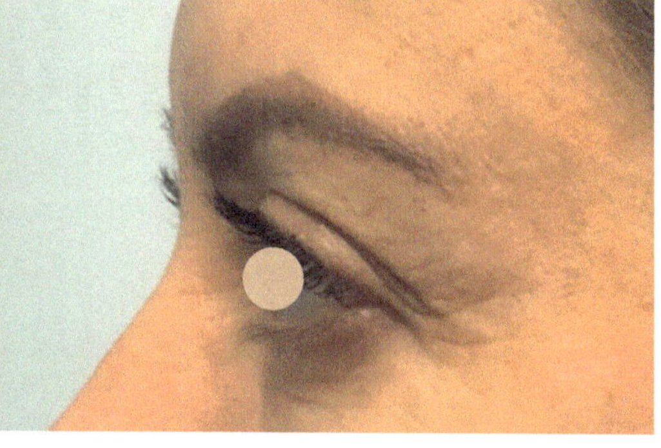

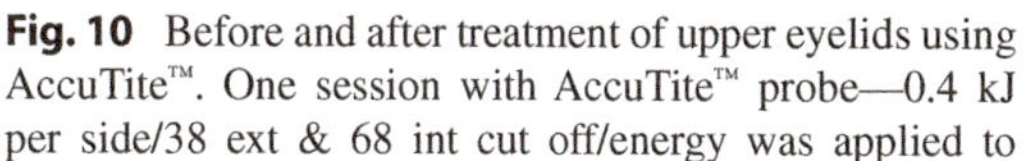
Fig. 10 Before and after treatment of upper eyelids using AccuTite™. One session with AccuTite™ probe—0.4 kJ per side/38 ext & 68 int cut off/energy was applied to tighten the skin of the upper eyelids. The result is 6 months after the procedure

Table 3 BodyTite™ treatment protocols for different areas of the body

Status	Area	Energy	Temperature (t°)	Technique	Depth
Ectomorph	– Abdomen – Breast – Inner and outer thighs – Lower legs – Flank area – Back	10 kJ/10 sq.cm	The purpose is to reach 40° ext. t	Tightening	1 cm depth
Mesomorph	-ll-	-ll-	The purpose is to reach 40° ext. t, and 70° int. t	Tightening, followed by melting, followed by liposuction	1–2 cm depth for tightening, followed by 2–4 cm melting of fat
Endomorph	-ll-	-ll-	The purpose is to reach 40° ext. t, and 70° int. t 2 cm tightening, followed by 6/4/2 cm melting, depending on the preoperative pinch test	-ll-	2 cm tightening, followed by 6/4/2 cm melting, depending on the preoperative pinch test

ties from previous liposuctions; lifting and tightening of residual skin excess; prevention of soft-tissue ptosis (gynecomastia). The author recommends the following treatment options, depending on the preoperative status of the patient and the goal of the intervention.

- **Ectomorph**—Usually aim to correct loose skin. The area is treated at a depth of 1 cm, with the aim of reaching a minimum of 10 kJ per 10 cm^2 treated area (Fig. 14b with video material attached to it).
- **Mesomorph**—In this case, it is recommended to first achieve the above-mentioned parameters to tighten the skin, then, if isolated fat accumulations are present, radiofrequency lipolysis is performed during the same procedure, with the aim of reaching 70 °C in the treated subcutaneous fat. The procedure ends with vibration associated liposuction. The radiofrequency precedes liposuction, and the author considers this sequence to be key to the potential of skin tightening (Fig. 14a).
- **Endomorph**—The aim is to achieve skin tightening by working superficially—2 cm. Reach 10–15 kJ of energy per 10 cm^2 of treated area, then it is proceeded to lipolysis of the deep layers. Depending on the pre-op pinch test for the specific patient, it is recommended to work at several levels, for example: pinch test 6 cm—the area is treated at the level of 6 cm, 3 cm, as it was previously treated at 1 cm for the purpose of tightening; pinch test 4 cm—the area is treated at 4 cm, as it was previously treated at 2 cm for the purpose of tightening. In this type of patient, regardless of the potential of radiofrequency-based skin tightening, the possibility of an excision technique at a subsequent stage should always be discussed preoperatively (Figs. 11, 12, 13, and 14c).

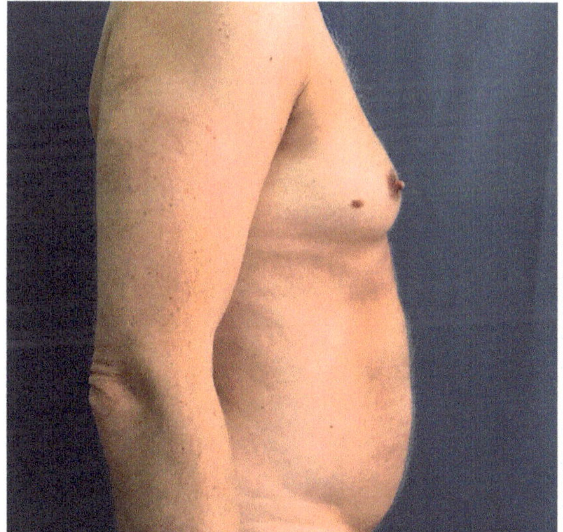
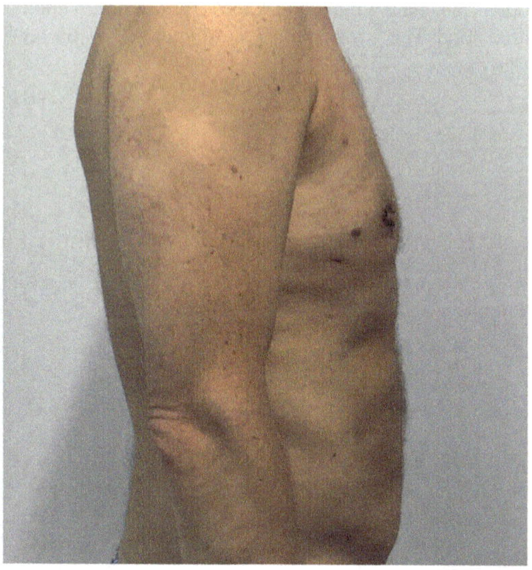
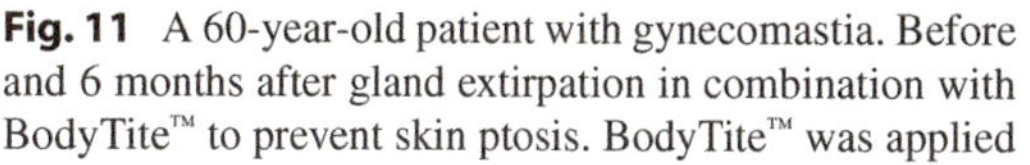

Fig. 11 A 60-year-old patient with gynecomastia. Before and 6 months after gland extirpation in combination with BodyTite™ to prevent skin ptosis. BodyTite™ was applied as follows: 20 W probe/40 ext and 70 int cut off/10 kJ per side at 2 cm depth

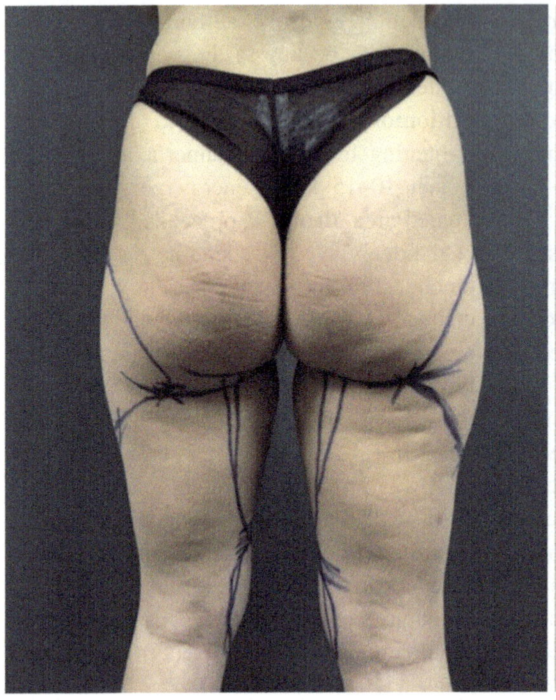
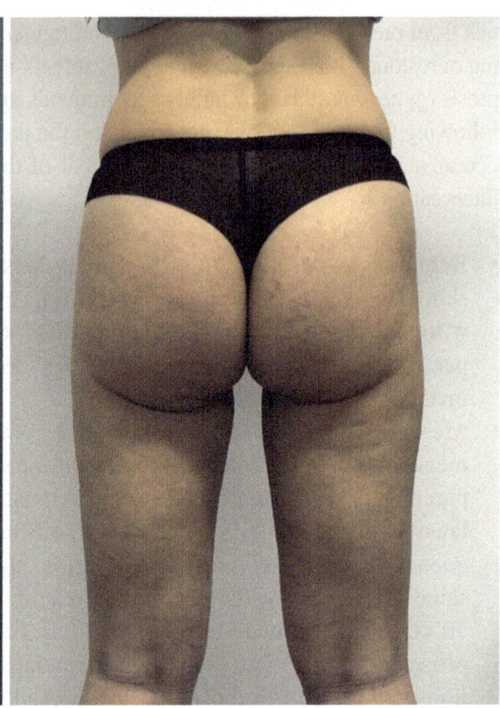

Fig. 12 BodyTite™ with vibration-assisted liposuction on outer and inner thighs and knees. Before and 6 months after. BodyTite™ was applied as follows: 20 W probe/40 ext and 70 int cut off/10 kJ in the outer thighs per side at 2 cm depth/10 kJ in the inner thighs per side at 2 cm depth/5 kJ in the knees per side at 2 cm depth

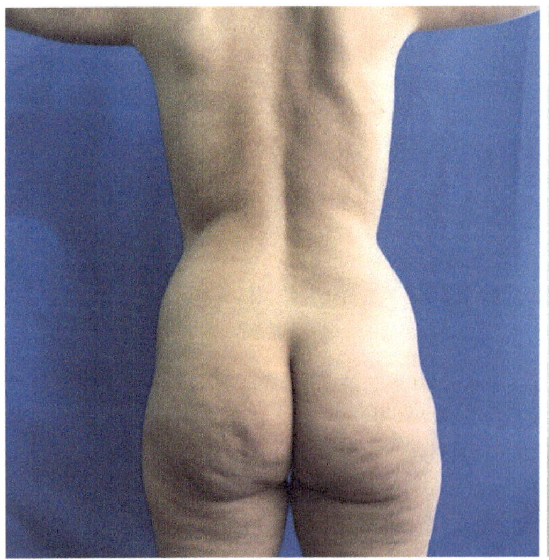
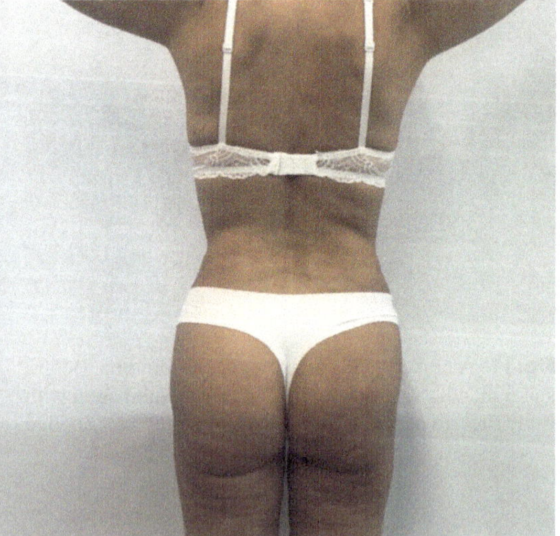

Fig. 13 BodyTite™ with vibration-assisted liposuction of the flanks, outer and inner thighs. Before and 6 months after. BodyTite™ was applied as follows: 20 W probe/40 ext and 70 int cut off/10 kJ in the flanks per side at 2 cm depth/10 kJ in the outer thighs per side at 2 cm depth/10kJ in the inner thighs per side at 2 cm depth

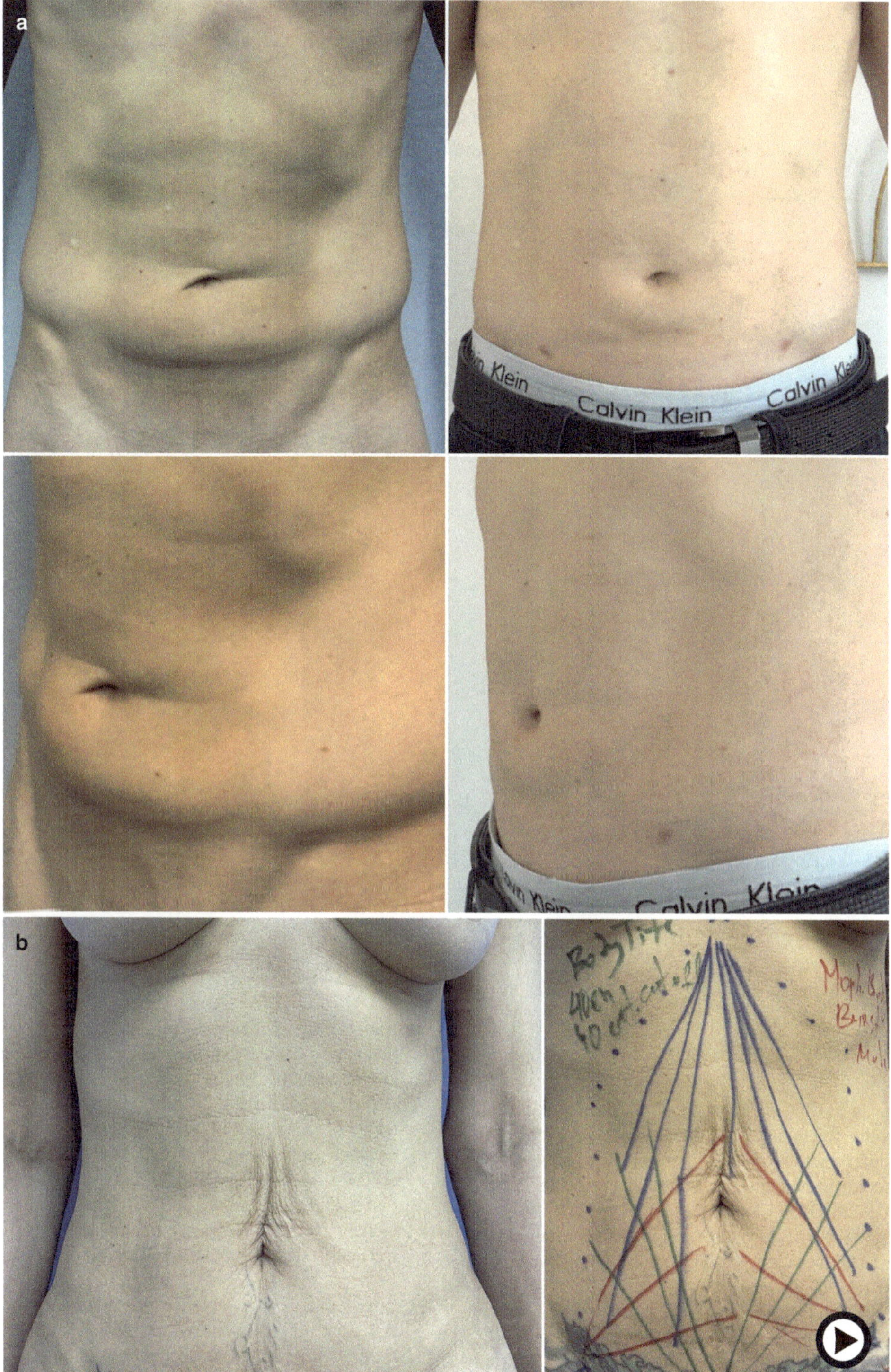

Fig. 14 (**a**) BodyTite™ for isolated fat accumulations in the abdominal area and skin excess in the area above the navel. Before and 6 months after. BodyTite™ was applied as follows: 20 W probe/40 ext and 70 int cut off/overall of 30 kJ at 2 cm depth were used. (**b**) Pre-op markings of BodyTite™ for treatment of loose skin in the abdominal area in combination with Morpheus8 Body™ on burst mode in the same procedure. (**c**) BodyTite™ with all the different applicators for radiofrequency therapy of different areas of the body—BodyTite™, FaceTite™, AccuTite™, Morpheus8™. Intraoperative demonstration of the procedure (▶ https://doi.org/10.1007/000-b0b)

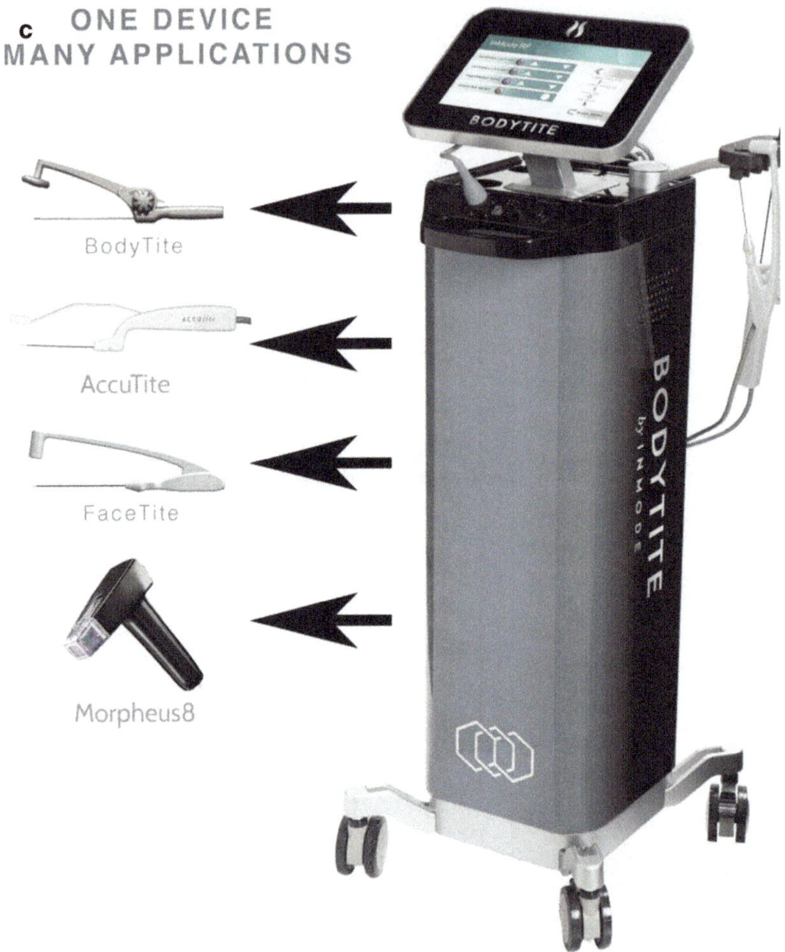

Fig. 14 (continued)

References

1. Dayan E, Chia C, Burns AJ, Theodorou S. Adjustable depth fractional radiofrequency combined with bipolar radiofrequency: a minimally invasive combination treatment for skin laxity. Aesthet Surg J. 2019;29(53):S112–5119.
2. Mulholland RS. Nonexcisional, minimally invasive rejuvenation of the neck. Clin Plast Surg. 2014;41:11–31.
3. Mulholland RS. The bodytite book, vol. 261. 2nd ed; 2021. p. 734–50.
4. Mulholland RS. Radiofrequency energy for non-invasive and minimally invasive skin tightening. Clin Plast Surg. 2011;38:437–48.
5. Dayan E, Burns AJ, Rohrich RJ, Theodorou S. The use of radiofrequency in aesthetic surgery. Plast Reconstr Surg Glob Open. 2020;8(8):e2861.
6. Elsaie ML. Cutaneous remodeling and photorejuvenation using radiofrequency devices. Indian J Dermatol. 2009;54:201.
7. Atiyeh BS, Dibo SA. Nonsurgical nonablative treatment of aging skin: radiofrequency technologies between aggressive marketing and evidence-based efficacy. Aesthet Plast Surg. 2009;33:283–94.
8. Fisher GH, Jacobson LG, Bernstein LJ, et al. Nonablative radiofrequency treatment of facial laxity. Dermatol Surg. 2005;31(9 pt 2):1237–41. discussion 1241
9. Ruiz-Esparza J. Nonablative radiofrequency for facial and neck rejuvenation. A faster, safer, and less painful procedure based on concentrating the heat in key areas: the thermalift concept. J Cosmet Dermatol. 2006;5:68–75.
10. Alexiades-Armenakas M, Dover JS, Arndt KA. Unipolar versus bipolar radiofrequency treat-

ment of rhytides and laxity using a mobile painless delivery method. Lasers Surg Med. 2008;40:446–53.
11. Alster TS, Lupton JR. Nonablative cutaneous remodeling using radiofrequency devices. Clin Dermatol. 2007;25:487–91.
12. Dierickx CC. The role of deep heating for noninvasive skin rejuvenation. Lasers Surg Med. 2006;38:799–807.
13. Narins DJ, Narins RS. Non-surgical radiofrequency facelift. J Drugs Dermatol. 2003;2:495–500.
14. Fitzpatrick R, Geronemus R, Goldberg D, et al. Multicenter study of noninvasive radiofrequency for periorbital tissue tightening. Lasers Surg Med. 2003;33:232–42.
15. Bassichis BA, Dayan S, Thomas JR. Use of a nonablative radiofrequency device to rejuvenate the upper one-third of the face. Otolaryngol Head Neck Surg. 2004;130:397–406.
16. Nahm WK, Su TT, Rotunda AM, et al. Objective changes in brow position, superior palpebral crease, peak angle of the eyebrow, and jowl surface area after volumetric radiofrequency treatments to half of the face. Dermatol Surg. 2004;30:922–8. discussion 928
17. Jacobson LG, Alexiades-Armenakas M, Bernstein L, et al. Treatment of nasolabial folds and jowls with a noninvasive radiofrequency device. Arch Dermatol. 2003;139:1371–2.
18. Alster TS, Tanzi E. Improvement of neck and cheek laxity with a nonablative radiofrequency device: a lifting experience. Dermatol Surg. 2004;30(4 pt 1):503–7. discussion 507
19. El-Domyati M, El-Ammawi TS, Medhat W, et al. Radiofrequency facial rejuvenation: evidence-based effect. J Am Acad Dermatol. 2011;64:524–35.
20. Theodorou SJ, Del Vecchio D, Chia CT. Soft tissue contraction in body contouring with radiofrequency-assisted liposuction: a treatment gap solution. Aesthet Surg J. 2018;38:S74–83.
21. Friedman DJ, Gilead LT. The use of hybrid radiofrequency device for the treatment of rhytides and lax skin. Dermatol Surg. 2007;33:543–51.
22. Bogle MA, Ubelhoer N, Weiss RA, et al. Evaluation of the multiple pass, low fluence algorithm for radiofrequency tightening of the lower face. Lasers Surg Med. 2007;39:210–7.
23. Levy AS, Grant RT, Rothaus KO. Radiofrequency physics for minimally invasive aesthetic surgery. Clin Plast Surg. 2016;43:551–6.

Minimally Invasive Ultrasound-Based Procedures: VASERlipo®: High-Definition Procedures

Introduction

VASERlipo® is widely used for the purpose of high definition in men and women, forming a six pack, contouring in the area of various muscle groups both in the area of the chest and back and in the area of upper and lower limbs [1]. The author combines the intervention with vibration assisted liposuction. To achieve optimal results in terms of definition and contouring in individual parts of the body, lipofilling techniques are also used [2–14]. If it is necessary to combine the above-mentioned techniques, the sequence is as follows: ultrasound treatment of the area, followed by a vibration assister liposucion for the purpose of definition; radiofrequency technique for the purpose of prevention of skin sagging and lipofilling in areas of specific muscle groups (Figs. 1, 2, 3, 4, 5, 6 and 7a–c). **When the area of treatment needs additional tightening after VASERlipo®, the author prefers to use Morpheus8 Body™, rather than BodyTite™ in the same procedure, however, when neighbouring area needs additional tightening, this will be treated by BodyTite™ or FaceTite™ or AccuTite™ depending on how large this area is.**

E. Sharkov, *Body Contouring Surgery*, https://doi.org/10.1007/978-3-031-33350-7_5

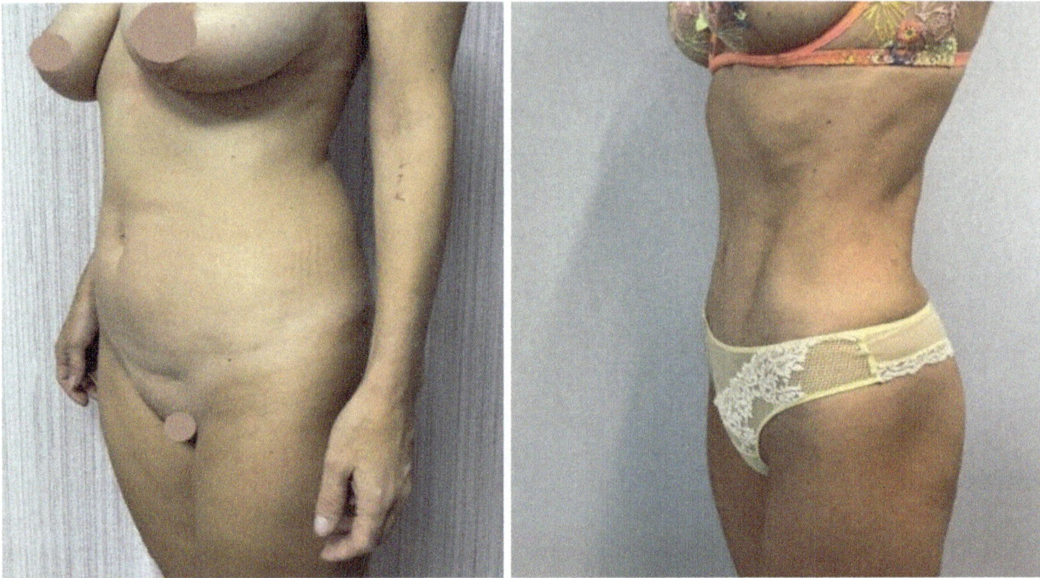

Fig. 1 Before and 6 months after ultrasound lipoplasty with vibration assisted liposuction. The used parameters of the ultrasound device are illustrated in Table 1

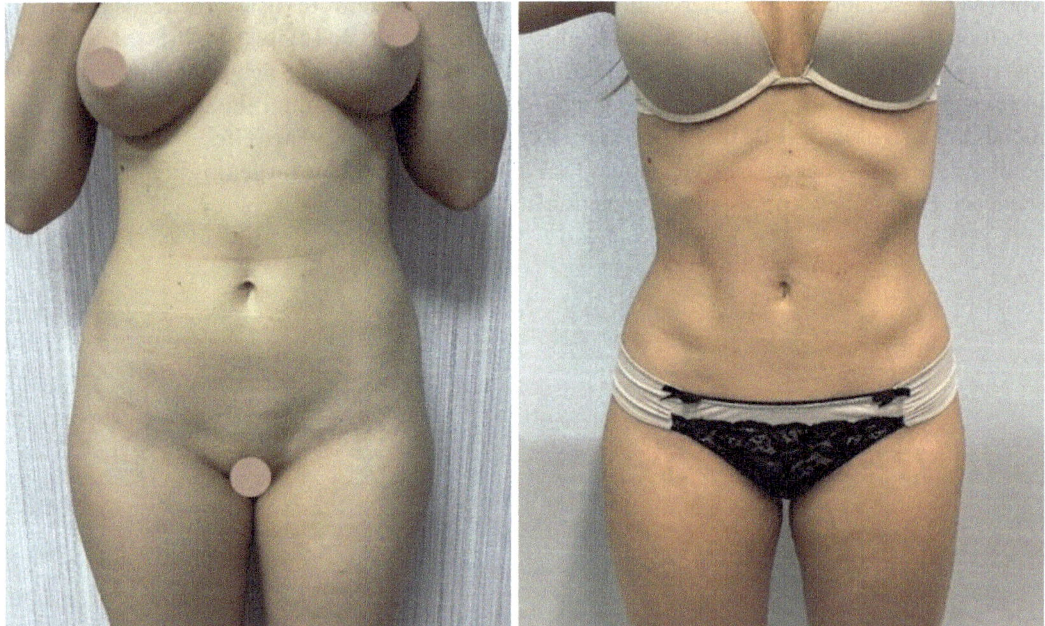

Fig. 2 Before and 6 months after ultrasound lipoplasty with vibration assisted liposuction. The used parameters of the ultrasound device are illustrated in Table 1

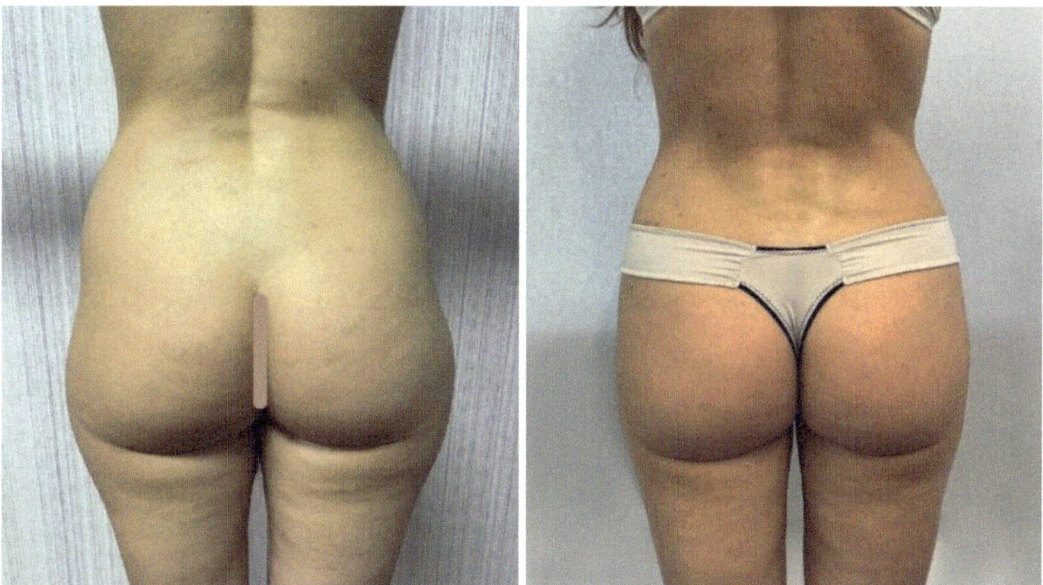

Fig. 3 Before and 6 months after ultrasound lipoplasty with vibration assisted liposuction. The used parameters of the ultrasound device are illustrated in Table 1

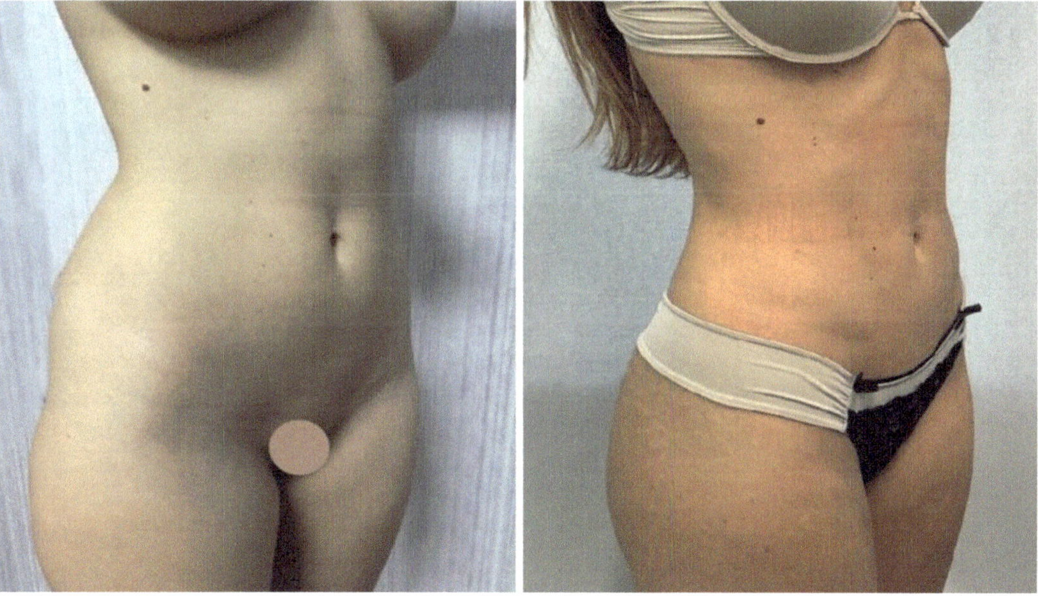

Fig. 4 Before and 6 months after ultrasound lipoplasty with vibration assisted liposuction. The used parameters of the ultrasound device are illustrated in Table 1

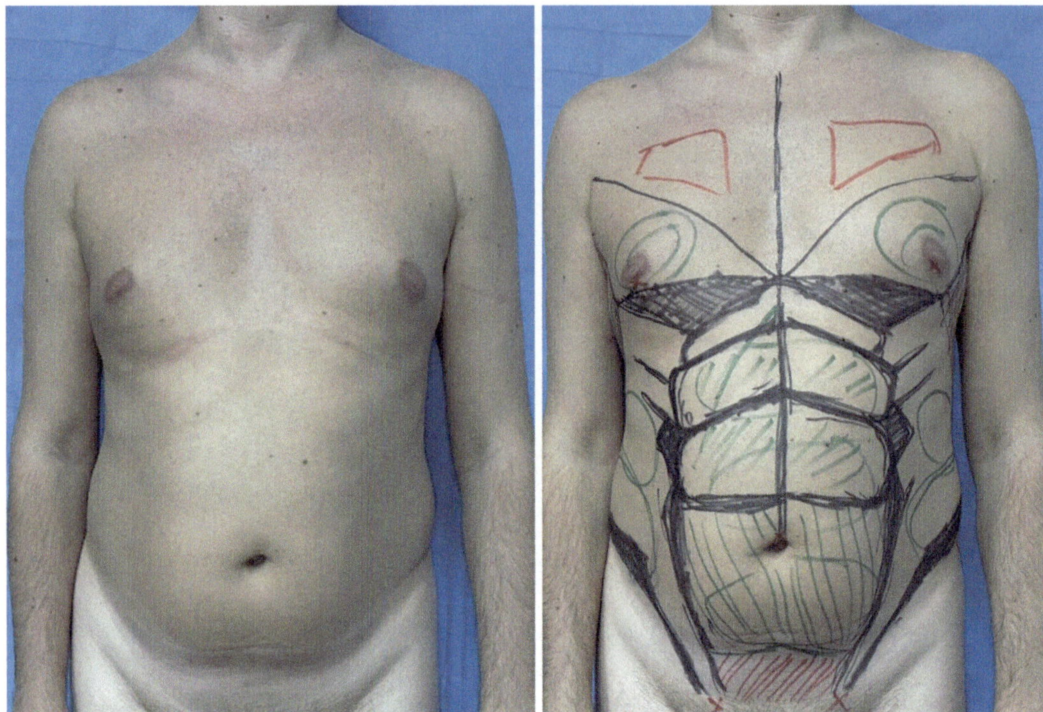

Fig. 5 A 39-year-old male patient for VASERlipo® ultrasound high definition of the abdomen, flanks and chest area. Pre-op status and marking for the procedure

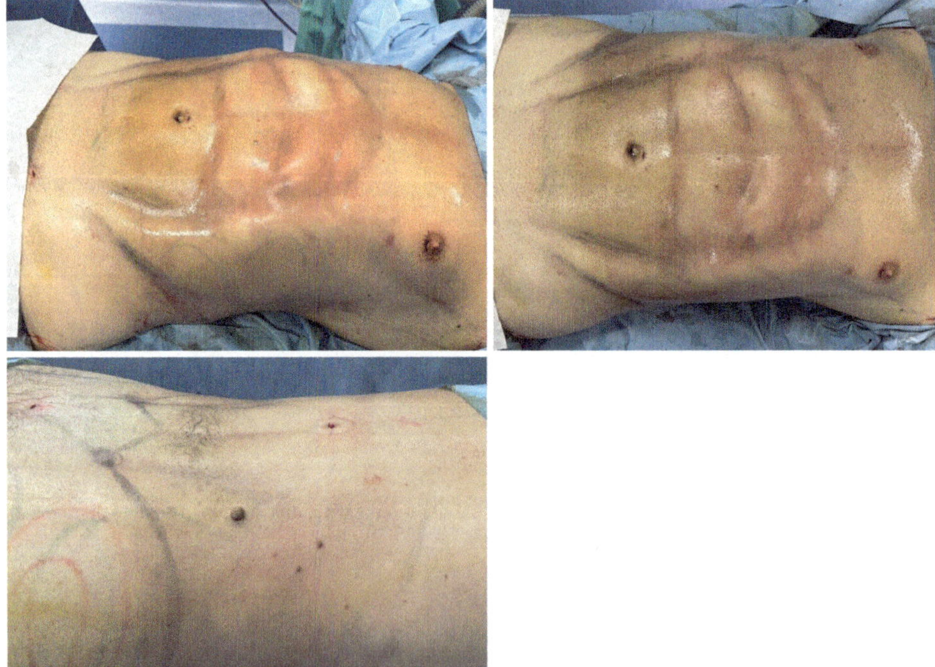

Fig. 6 Immediately after the procedure—pictures of the abdomen, chest and the area of the lower back and flanks. VASERlipo® and vibrational liposuction were done as described in Table 1 of Chapter "Vibrational Type of Liposuction".

Fig. 7 (**a**) Before and 6 months after VASERlipo® and vibrational liposuction were done as described in Table 1 of Chapter "Vibrational Type of Liposuction". (**b**) Patient with abdominoplasty done by another clinic years ago. Before 3 months and 6 months after VASERlipo® and vibrational liposuction done as described in Table 1 of Chapter "Vibrational Type of Liposuction". (**c**) VASERlipo® system and the different type of probes for ultrasound delivery

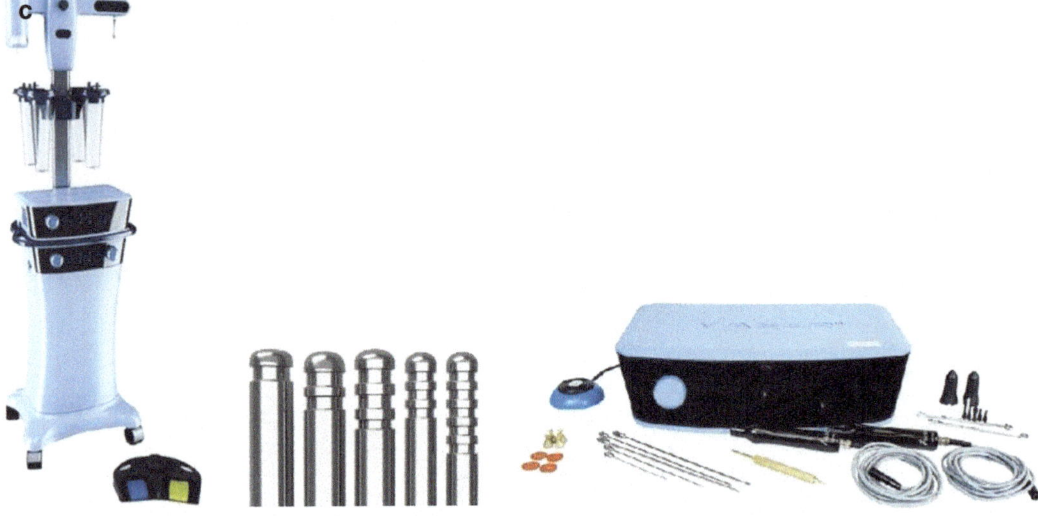

Fig. 7 (continued)

Table 1 Author's preferable parameters, also described for the first time by Alfredo E. Hoyos MD

Area	Type of sample	Mode of operation	Duration of treatment
Abdomen	2-ring probe (energy facing forward) Athletic patients 3-ring probe (energy spreading in these patients)	First VASER mode on 80% superficially and then continuous C mode on 80% deep	1 min per 100 mL infiltrated solution
Breasts	2-ring people	-||-	-||-
Arms and legs (thighs, lower legs and knees)	2-ring people	60% V mode, superficially and then 60% C mode deep	-||-
Back, including flanks	-||-	80% V mode, superficially, 80% C mode deep	

References

1. Hoyos AE, Prendergast PM. High definition body sculpting; 2014. p. 73–80.
2. Cimino WW. History of ultrasound-assisted lipoplasty. In: Shiffman MA, Di Giuseppe A, editors. Body contouring: art, science, and clinical practice. Berlin: Springer; 2010. p. 399.
3. Cimino WW. The physics of soft tissue fragmentation using ultrasonic frequency vibrations of metal probes. Clin Plast Surg. 1999;26:447–61.
4. Ogawa T, Hattori R, Yamamoto T, Gotoh M. Safe use of ultrasonically activated devices based on current studies. Expert Rev Med Devices. 2011;8(3):319–24.
5. Scuderi N, Devita R, D'Andrea F, Vonella M. Nuove prospettive nella liposuzione la lipoemulsificazone. Giorn Chir Plast Ricostr ed Estetica. 1987;2(1):33–9.
6. Zocchi ML. Clinical aspects of ultrasonic liposculpture. Perspect Plast Surg. 1993;7:153–74.
7. Zocchi ML. Ultrasonic assisted lipoplasty. Clin Plast Surg. 1996;23(4):575–98.
8. Troilius C. Ultrasound-assisted lipoplasty: is it really safe? Aesthet Plast Surg. 1999;23(5):307–11.
9. Baxter RA. Histologic effects of ultrasound-assisted lipoplasty. Aesthet Surg J. 1999;19:109–14.
10. Cimino WW. Ultrasonic surgery: power quantification and efficiency optimization. Aesthet Surg J. 2001;21(3):233–40.
11. Cimino WW. Ultrasound-assisted lipoplasty: basic physics, tissue interactions, and related results/complications. In: Shiffman MA, Di Giuseppe A, editors. Body contouring: art, science, and clinical practice. Berlin: Springer; 2010. p. 392.
12. Nagy MW, Vanek PF Jr. A multicenter, prospective, randomized, single-blind, controlled clinical trial comparing VASER-assisted lipoplasty and suction-assisted lipoplasty. Plast Reconstr Surg. 2012;129(4):681e–9e.
13. Cimino WW. VASER-assisted lipoplasty: technology and technique. In: Shiffman MA, Di Giuseppe A, editors. Liposuction principles and practice. Berlin Heidelberg: Springer; 2006. p. 239–44.
14. Jewell ML, Fodor PB, de Souza Pinto EB, Al Shammari MA. Clinical application of VASER-assisted lipoplasty: a pilot clinical study. Aesthet Surg J. 2002;22(2):131–46.

Vibrational Type of Liposuction

Introduction

Vibrational type of liposuction in combination with **VASERlipo®** allows for optimal definition, minimal physical strain on the part of the operator and a high degree of survival of the extracted fat for the purpose of using it for lipofilling (Table 1) [1–7]. The combination with **BodyTite™** radiofrequency enables prevention of skin sagging. It should be clear that if the extracted fat will be used for lipofilling, then the donor area can be treated with **BodyTite™** only after harvesting. In all other circumstances, it is recommended to first treat with radiofrequency energy and then perform vibration-assisted liposuction (Figs. 1, 2 and 3a, b).

Table 1 Author's preferred types of cannulas for vibrational lipoaspiration, also described for the first time by Alfredo E. Hoyos, MD

Area	Purpose	Cannula type—always 'Mercedes' type
Abdomen	– definition (framing) – Lipoaspiration to 'empty'	3 mm superficial and deep treatment, followed by 4 mm -II-, as the author uses 'curved cannula'
Breasts	Definition	-II- and 3 and 4 mm 45° angled cannula
Hips	Lipoaspiration and definition	4 mm long curved cannula and 4 mm angled cannula; 3 mm long similar cannulas may also be used. Curved and angled cannulas in patients with more serious fat accumulations
Arms	Definition AND lipoaspiration	3 mm, followed by 4 mm long curved cannula
Inner thigh	Definition AND liposuction	4 mm long curved cannula
Knees	Lipoaspiration	4 mm and sometimes also 3 mm angled cannulas
Outer thighs	Lipoaspiration and definition	4 mm and 3 mm long curved cannula
Lower legs	-II-	4 mm long curved cannula

E. Sharkov, *Body Contouring Surgery*, https://doi.org/10.1007/978-3-031-33350-7_6

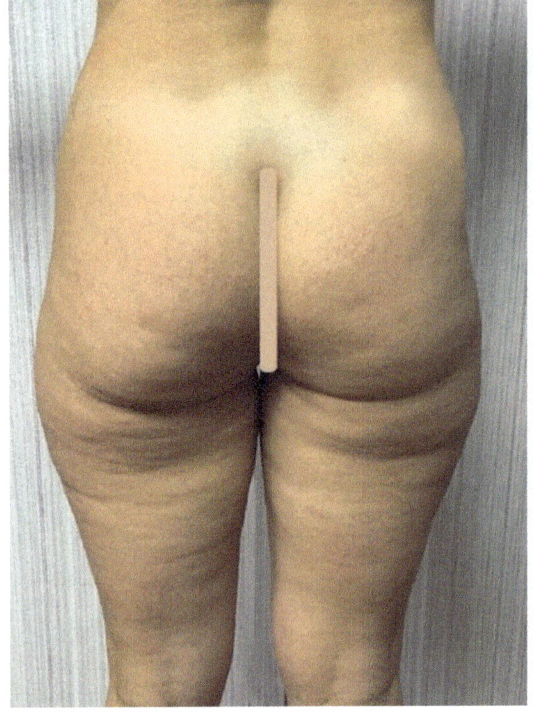

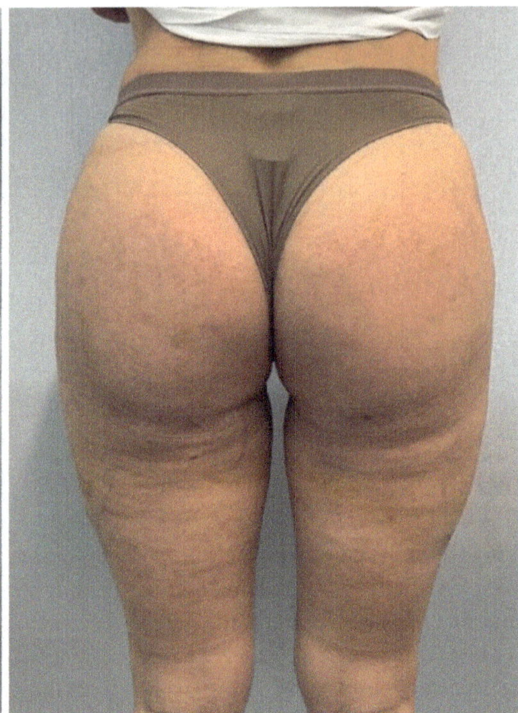

Fig. 1 Vibration-assisted liposuction of inner and outer thighs, followed by a radiofrequency procedure in the same areas and BBL of buttocks (250 cc per side). 4 mm Mercedes type curved cannulas for the inner thighs; 3 and 4 mm Mercedes type curved cannulas for the outer thighs. Early results—1 month post-operative

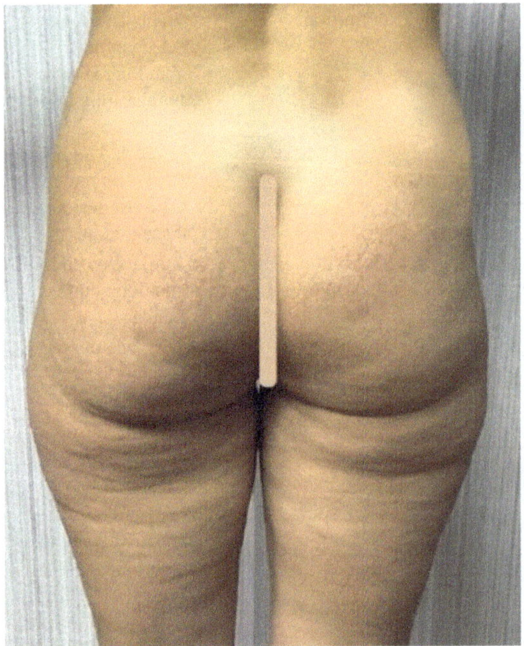

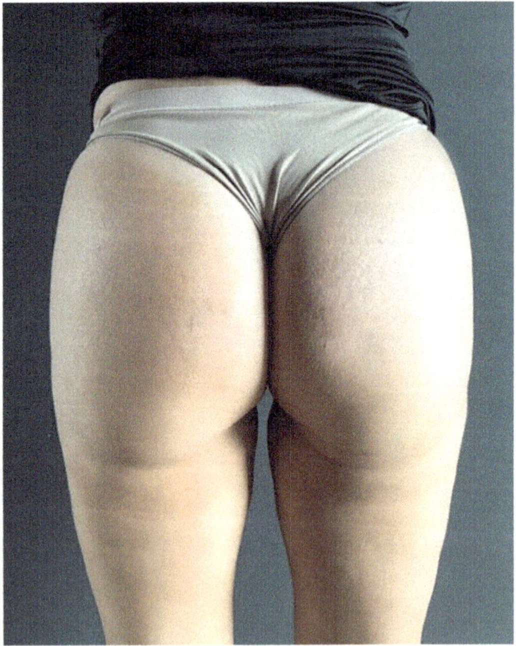

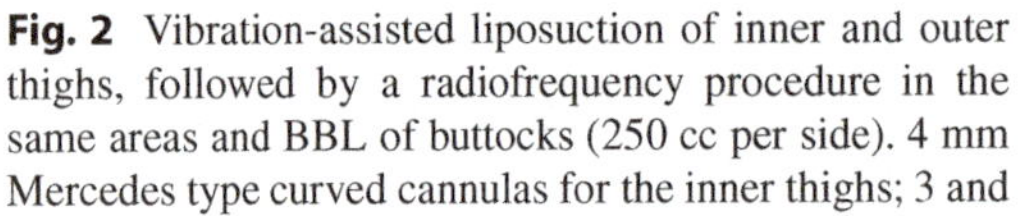

Fig. 2 Vibration-assisted liposuction of inner and outer thighs, followed by a radiofrequency procedure in the same areas and BBL of buttocks (250 cc per side). 4 mm Mercedes type curved cannulas for the inner thighs; 3 and 4 mm Mercedes type curved cannulas for the outer thighs. The result is 1 year after the procedure. Early result of the same patient is shown in Fig. 1.

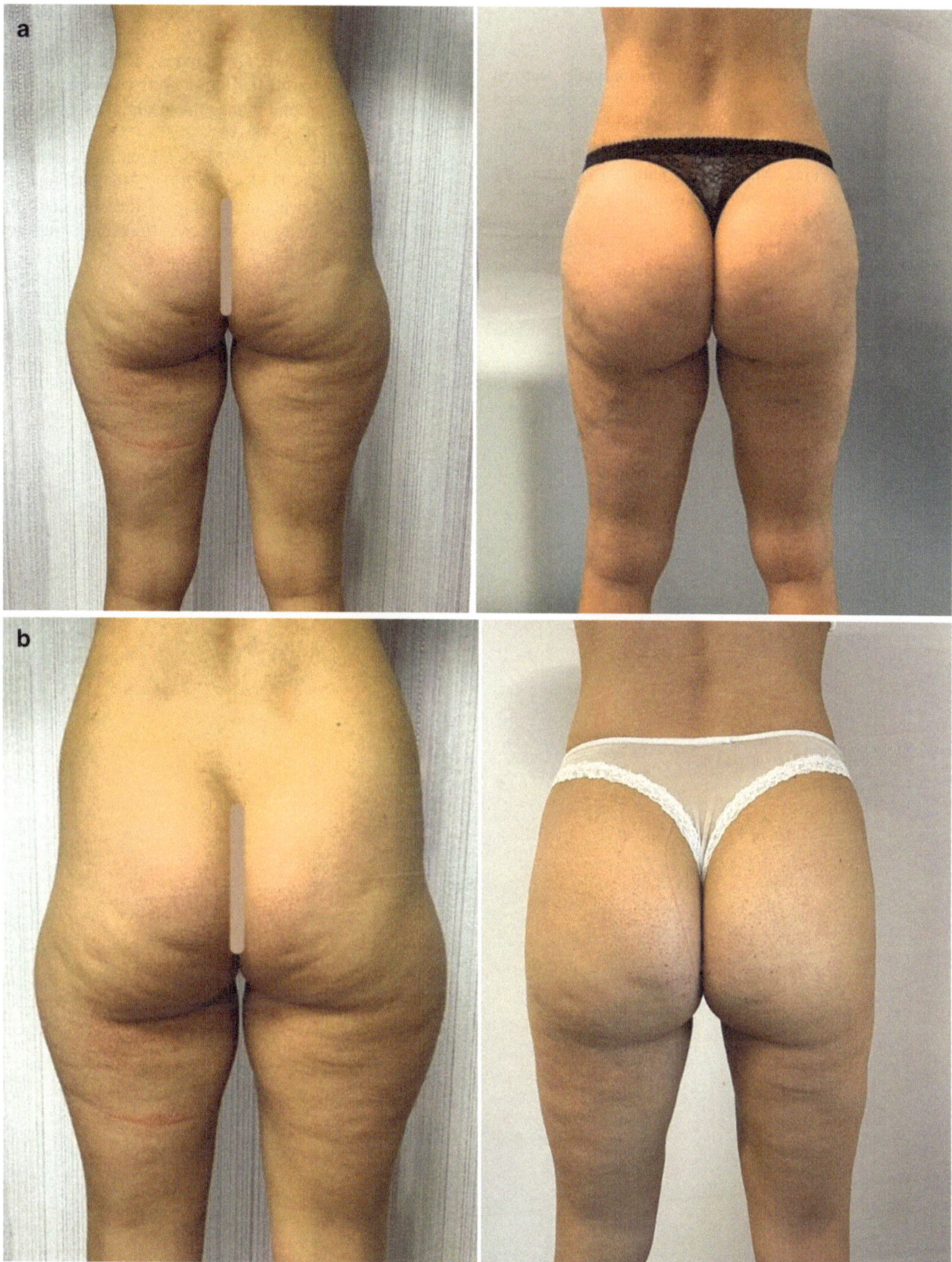

Fig. 3 (**a**) Vibration-assisted liposuction of inner and outer thighs, followed by a radiofrequency procedure in the same areas and BBL of buttocks (300 cc per side). 4 mm Mercedes type curved cannulas for the inner thighs; 3 and 4 mm Mercedes type curved cannulas for the outer thighs. Early post-operative results—1 month after the procedure (**b**) Vibration-assisted liposuction of inner and outer thighs, followed by a radiofrequency procedure in the same areas and BBL of buttocks (300 cc per side). 4 mm Mercedes type curved cannulas for the inner thighs; 3 and 4 mm Mercedes type curved cannulas for the outer thighs. The result is 1 year after the procedure. Early result of the same patient is shown in Fig. 3a

References

1. Hoyos A, Perez M. Dynamic-definition male pectoral reshaping and enhancement in slim, athletic, obese, and gynecomastic patients through selective fat removal and grafting. Aesthet Plast Surg. 2012;36(5):1066–77.
2. Hoyos A, Perez M. Arm dynamic definition by liposculpture and fat grafting. Aesthet Surg J. 2012;32(8):974–87.
3. Hoyos AE. High definition liposculpture. Bucaramanga, Colombia: XIII International Course of Plastic Surgery; 2003.
4. Ersek RA, Salisbury AV. Abdominal etching. Aesthet Plast Surg. 1997;21(5):328–31.
5. Hoyos AE, Perez ME, Domínguez-Millán R. Variable sculpting in dynamic definition body contouring: procedure selection and management algorithm. Aesthet Surg J. 2021;41(3):318–32.
6. Hoyos AE, Millard JA. VASER-assisted high-definition liposculpture. Aesthet Surg J. 2007;27(6):594–604.
7. Illouz YG. Surgical remodeling of the silhouette by aspiration lipolysis or selective lipectomy. Aesthet Plast Surg. 1985;9(1):7–21.

Part III

The Role of Non- and Minimally Invasive Techniques in Open Surgery Procedures

Abdominoplasties in Combination with Radiofrequency, Ultrasound Procedures, Vibrational Lipoaspiration and Myostimulation Procedures

Introduction

The surgical technique is used in the following types of patients [1–8]:

- Patients who have lost a lot of weight, the skin of the abdomen cannot be retracted completely and hangs (so-called apron)
- Patients without an 'apron', but with soft and loose skin of the abdomen, stretch marks (striae) and caudally dislocated navel
- Female patients after caesarean section

Historically, world famous surgeons have contributed to the process of improving this type of surgical technique: Kelly/1899/—the first attempt to remove excess skin and fatty tissue from the abdominal wall; Jolly/1911/—the first low-positioned transversal cut; Thorek—navel preservation technique; Babcock/1916/—the first vertical resection; Pitanguy/1967/—described 300 cases of lipectomy [9]; Regnault/1972/—W—technique; Grazer/1973/—'bikini—line—incision'; Callia/1967/—'low-incision' with extension behind the inguinal fold; Grazer and Goldwyn/1977/—the first vertical plication of m. rectus abdominis; Rebello/1977/—the first reverse abdominoplasty; Psillakis/1978/—proposed a plication of m. obliquus abd. Ext. in order to reduce the circumference of the hips; Matarasso/1988/—the first to perform additional contour liposuction; Lockwood/1995/—'high-lateral-tension abdominoplasty'. Francisco Villegas is the first to describe the Tulua abdominoplasty—removing excess skin in the infraumbilical area with transversal plication of the abdominal muscles, creating a new navel and performing liposuction of the entire body contour.

Knowledge of the anatomical features of the area is the basis of good surgical practice. In our practice, we have come to the conclusion that the most important thing is respect for blood supply vessels. Huger divided the blood supply into 3 zones [10]:

- Zone I: zone fed by the deep epigastric arcade/perforators of m.rectus abdominis/
- Zone II: zone of lower abdominal circulation—a. epigastrica inf. Superficialis, a. pudenda externa, a. circumflexa ilium superficialis
- Zone III: lateral zone—6 lateral intercostal and 4 lumbar arteries

In most cases, one or more sources of blood supply are affected.

- In plication, the perforants from the deep epigastral vessels/a.epigastrica superior et infe-

Supplementary Information The online version contains supplementary material available at https://doi.org/10.1007/978-3-031-33350-7_7. The videos can be accessed individually by clicking the DOI link in the accompanying figure caption or by scanning this link with the SN More Media App.

E. Sharkov, *Body Contouring Surgery*, https://doi.org/10.1007/978-3-031-33350-7_7

rior profunda, a.circumflexa ilium profunda/ are always affected
- In extended abdominoplasty, circumferential abdominoplasty, etc., a.epigastrica inf. Superficialis, a. circumflexa ilium superficialis are most often affected

With a view to the above, the preservation of intercostal and subcostal perforants is paramount to the survival of the flap.

Preoperative assessment is paramount in choosing the appropriate technique, taking into account the possible contraindications, either absolute and/or relative. From an anamnestic point of view, it is important to provide information regarding previous births, previous surgical interventions on the abdominal wall, periods of excessive weight gain and weight loss, desire for future pregnancy, severe general conditions—cardiovascular diseases (CVD), TE, etc., tendency to form cicatrices and keloids, smoking. When evaluating the patient's status, the following are taken into account: visible scars, presence of abdominal hernia, diastasis of the abdominal muscles, quantity, quality, and elasticity of the skin of the abdominal wall. The possible contraindications are severe general conditions, desire for future pregnancy; TE—anamnestically, BMI >40/severe degree of obesity/, unrealistic patient expectations, tendency to keloids and abnormal cicatrization [11, 12].

Types of Abdominoplasty

Classic Abdominoplasty/with or Without Plication

It provides correction of the excessive skin and accumulated excess of subcutaneous fat in the area of the abdominal wall, the diastasis of abdominal muscles and the skin stretch marks (striae) [13–15] (Figs. 1a, b, 2 and 3). The surgical technique consists of the following sequence of actions:

- Selection of incision/according to the patient's habitus, the type of underwear/
- Elevation of the skin and subcutaneous flap with preservation of the umbilical stock
- If necessary, plication of available diastasis of m.rectus abdominis, m.obliqus abdominis, 'low horizontal plication'
- Excision of the excessive skin and subcutaneous fat excess
- Suturing the navel
- Baroudi sutures
- Closure of the surgical incision with adequate redistribution of tension, drainage

Application of Non-invasive and Minimally Invasive Techniques in Classic Abdominoplasty

(a) Intraoperatively
  - **Radiofrequency procedures:**
    - **BodyTite™:** Internal radiofrequency treatment in the area cranial to a planned excision is not recommended due to the coagulation effect and possible complications along the postoperative wound. It is possible to apply radiofrequency in adjacent areas, for example the flanks, with the ultimate goal of achieving 360 degree definition in the lower torso. This type of combination, together with the subsequent vibration-assisted liposuction of the same areas and/or vibration-assisted liposuction of the abdomen refers as 3D abdominoplasty. BodyTite™ leads to a permanent fat destruction in the flanks, providing lasting results. In addition, significant skin contraction is expected.
    - **Morpheus8 Body™:** At the end of the surgery radiofrequency microneedling could be applied to improve skin elasticity. The procedure parameters are as follows:

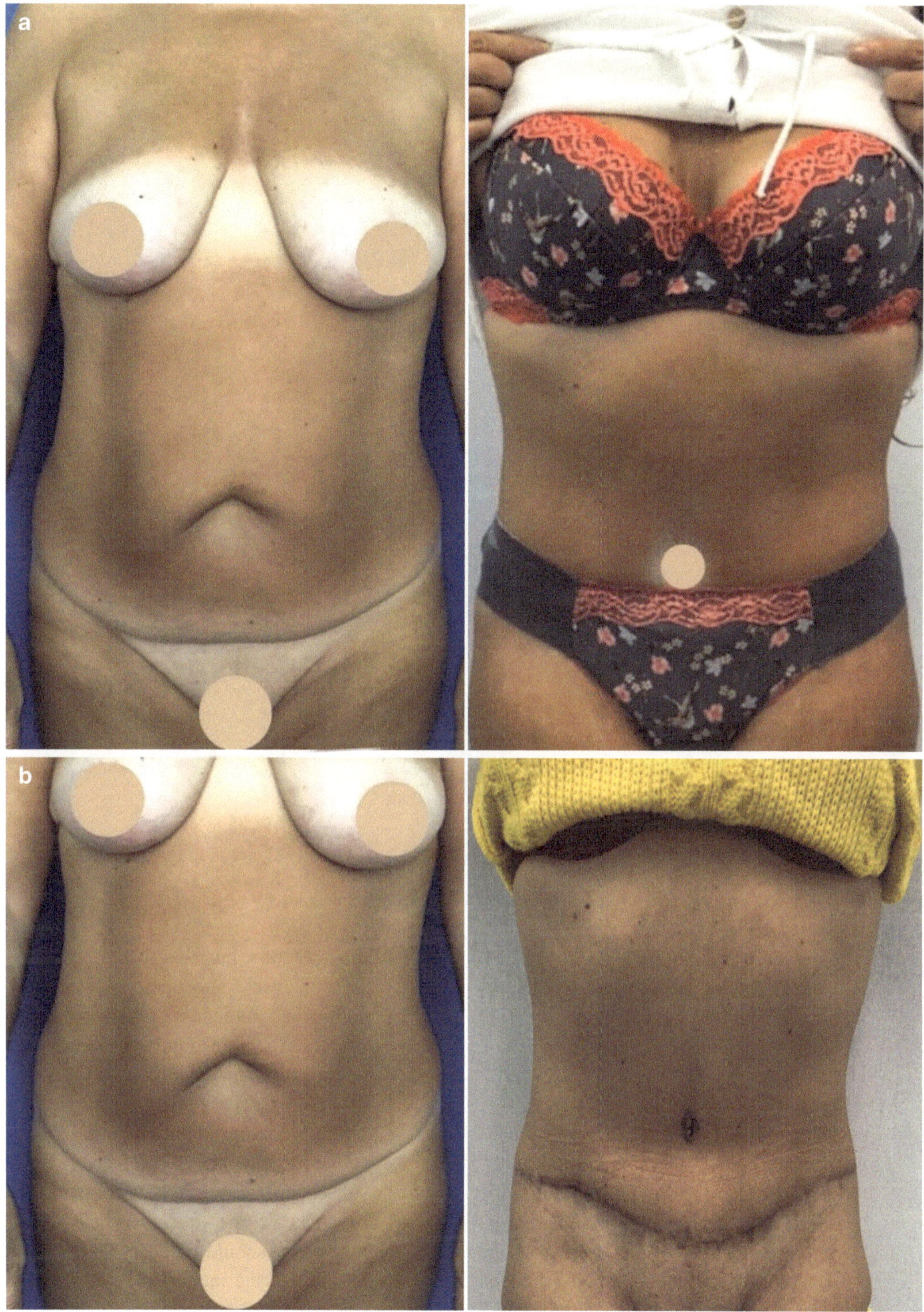

Fig. 1 (**a**) and (**b**) A 42-year-old female patient. Before and 6 months after classic abdominoplasty

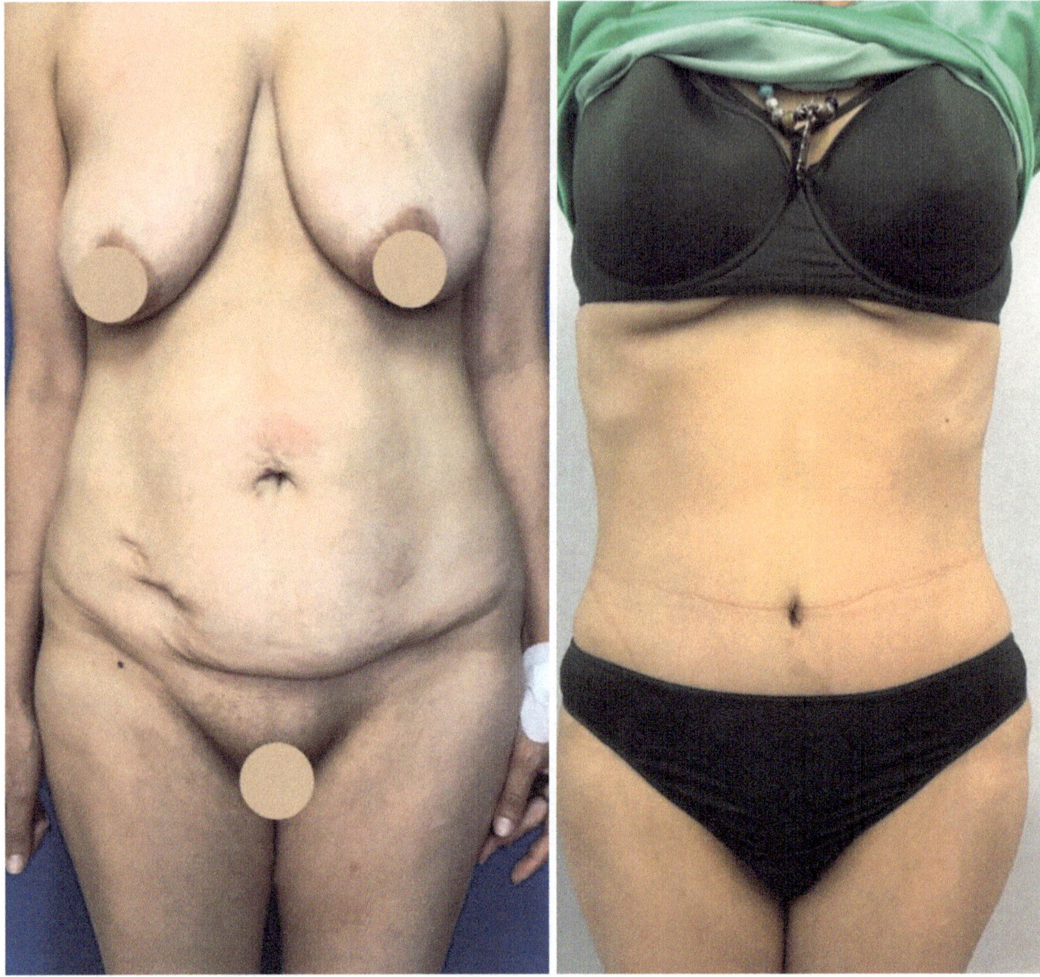

Fig. 2 A 40-year-old female patient. Before and 1 year after classic abdominoplasty

7–5–3 mm burst mode depth with 30 kJ, 3 stacks per place, and procedure can be repeated on the 45th postoperative day, again in 45 more days.

- **Ultrasound procedures**
  - **VASERlipo®:** Ultrasound lipoplasty is possible both in the area cranial to the excision and in the flanks area. The ultrasound technique is vascular sparing; therefore, it is believed that the combination with an open excision technique does not increase the risk regarding the repair of the operative defect [16]. **VASERlipo®** and the subsequent vibration-assisted liposuction may precede, but also follow, the excision of excess subcutaneous skin. The author recommends that the excision precedes the ultrasound treatment, when talking about the abdominal area, due to the more precise evaluation in the definition process, and in cases where ultrasound treatment is performed with subsequent vibration-assisted aspiration of areas on the dorsal surface of the body, they should precede the excision, because of the increased risk of excess compression on the flap in a presumed previous excision of the excess from the abdominal area. This type of combination (together with a subsequent

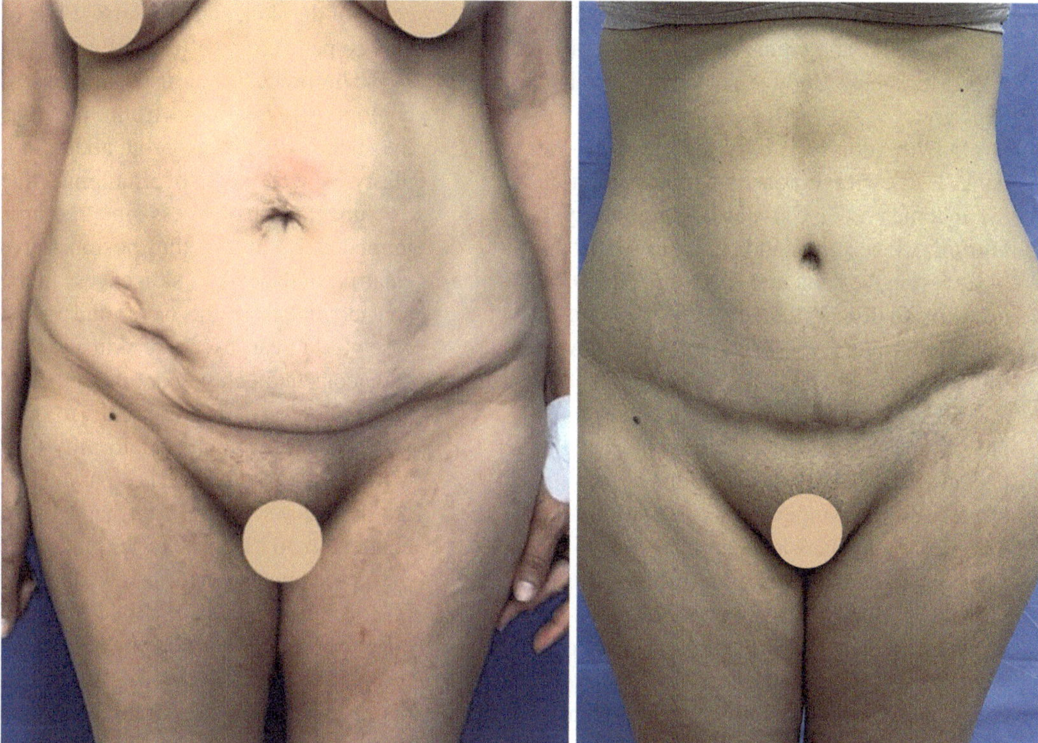

Fig. 3 A 40-year-old female patient. Before and 2 years after classic abdominoplasty

vibration-assisted liposuction of the areas) refers the technique to a subtype of 4D abdominoplasty, in which the desired effect is excision of excess subcutaneous skin and high definition in the abdomen and flanks area.

- **Vibration-assisted liposuction**
  - Vibration-assisted liposuction is used in the following options:

    As part of 3D abdominoplasty, where after BodyTite™ in the flanks area, vibration-assisted liposuction is performed on the same area ± vibration-assisted liposuction in the area cranial to the abdominal excision.

    As part of 4D Abdominoplasty, in which ultrasound treatment is performed, followed by aspiration and definition of the flanks, after which excision of the excess of skin and subcutaneous fat from the abdomen is performed, followed by ultrasound definition of the overlying flap and flanks.
- **Radiofrequency procedures in combination with ultrasound procedures and vibration-assisted liposuction**

The following combinations are possible intraoperatively, depending on the preoperative status and desired effect, in the following sequence:

- **A** (1). BodyTite™ on the flanks with vibration-assisted liposuction on the flanks ± (2). Classic abdominoplasty ± (3). Vaserlipo® on the abdomen with vibration-assisted liposuction on the abdomen and flanks
- **B** (1). BodyTite™ on the flanks with vibration-assisted liposuction on the flanks ± (2). Classic abdominoplasty ± (3). Morpheus8 Body™ on the abdomen and flanks
- **C** (1). VaserLipo® on the flanks with vibration-assisted liposuction on the flanks ± (2). Classic abdominoplasty ± (3A). Vaserlipo® in the

abdominal area with vibration-assisted liposuction in the abdominal and flanks area or (3B). Morpheus8 Body™ in the abdominal and flank area

- **D** (1). Vibration-assisted liposuction on the flanks ± (2). Vibration-assisted liposuction on the abdomen ± (3). Classic abdominoplasty
- **Option A** is recommended in cases where the pinch test in the flank area is ≥6 cm, due to the need for additional tightening of the skin. In an endomorphic type of patient, step 2 will follow, but not step 3, which is recommended at a subsequent surgical stage. In a mesomorphic type of patient, step 3 is feasible, if the patient wishes additional definition.
- **Option B** is recommended in cases where the pinch test in the flank area is ≥6 cm, due to the need for additional tightening of the skin. In this case, point 3 is recommended after the excision, if there is a need to stimulate collagenogenesis due to reduced elasticity in the area cranial from the removed excess, which is a possible option for ecto-, as well as meso- and endomorphic types of patients.
- **Option C** is recommended for ecto- and mesomorphic types of patients with a pinch test <6 cm in the flank area, in which 360° definition is aimed for.
- **Option D** is recommended for endo- and mesomorphic types of patients, where there is an additional risk of complications due to existing comorbidities and/or harmful habits.

(b) Secondary procedures

- **Radiofrequency procedures:**
  - **BodyTite™, FaceTite™, AccuTite™** are used to correct residual contour irregularities and skin laxity. Use the specified tip depending on the area of the surgical defect. For the large deformity—the BodyTite cannula is used and small deformity—the FaceTite and AccuTite cannulas are used. The goal is to reach parameters as follows: 70 °C for the internal probe for destruction of subcutaneous fat accumulation and 40 °C for the external probe for additional tightening of the skin, and deposit 8–10 kJ of energy per 10 cm^2 of treated area [17–19]. The procedure is used in areas of contour irregularities from previous liposuction in 3D and 4D abdominoplasty, as well as in 'overjumping' due to subcutaneous excess in the area immediately above the postoperative cicatrix; in the case of skin excess in the area cranial from the navel and in the case of 'dog-ear' excess of skin and subcutaneous fat in classic or other types of abdominoplasty. Wait 6 months to optimally assess the contour deformity.
  - **Morpheus8 Body™:** The parameters are as follows: 7–5–3 mm burst mode depth with 30 kJ, 3 stacks per place, and the procedure is performed in the late postoperative period, on the 45th day, after which a third one can be performed for optimal effect, again in 45 days. It is mainly used in the area cranial from the navel.
  - **EVOLVE X™:** A non-invasive technique with radiofrequency energy that provides skin tightening, fat melting, and stimulation of the underlying musculature [20]. The procedure requires a cycle of several sessions and the expected improvement is 15–20% with a mostly supportive effect. The author recommends this type of interventions to start after the 45th postoperative day when looking for a positive effect, when the previous interventions included an open surgical technique.
- **Ultrasound Procedures**
  - An ultrasound massage with parameters 1.5 W/cm^2, frequency 3 MHz and duration of treatment of the respective area of 5 min, for a period of 10 days, starting from the second postoperative day, is recommended in each area with previous liposuction, respectively, areas of liposuction in 3D and 4D abdominoplasty. The process accelerates the drainage of oedema and improves

venous outflow, thereby accelerating the recovery period and improving the final results.

- **Myostimulation**
  - **TrueSculptFlex®** rely on electrical muscle stimulation and allows toning and tightening of the muscles in up to 8 areas at the same time. Electrostimulation of individual muscle groups is recommended after the fourth to sixth postoperative month, due to the need for complete resorption of primary and secondary oedema in the area of the surgical intervention. The procedure aims to optimize results in terms of muscle definition. The procedure requires a cycle of several sessions and the expected improvement is 10–15% with a mostly supportive effect.
  - Mini Abdominoplasty/with or Without Plication/

This type of intervention is an ideal option for patients with skin and/or subcutaneous fat excess located in the lower third of the abdomen. This type of intervention is increasingly used in patients after caesarean section. The technique is analogous to that of a classic abdominoplasty, except that there is no transposition of the navel.

Application of Non-invasive and Minimally Invasive Techniques

(a) Intraoperatively

- **Radiofrequency procedures:**
  - **BodyTite™:** Radiofrequency treatment in the area cranial from the marked area to be excised is not recommended, due to the coagulation effect. It can be applied in adjacent areas, for example, the flank area, with the ultimate goal of achieving 360° definition in the hip and abdomen area (Figs. 4 and 5). The parameters are described in detail in Section: 3D Abdominoplasty.
  - **Morpheus8 Body™:** At the end of the surgical intervention a radiofrequency microneedling procedure could be applied in order to improve the elasticity of skin in the abdominal area. The procedure parameters are as follows: 7–5–3 mm burst mode depth with 30 kJ, 3 stacks per place.
- **Ultrasound procedures**
  - **Vaserlipo®:** Ultrasound lipoplasty is possible both in the area cranial to the excision and in the flanks area. The ultrasound technique is vascular sparing; therefore, it is believed that the combination with an open excision technique does not increase the risk regarding the repair of the operative defect. Vaserlipo® and the subsequent vibration-assisted liposuction may precede, but also follow, the excision of excess subcutaneous skin. The author recommends that the excision precedes the ultrasound treatment, when talking about the abdominal area, due to the more precise evaluation in the definition process, and in cases where ultrasound treatment is performed with subsequent vibration-assisted aspiration of areas on the dorsal surface of the body, they should precede the excision, because of the increased risk of excess compression on the flap in a presumed previous excision of the excess from the abdominal area. The parameters are described in detail in Section: 4D Abdominoplasty.
- **Vibration-assisted liposuction**
  - Vibration-assisted liposuction is used in the following options:

    After BodyTite™ in the flank area, vibration-assisted liposuction is performed on the same area ± vibration-assisted liposuction in the area cranial to the excision.

    After ultrasound treatment is performed, followed by subsequent aspiration and definition of the flank, excision of the excess skin and subcutaneous fat from the abdominal area is performed, followed by ultrasound treatment and definition of the overlying flap and flanks.

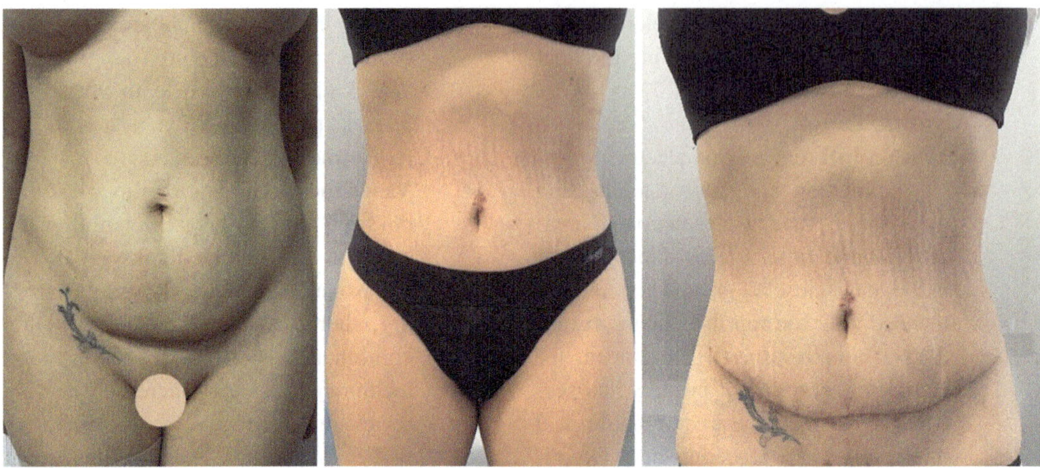

Fig. 4 Before and 6 months after mini abdominoplasty with BodyTite™ and vibration-assisted liposuction on the flanks

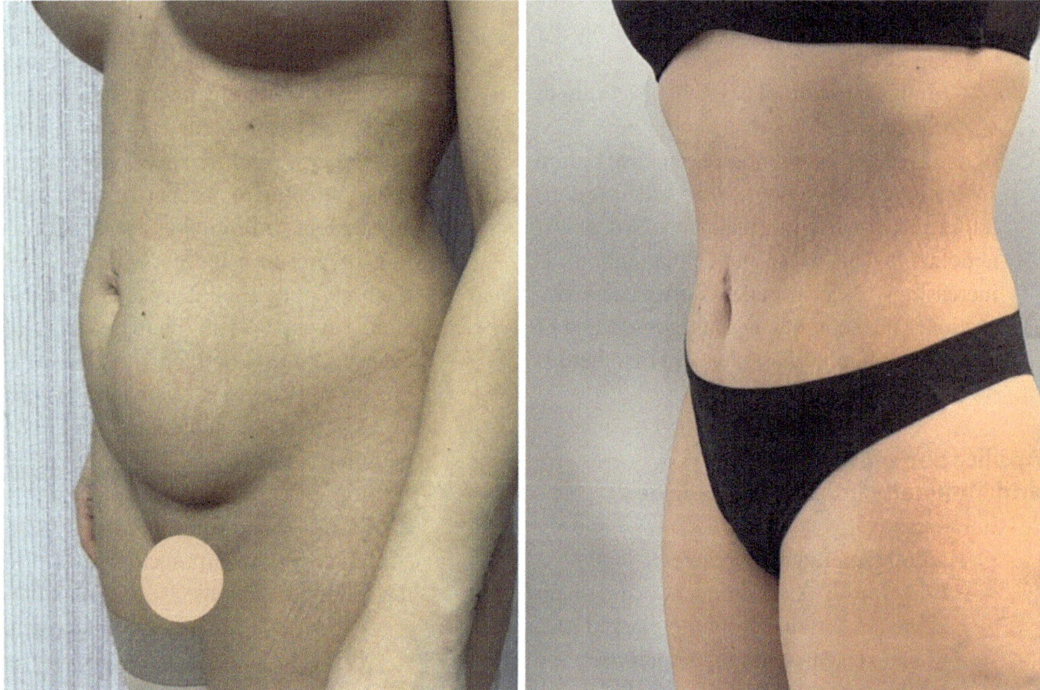

Fig. 5 Before and 6 months after mini abdominoplasty with BodyTite™ and vibration-assisted liposuction on the flanks

- **Radiofrequency procedures in combination with ultrasound procedures and vibration-assisted liposuction**

The following combinations are possible, depending on the preoperative status and desired effect, in the following sequence during the operative process:

- **A** (1). BodyTite™ on the flanks with vibration-assisted liposuction on the flanks ± (2). Mini abdominoplasty +/− (3). Vaserlipo® on the abdomen with vibration-assisted liposuction on the abdomen and flanks
- **B** (1). BodyTite™ on the flanks with vibration-assisted liposuction on the flanks

± (2). Mini abdominoplasty ± (3). Morpheus8 Body™ on the abdomen and flanks
  - **C** (1). Vaserlipo® on the flanks with vibration-assisted liposuction on the flanks ± (2). Mini abdominoplasty ± (3A). Vaserlipo® in the abdominal area with vibration-assisted liposuction in the abdominal and flank area or (3B). Morpheus8 Body™ in the abdominal and flank area
  - **D** (1). Vibration-assisted liposuction on the flanks ± (2). vibration-assisted liposuction on the abdomen ± (3). Mini abdominoplasty.

(b) Secondary procedures

- **Radiofrequency procedures:**
  - **BodyTite™, FaceTite™, AccuTite™** are used to correct residual contour irregularities and skin laxity [21]. Use the specified tip depending on the area of the surgical defect. For large deformity—the BodyTite cannula is used and small deformity—the FaceTite and AccuTite cannulas are used. The goal is to reach parameters as follows: 70 °C for the internal probe for destruction of subcutaneous fat accumulation and 40 °C the external probe for additional tightening of the skin, and deposit 8–10 kJ of energy per 10 cm^2 of treated area. The procedure is used in areas of contour irregularities from previous liposuction in 3D and 4D abdominoplasty, as well as in 'overjumping' due to subcutaneous excess in the area immediately above the postoperative cicatrix; in the case of skin excess in the area cranial from the navel and in the case of 'dog-ear' excess of skin and subcutaneous fat in classic or other types of abdominoplasty. Wait sixth months to optimally assess the contour deformity.
  - **Morpheus8 Body™:** The parameters are as follows: 7–5–3 mm burst mode depth with 30 kJ, 3 per place, and the procedure is performed in the late postoperative period, on the 45th day, after which a third one can be performed for optimal effect, again in 45 days. It is mainly used in the area cranial from the navel.
  - **EVOLVE X™:** A non-invasive technique with radiofrequency energy that provides skin tightening, fat melting and stimulation of the underlying musculature. The procedure requires a cycle of several sessions and the expected improvement is 15–20% with a mostly supportive effect. The author recommends this type of interventions to start after the 45th postoperative day when looking for a positive effect, when the previous interventions included an open surgical technique.
- **Ultrasound procedures**
  - An ultrasound massage with parameters 1.5 W/cm^2, frequency 3 MHz and duration of treatment of the respective area of 5 min, for a period of 10 days, starting from the second postoperative day, is recommended in each area with previous liposuction, respectively, areas of liposuction in 3D and 4D abdominoplasty. The process accelerates the drainage of oedema and improves venous outflow, thereby accelerating the recovery period and improving the final results.
- **Myostimulation**
  - **TrueSculptfleX®** electrostimulation of individual muscle groups is recommended after the fourth to sixth postoperative month, due to the need for complete resorption of primary and secondary oedema in the area of the surgical intervention. The procedure aims to optimize results in terms of muscle definition. The procedure requires a cycle of several sessions, and the expected improvement is 10–15% with a mostly supportive effect.

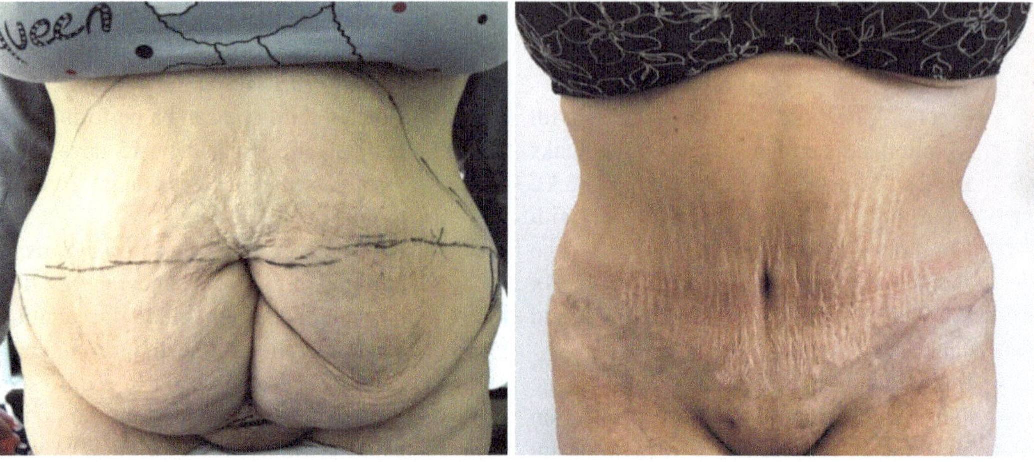

Fig. 6 Before and 6 months after High-Lateral-Tension (HLT) abdominoplasty

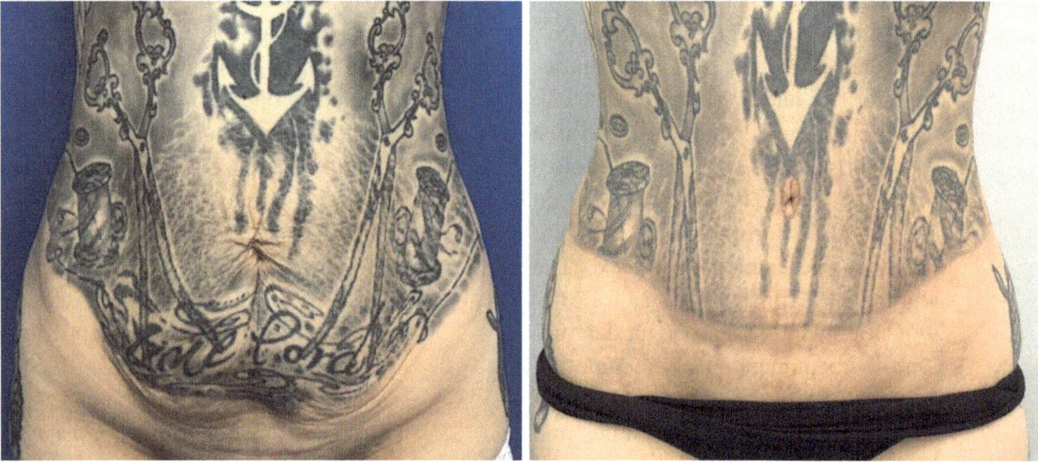

Fig. 7 Before and 6 months after High-Lateral-Tension (HLT) abdominoplasty

High-Lateral-Tension (HLT) Abdominoplasty

Provides correction of excess skin and accumulated excess of subcutaneous fat in the area of the abdominal wall. Lockwood introduced the technique in order to redistribute the main stress laterally, which restricts the dislocation and expansion of the postoperative scar [22, 23] (Figs. 6, 7 and 8).

Application of non-invasive and minimally invasive techniques: The intra- and postoperative application of non-invasive and minimally invasive techniques aimed at achieving an additional positive effect in terms of optimal contouring of the treated area, overlap with the techniques described for classic and mini abdominoplasty.

Extended Abdominoplasty

This type of abdominoplasty is suitable for patients with excessive skin and subcutaneous fat in the abdomen and flanks area. The technique is similar to that of the classic abdominoplasty, but the incision reaches or passes behind the mid-axillary line, which allows, despite the excessive skin and subcutaneous fat, to prevent 'dog-ear' postoperative deformities [24].

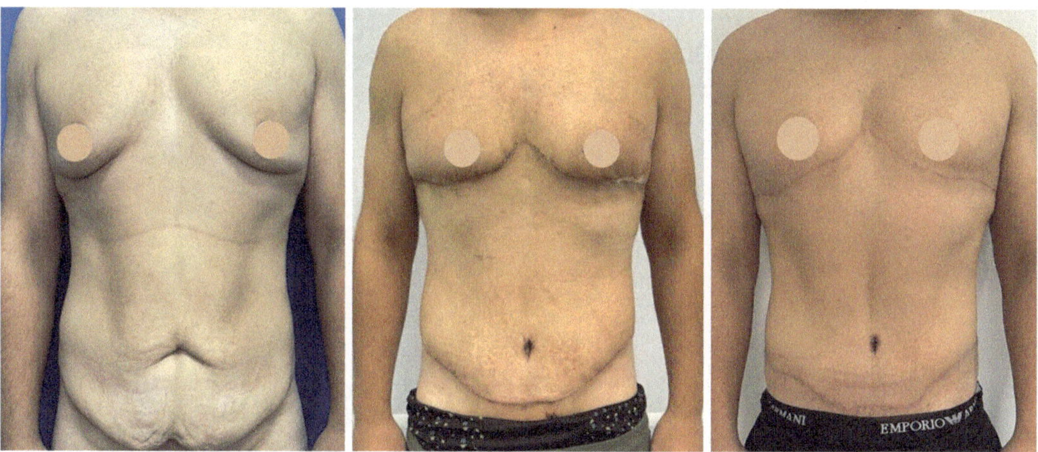

Fig. 8 Before 2 months and 1 year after High-Lateral-Tension (HLT) abdominoplasty in combination with upper-body lift with free nipple transfer

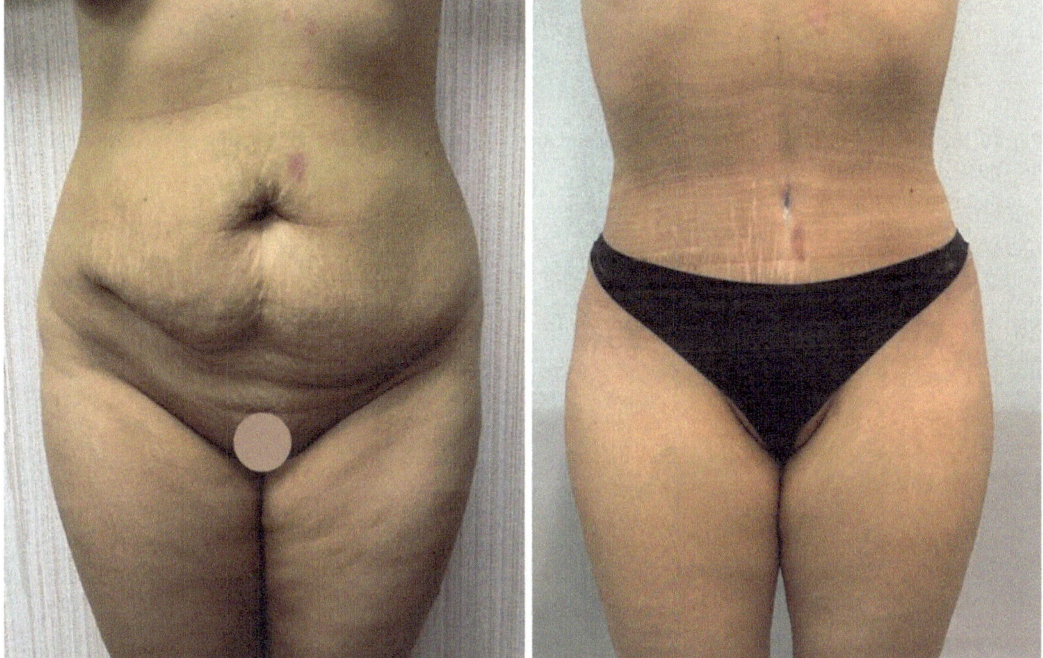

Fig. 9 Before and 6 months after extended 3D abdominoplasty with BodyTite™ and vibration-assisted liposuction of the flanks

Application of non-invasive and minimally invasive techniques: The intra- and postoperative application of non-invasive and minimally invasive techniques, aimed at achieving an additional positive effect in terms of optimal contouring of the treated area, overlap with the techniques described for classic and mini abdominoplasty (Figs. 9, 10, 11, 12, 13 and 14).

Circumferential Abdominoplasty (Belt Lipectomy)

It is used in patients after massive weight loss, which has led to excessive skin and subcutaneous fat along the entire circumference of the abdominal wall. Allows full correction of excess in the area of hip, buttocks, lateral and front surface of

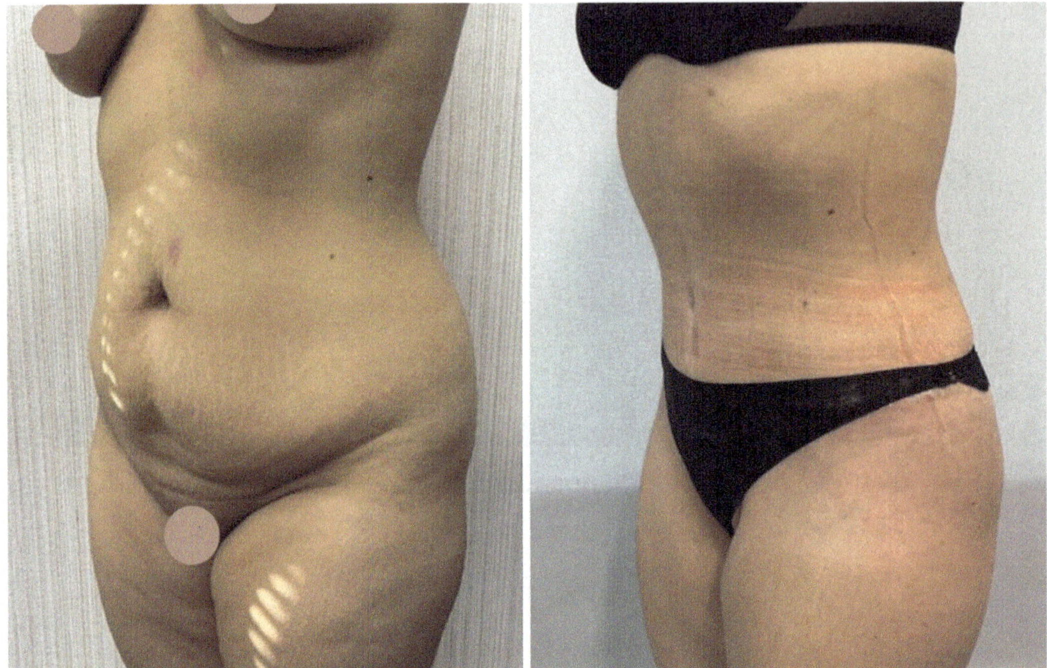

Fig. 10 Before and 6 months after extended 3D abdominoplasty with BodyTite™ and vibration-assisted liposuction of the flanks

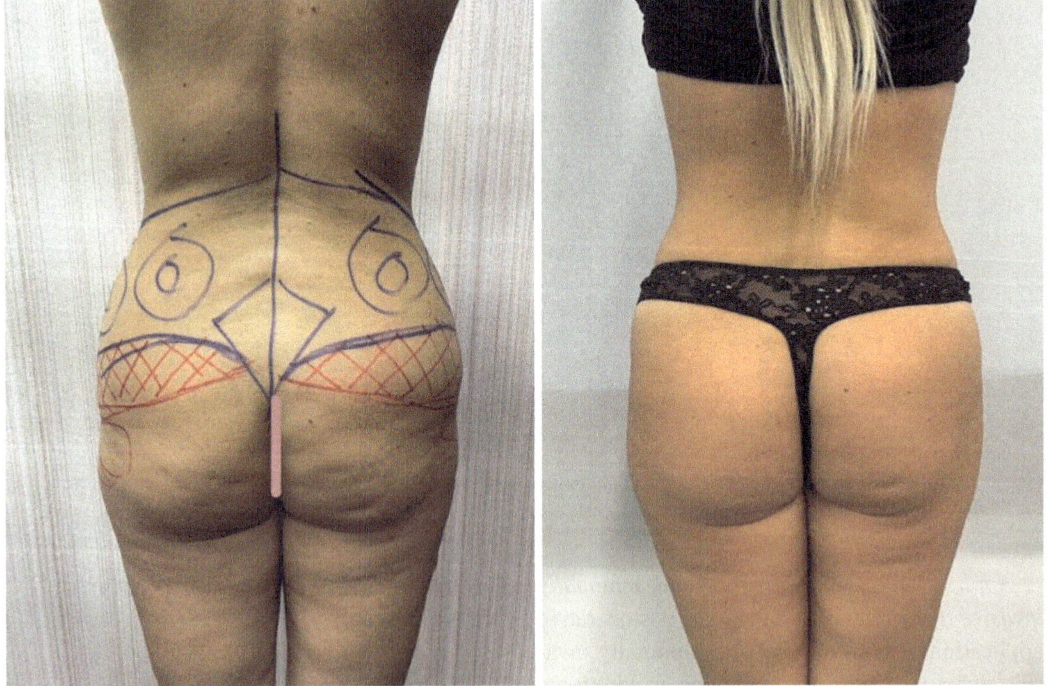

Fig. 11 Before and 6 months after extended 3D abdominoplasty with BodyTite™ and vibration-assisted liposuction of the flanks

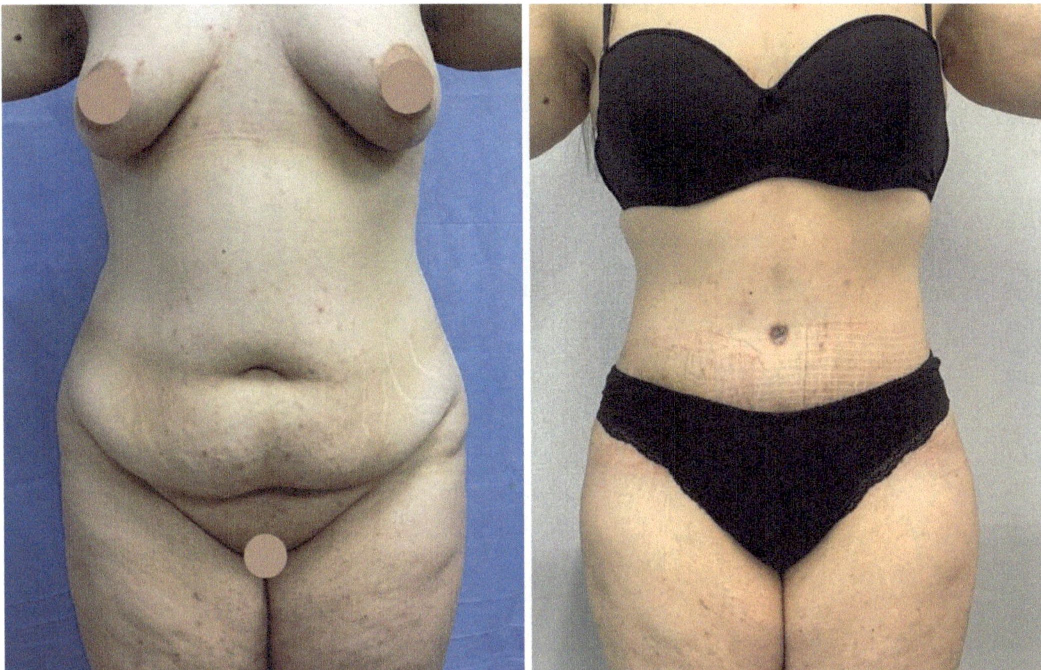

Fig. 12 Before and 6 months after extended 3D abdominoplasty with BodyTite™ and vibration-assisted liposuction of the flanks

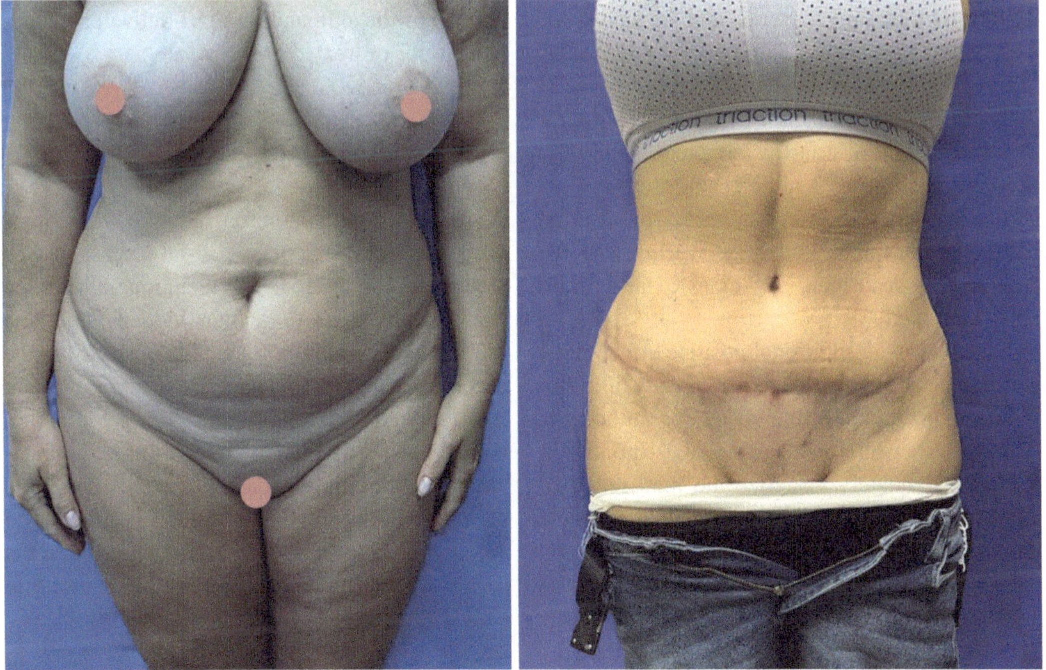

Fig. 13 Before and 6 months after extended 3D abdominoplasty with BodyTite™ and vibration-assisted liposuction of the flanks

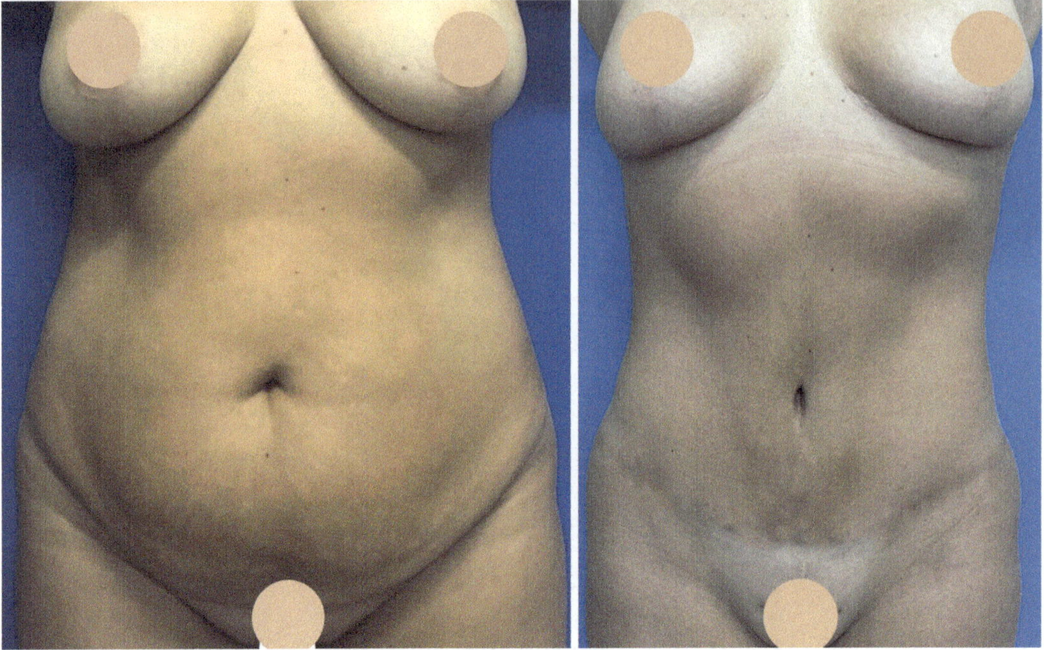

Fig. 14 Before and 1 year after extended 3D abdominoplasty with BodyTite™ and vibration-assisted liposuction of the flanks

the thighs, abdominal ptosis and ptosis of the mons pubis [25] (Figs. 15 and 16).

Application of non-invasive and minimally invasive techniques: The intra- and postoperative application of non-invasive and minimally invasive techniques, aimed at achieving an additional positive effect in terms of optimal contouring of the treated area, overlap with the techniques described in classic and mini abdominoplasty.

In this case, an additional positive effect in the buttock area can be expected by means of radiofrequency treatment of the same. The author recommends to wait for a period of 9 months in order to adequately visualize the final result of the surgical technique and adequately evaluate the possibilities to improve the final result by means of BodyTite™ radiofrequency therapy. The goal is to achieve a temperature of 40 °C on the surface of the skin and 8–10 kJ delivered energy per 10 cm^2 of treated area.

Reverse Abdominoplasty

A specific operative approach applied to patients with skin and subcutaneous fat excess in the upper abdominal area. The technique allows the postoperative scar to remain hidden under the inframammary (IMF) folds. In most cases, the umbilical ring does not need repositioning, and the technique itself is often used in combination with 'bra-line back lift'—intervention, augmentation mammoplasty, mastopexy, etc. This type of intervention is widely used in combination with upper-body lift and breast contouring in the second or subsequent stage of a body contouring plan (Fig. 17, 18 and 19).

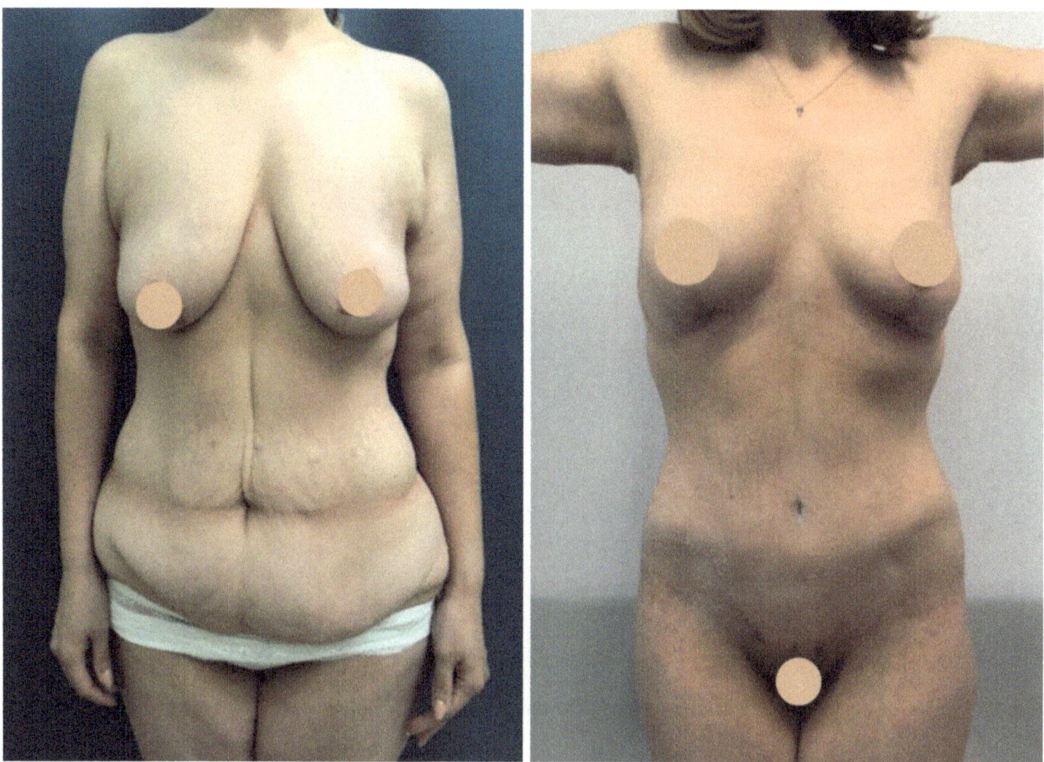

Fig. 15 Before and 1 months after belt Lipectomy and 18 months after inverted-T mastopexy with L-type brachioplasty

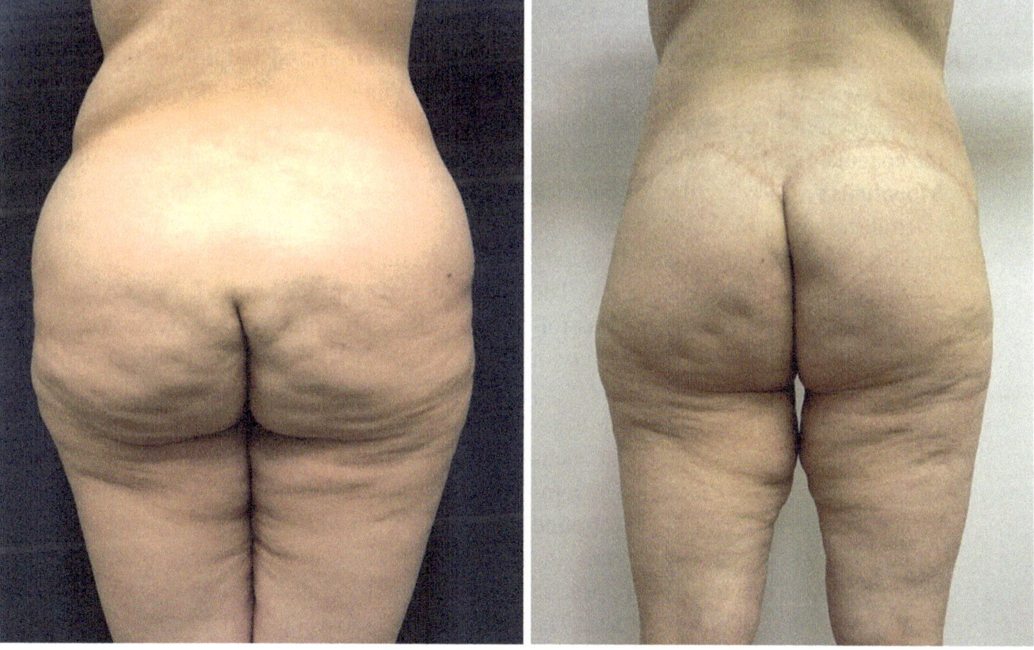

Fig. 16 Before and 1 year after belt lipectomy. Same patient from Fig. 15

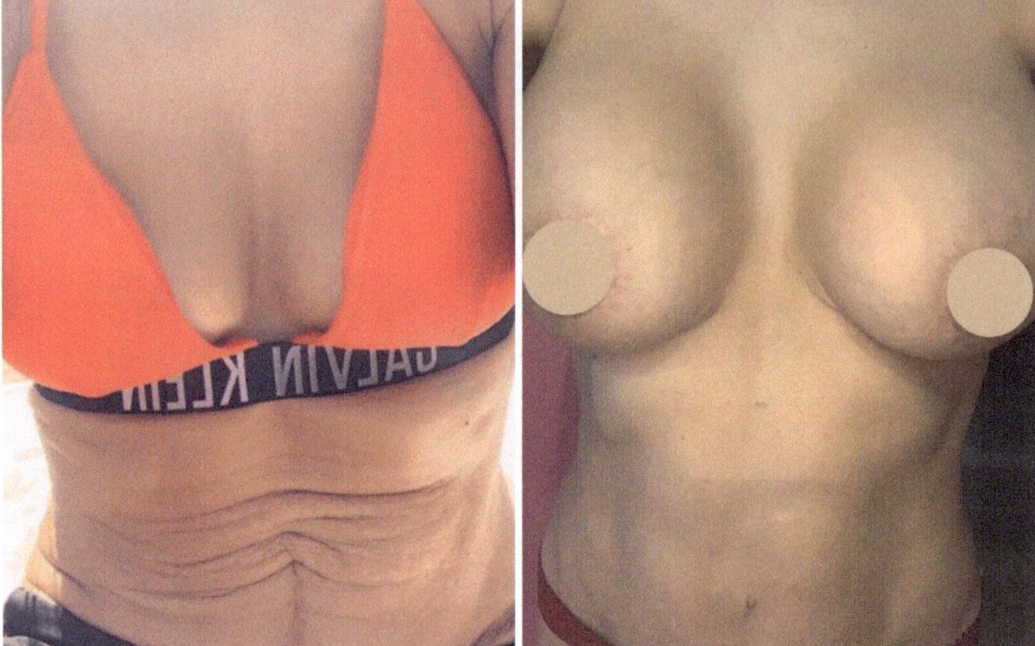

Fig. 17 A 35-year-old female patient—before and 6 months after reverse abdominoplasty with separate inframammary excisions

Application of Non-invasive and Minimally Invasive Techniques

(a) Intraoperatively
- **Radiofrequency procedures:**
  - **BodyTite™:** Radiofrequency treatment is not recommended in the area, due to the coagulation effect
  - **Morpheus8 Body™:** Radiofrequency microneedling procedure could be applied in order to improve the elasticity of skin in the abdominal area. The parameters of the procedure are as follows: 7-5-3 mm burst mode depth with 30 kJ, 3 stack per place.
- **Ultrasound procedures**
  - **Vaserlipo®:** The ultrasound technique is vessel sparing [26]. The author recommends excision to precede ultrasound treatment, when talking about the abdominal area, due to the more precise evaluation in the definition process. The parameters are described in detail in Section: 4D Abdominoplasty (Fig. 18 video attached to Fig. 18).
- **Vibration-assisted liposuction**
  - Vibration-assisted liposuction is used after excision of the skin and subcutaneous fat excess from the abdominal area, followed by ultrasound treatment and definition of the overlying flap and flanks.

(b) Secondary procedures
- **Radiofrequency procedures:**
  - **BodyTite™, FaceTite™, AccuTite™** are used to correct residual contour irregularities and skin laxity.
  - **Morpheus8 Body™:** The parameters are as follows: 7–5–3 mm burst mode depth with 30 kJ, 3 stacks per place, and the procedure is performed in the late postoperative period, on the 45th postoperative day, after which a third one

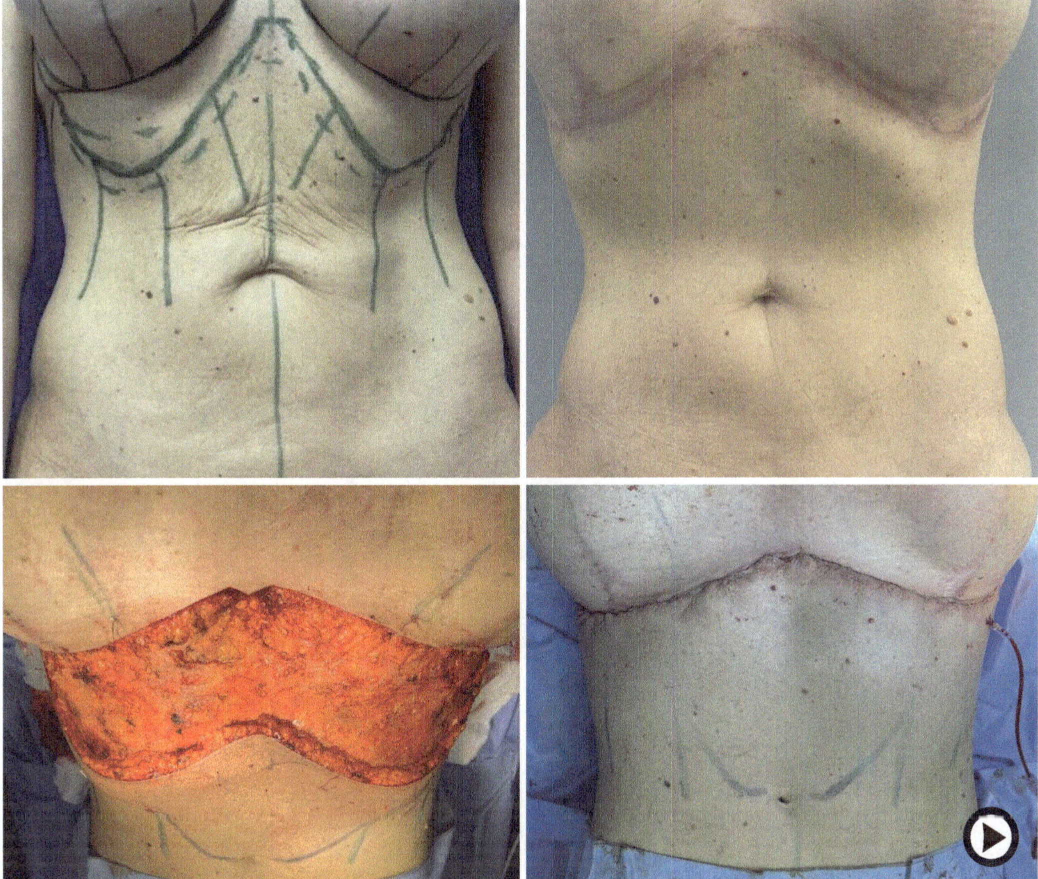

Fig. 18 A 40-year-old female patient—before and 6 months after, also intraoperative illustration of the excision and immediately after reverse abdominoplasty with submammary scars crossing the midline. Endoscopic illustration of the subcutaneous tunnel above the umbilicus during endoscopic reverse abdominoplasty, which is done in order to lift the skin and reduce the soft tissue redundancy in this area (▶ https://doi.org/10.1007/000-b0d)

can be performed for optimal effect, again in 45 days. It is mainly used in the area cranial from the navel.

- **EVOLVE X™:** A non-invasive technique with radiofrequency energy that provides skin tightening, fat melting, and stimulation of the underlying musculature. The procedure requires a cycle of several sessions, and the expected improvement is 15–20% with a mostly supportive effect. The author recommends this type of interventions to start after the 45th postoperative day when looking for a positive effect, when the previous intervention included an open surgical technique.
- **TrueSculptFlex®** Electrostimulation of individual muscle groups is recommended after the fourth to the sixth postoperative month, due to the need for complete resorption of primary and secondary oedema in the area of the surgical intervention. The procedure aims to optimize results in terms of muscle definition. The procedure requires a cycle of several sessions, and the expected improvement is 10–15% with a mostly supportive effect.

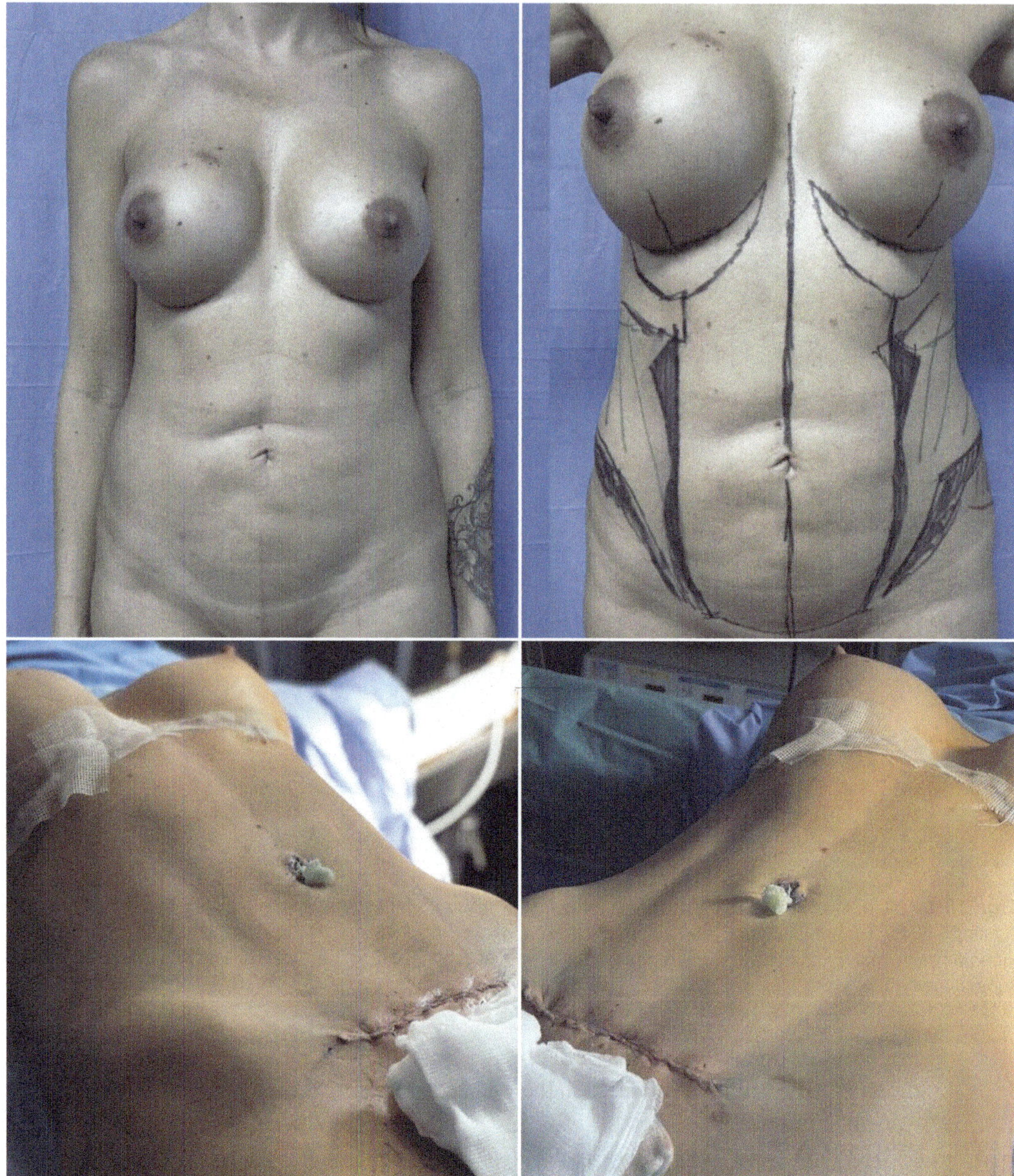

Fig. 19 A 40-year-old female patient—preoperative markings; intraoperative view; before (3rd without underwear) and sixth month (with underwear) after endoscopic reverse abdominoplasty with miniabdominoplasty and umbilical hernia repairment in combination with ultrasound VASERlipo® assisted definition of the abdomen and flanks. Postoperative scars are well hidden with the underwear

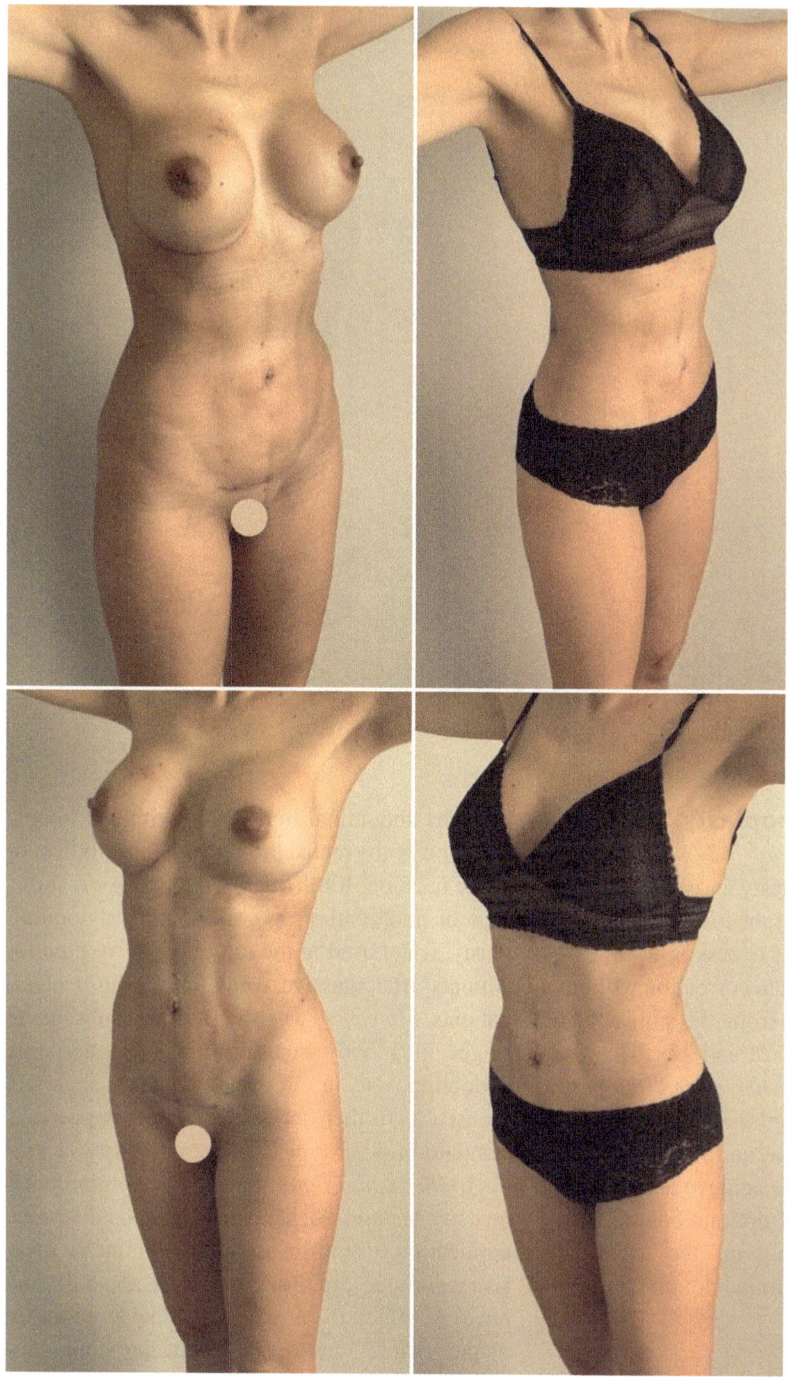

Fig. 19 (continued)

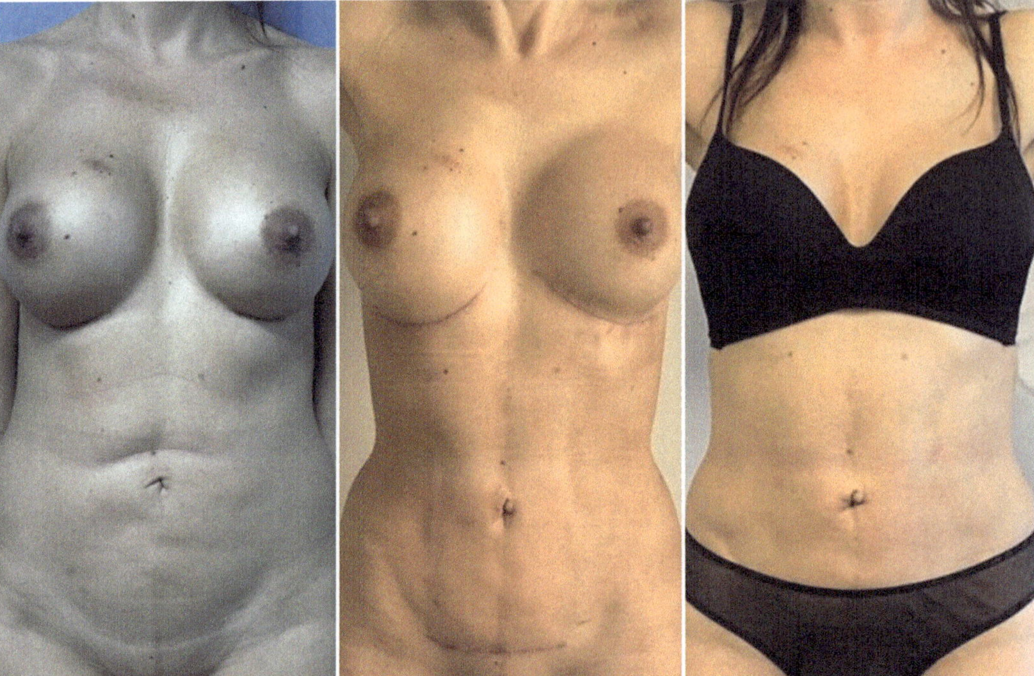

Fig. 19 (continued)

Fleur de Lys Abdominoplasty

This type of abdominoplasty is widely used in patients after massive weight loss, in whom the skin and subcutaneous fat excess is to a degree that does not allow adequate correction without a vertical midline incision from the pubis to the subxiphoid [27] (Figs. 20, 21 and 22).

Application of non-invasive and minimally invasive techniques: The intra- and postoperative application of non-invasive and minimally invasive techniques in order to achieve an additional positive effect in terms of optimal contouring of the treated area overlap with the techniques described in classic and mini abdominoplasty.

Endoscopic Abdominoplasty

A variant of conventional techniques that is applicable to patients with a weight close to the perfect for their habitus, with minimal accumulation of subcutaneous fat, muscle diastasis, without skin laxity. The nature of the intervention includes abdominal liposuction with endoscopic plication of the rectus through a transumbilical or pubic incision. It follows from the above that this type of intervention, as well as mini abdominoplasty, is not used in the initial operative plan for patients after massive weight loss and/or obese patients. However, when performing subsequent stages in a body contouring plan, endoscopic abdominoplasty, as an operative approach, could be used to further correct the area of a previous standard or other type of abdominoplasty.

Application of non-invasive and minimally invasive techniques: The intra- and postoperative application of non-invasive and minimally invasive techniques, in order to achieve an additional positive effect in terms of optimal contouring of the treated area, overlap with the techniques described in the classic and mini abdominoplasty. Ultrasound treatment is widely used in the area of the hip and/or abdomen and/or adjacent areas of the body with the aim of 360° definition and/or total body contouring. In the case of the mentioned preoperative status, procedures for additional tightening of the skin such as radio-

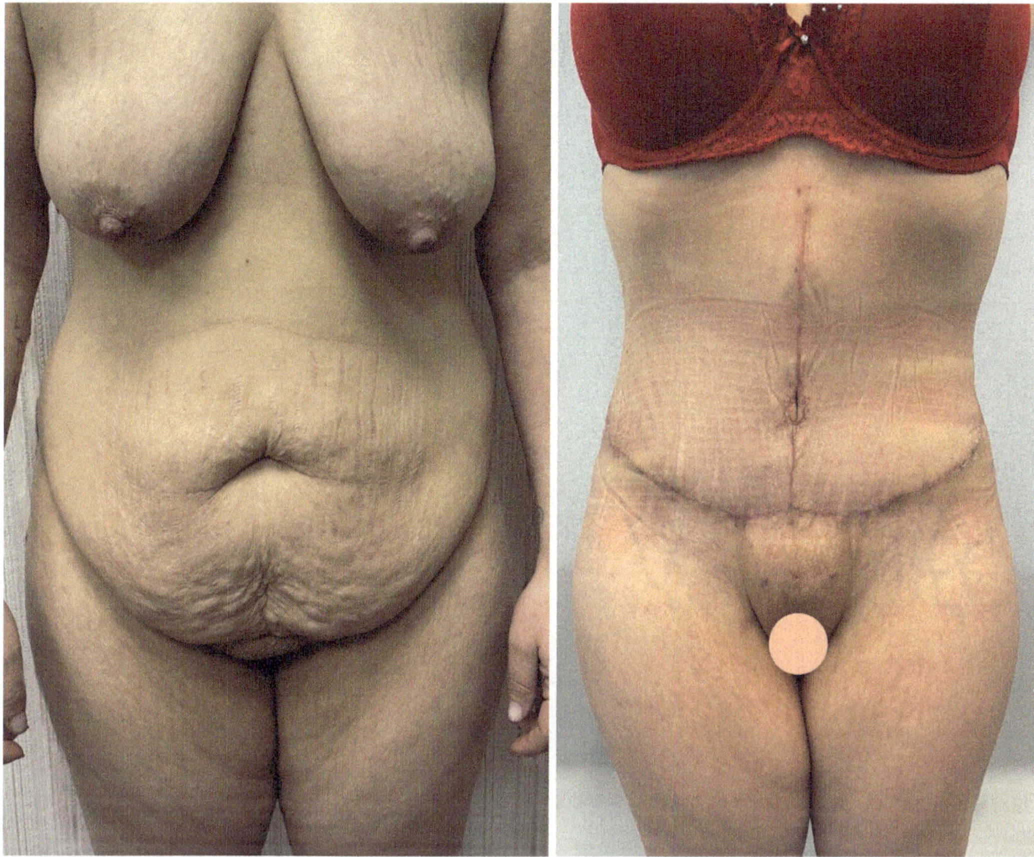

Fig. 20 Before and 6 months after Fleur De Lys Abdominoplasty in a 40-year-old massive weight loss patient

frequency interventions (Morpheus8 Body™ at the end of the surgical intervention, as well as EVOLVE X™ in the postoperative period) and electrical myostimulation procedures for additional definition (TrueSculptFlex®) are also widely used.

3D Abdominoplasty

An abdominoplasty variation, which, improves the aesthetics. BodyTite™ and vibration-type of liposuction in the flanks with/without vibrational liposuction in the abdomen area is added to classic and extended or high lateral tension abdominoplasty [9, 28–39]. Best candidates for 3D abdominoplasty—patients with subcutaneous excess in the abdomen and flanks with a compromised skin elasticity. These most often include patients above average age. To optimize lasting aesthetics, the preferred approach follows:

In prone position and after infiltration of Klein's solution, radiofrequency lipolysis is performed on the deep layer of subcutaneous fat, at a depth of 3 or 4 or 5 or 6 cm, depending on the preoperative pinch test, in the area of the lower back and flanks, the purpose being to achieve 70 °C heating to permanently destroy fat deposits (in the presence of 100% fat cells in 10 cm^2, even reaching a destruction of 50% of the fat cells will enable the patient to accumulate 50% less fat deposits in the area). It is followed by radiofrequency treatment at a depth of 1–2 cm, depending on the preoperative pinch test, for skin contraction, the purpose being to reach 40 °C superficial heating. The optimal energy recommended by the author is 8–10 kJ per 10 cm^2 of treated area.

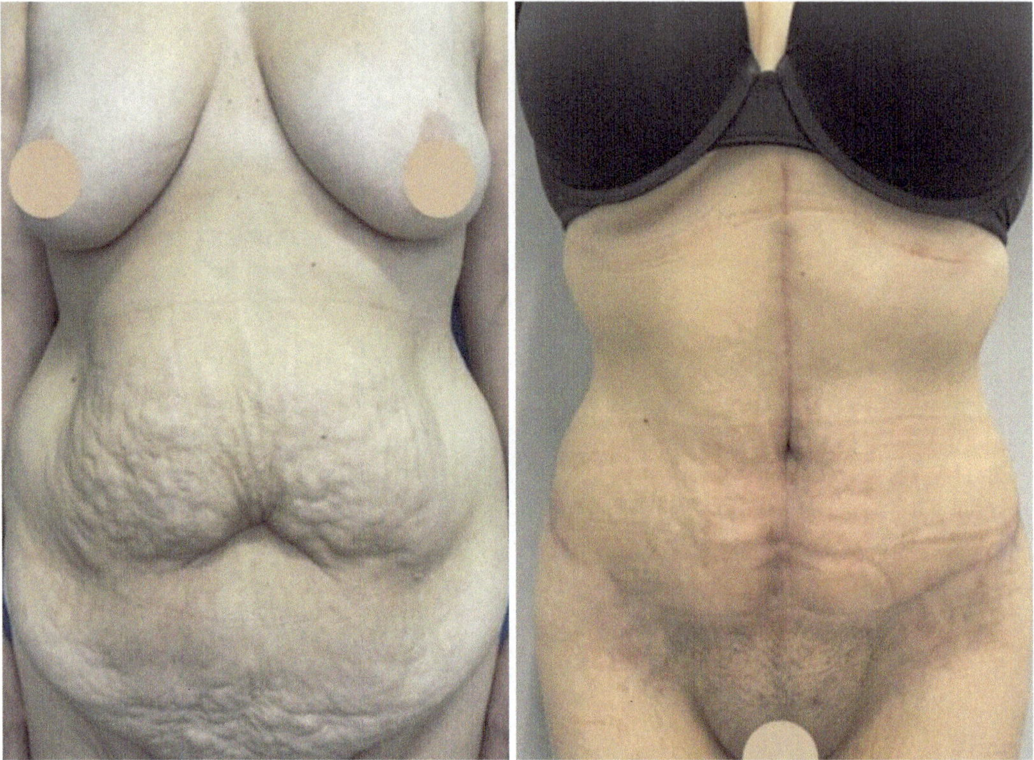

Fig. 21 Before and 6 months after Fleur De Lys Abdominoplasty

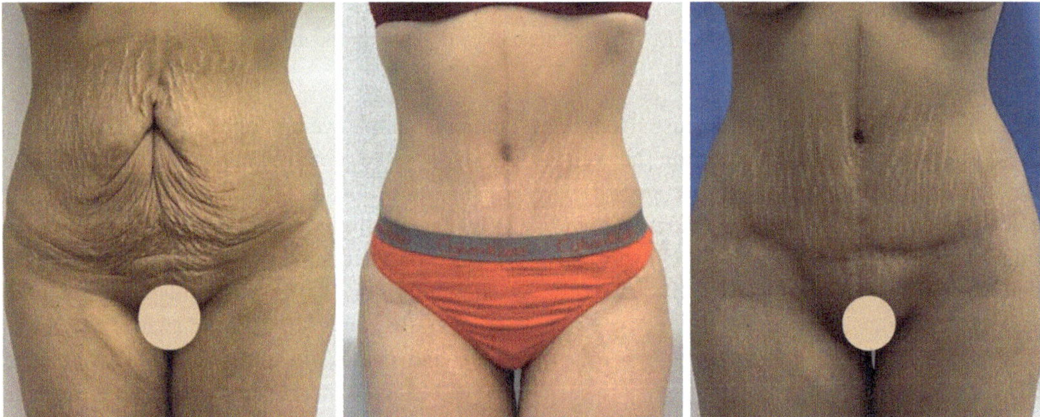

Fig. 22 Before and 6 months after Fleur De Lys Abdominoplasty in a 40-year-old patient. The picture showing the scar position and quality is 1 year after the procedure

Vibration assisted liposuction is performed in order to aspirate the already melted subcutaneous fat. The author recommends 3 and 4 mm straight and curved Mercedes type of cannulas.

Repositioning the patient supine and proceed as follow:

- Skin incision according to the preoperative marking/depending on the patient's habitus, the type of underwear
- *Infiltration of Klein's solution, followed by vibration-assisted liposuction with N4 straight and curved cannula in the flanks area and, if necessary, cranially from the navel*

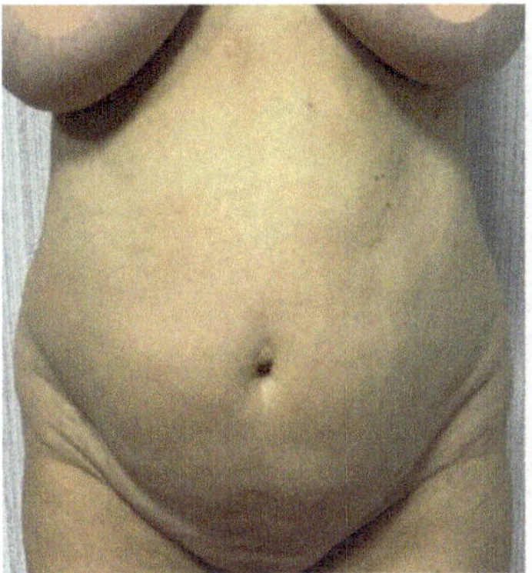
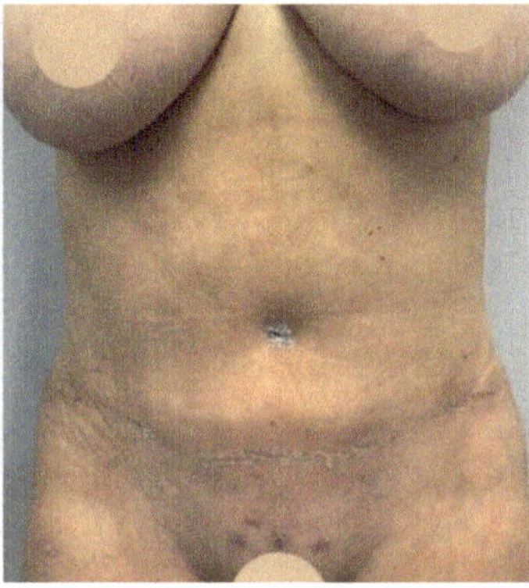
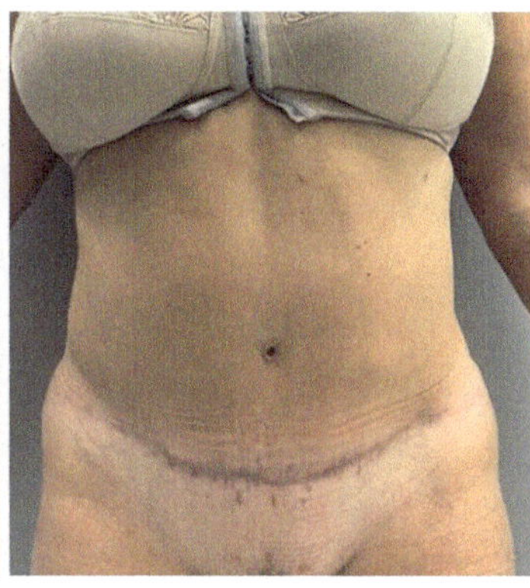

Fig. 23 Before and 3 months and 1 year after 3D abdominoplasty—abdominoplasty with muscle plication + BodyTite™ radiofrequency lipolysis of the flanks and vibration-assisted liposuction of the flanks and abdomen (cranially from the navel, the liposuction is 'sparing' with N4 long curved cannula of Mercedes type)

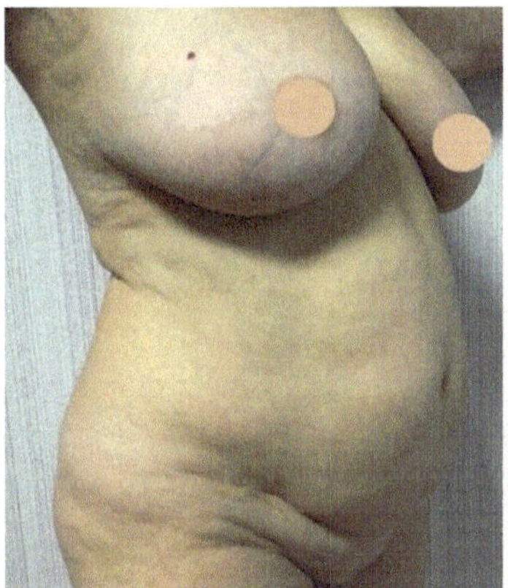
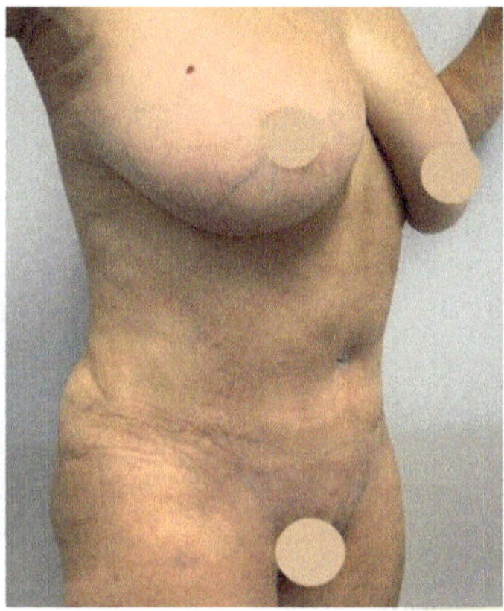
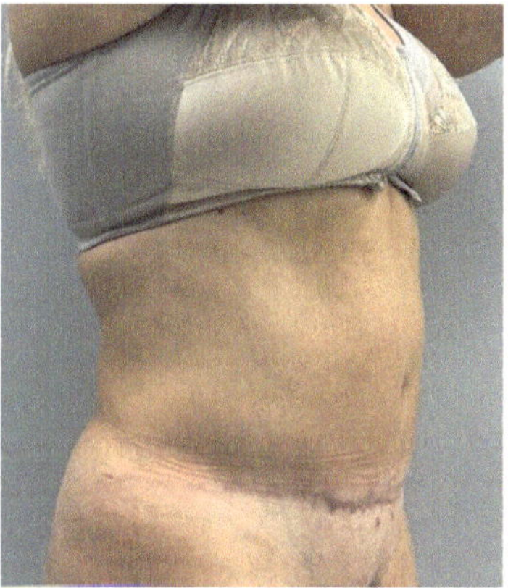

Fig. 24 Before 3 months and 1 year after 3D abdominoplasty—abdominoplasty with muscle plication + BodyTite™ radiofrequency lipolysis of the flanks and vibration-assisted liposuction of the flanks and abdomen (cranially from the navel, the liposuction is 'sparing' with N4 long curved cannula of Mercedes type)

- Elevation of the skin-subcutaneous flap with preservation of the umbilical stock
- If necessary, plication of available diastasis of m.rectus abdominis, m.obliqus abdominis, 'low horizontal plication'
- Excision of the excessive skin and subcutaneous fat excess
- Suturing the navel
- Additional Baroudi sutures
- Closure of the surgical incision with adequate redistribution of tension, drainage

Application of non-invasive and minimally invasive techniques: The intraoperative combination is the preferred one described by the author above. The postoperative application of non-invasive and minimally invasive techniques in order to achieve an additional positive effect in terms of optimal contouring of the treated area overlap with the techniques described in classic and mini abdominoplasty (Figs. 23, 24, 25 and 26).

4D Abdominoplasty

- In this case, high-definition Vaserlipo® sculpting in the abdominal area with/without the flanks area is added to procedure of abdominoplasty [40]. Best candidates for 4D abdominoplasty are patients with subcutaneous excess in the abdomen and flanks, pre-

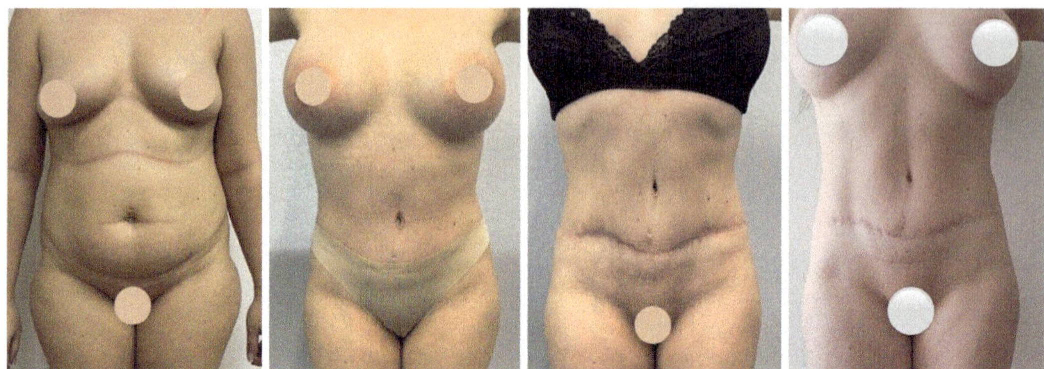

Fig. 25 Before 3 months and 1 year after 3D abdominoplasty—abdominoplasty with muscle plication + BodyTite™ radiofrequency lipolysis of the flanks and vibration-assisted liposuction of the flanks and abdomen (cranially from the navel, the liposuction is 'sparing' with N4 long curved cannula of Mercedes type). One-stage augmentation mammoplasty was performed with BodyTite™ radiofrequency lipolysis and vibration-assisted liposuction of the hips with N3 and N4 long curved cannula of Mercedes type

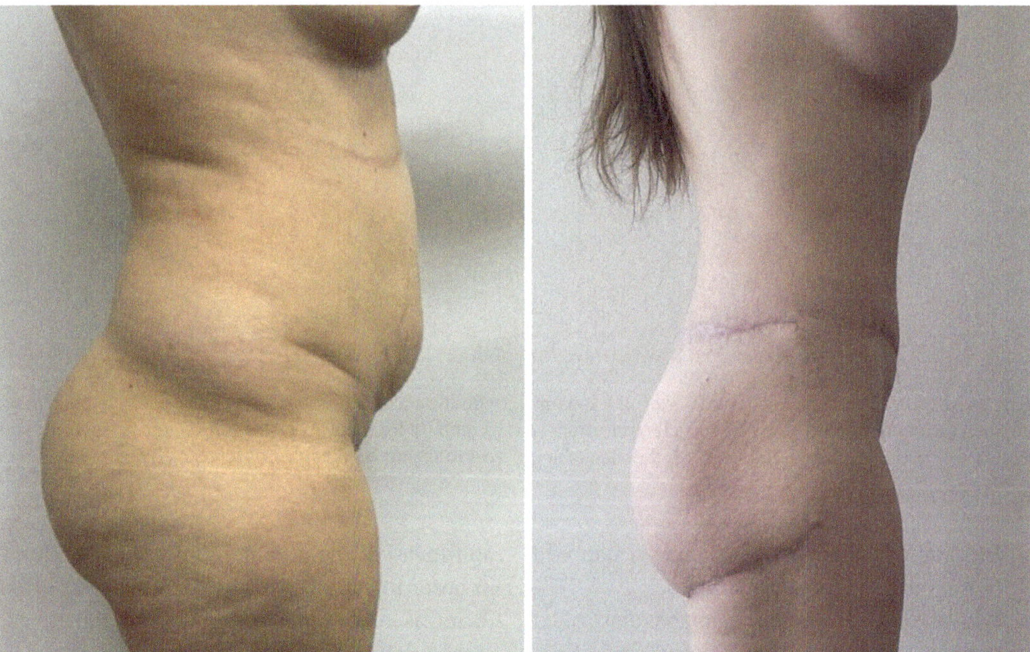

Fig. 26 Before and 1 year after 3D Abdominoplasty—abdominoplasty with muscle plication + BodyTite™ radiofrequency lipolysis of the flanks and Vibration-assisted liposuction of the flanks and abdomen. One-stage augmentation mammoplasty was performed with BodyTite™ radiofrequency lipolysis and vibration-assisted liposuction of the hips with N3 and N4 long curved cannula of Mercedes type. Postoperative scars in the lower back and buttock area from gluteoplasty procedure done 6 months after the combination of procedures from above

served skin elasticity and desired definition. These most often include young patients without serious accompanying diseases. To optimize the results and ensure longevity, the approach is as follows:

- In prone position, after infiltration of Klein's solution, it is proceeded to ultrasound treatment of the flank area as follows:
  - *Vaserlipo® with 2-ring cannula on 80% VASER MODE surface treatment of the*

tissues, as the duration of treatment of the area is 1 min per 100 mL of infiltrated solution and/or until overcoming the resistance while the cannula is moving subcutaneously. It is switched to 80% CONTINUOUS MODE with 2-ring cannula in order to treat the deep layer of subcutaneous fat tissue [26, 41–45].
  - *Vibration-assisted liposuction for definition and lipoaspiration, as the author recommends the use of straight, curved, and angled 3 and 4 mm cannulas of Mercedes type.*
- Repositioning the patient on his back, thoroughly covering and cleaning of the surgical field with subsequent actions are as follows:
  - Skin incision according to the preoperative marking/depending on the patient's habitus, the type of underwear
  - Elevation of the skin-subcutaneous flap with preservation of the umbilical stock—up to the level of the costal rim and 4–5 cm "tunnel" from the umbilicus up to the xyphoid bone
  - If necessary, plication of available diastasis of m.rectus abdominis, m.obliqus abdominis, 'low horizontal plication'
  - Excision of the excessive skin and subcutaneous fat excess
  - Suturing the navel
  - *Infiltration of Klein's solution, followed by ultrasound treatment analogous to that described above in the hip area. Vibration-assisted liposuction with N4 and N3 straight and curved cannula in the hip and abdomen area*
  - Additional deep Baroudi sutures
  - Closure of the surgical incision with adequate redistribution of tension, drainage

Application of non-invasive and minimally invasive techniques: The intraoperative combination is the preferred one described by the author above. The postoperative application of non-invasive and minimally invasive techniques for the purpose of achieving an additional positive effect in terms of optimal contouring of the treated area overlaps with the techniques described in the classic and mini abdominoplasty (Figs. 27, 28, 29 and 30).

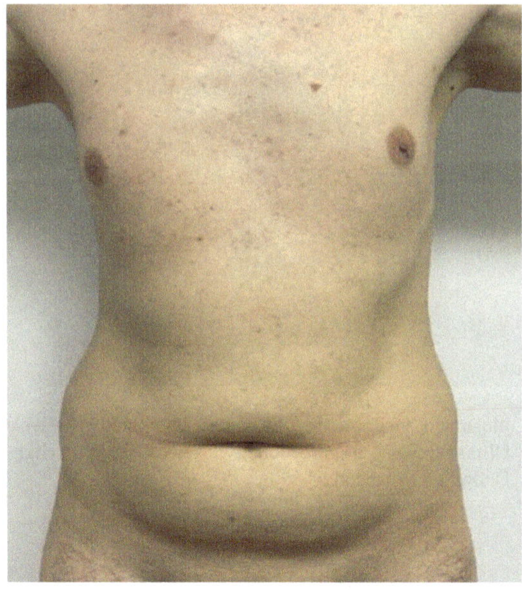

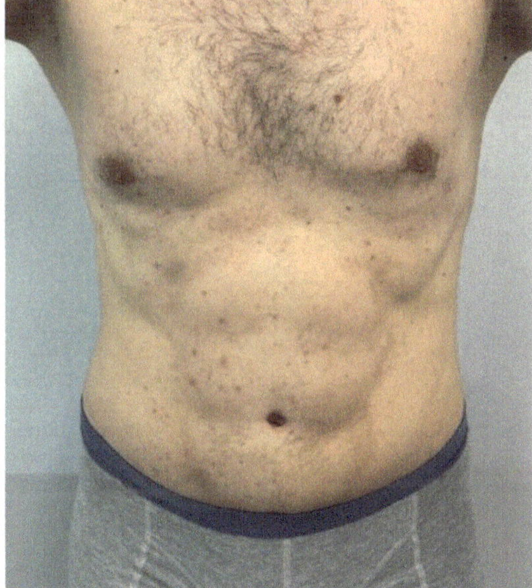

Fig. 27 Before and 3 months after ultrasound liposuction with abdominoplasty—4D Abdominoplasty. The used parameters of the ultrasound device are illustrated in Table 1 of Chapter "Minimally Invasive Ultrasound-Based Procedures: VASERlipo®: High-Definition Procedures"

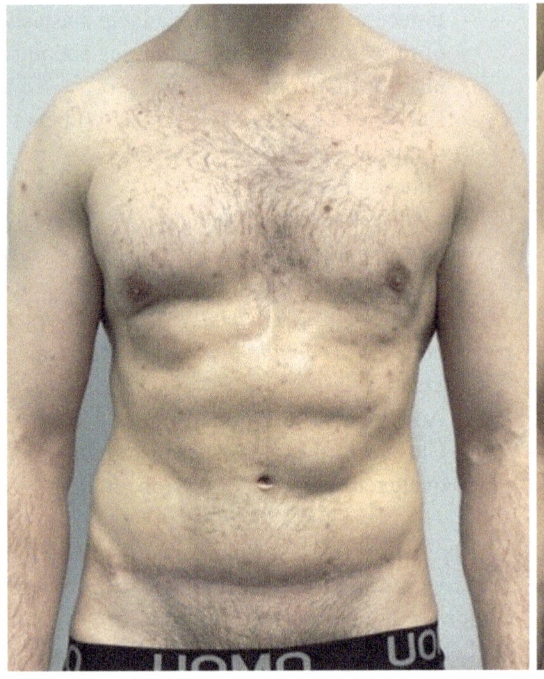

Fig. 28 1 year after and 1 year after ultrasound liposuction with abdominoplasty—4D abdominoplasty. The used parameters of the ultrasound device are illustrated in Table 1 of Chapter "Minimally Invasive Ultrasound-Based Procedures: VASERlipo®: High-Definition Procedures"

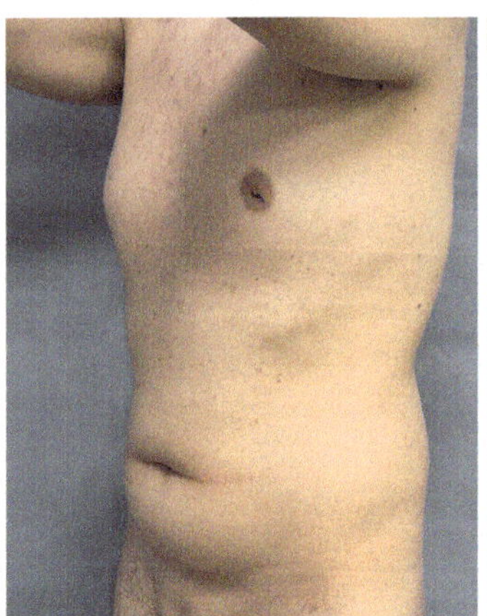

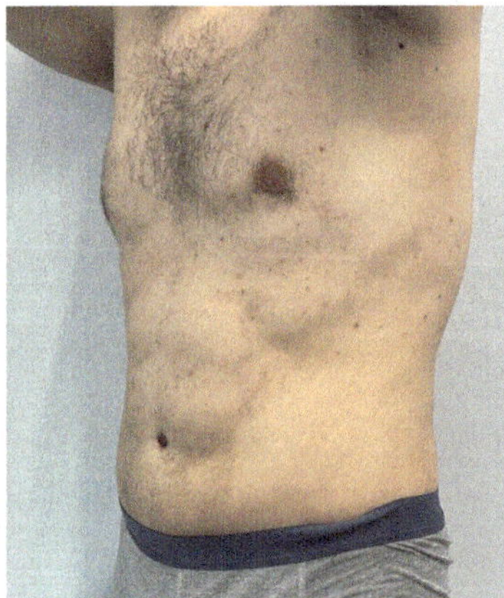

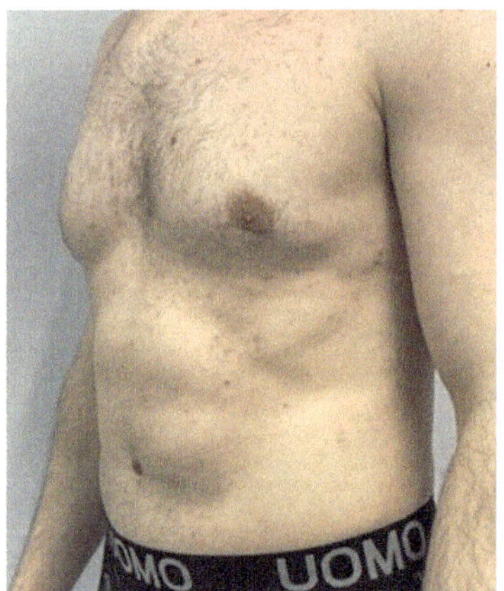

Fig. 29 Before, 3 months after and 1 year after ultrasound liposuction with abdominoplasty—4D abdominoplasty. The used parameters of the ultrasound device are illustrated in Table 1 of Chapter "Minimally Invasive Ultrasound-Based Procedures: VASERlipo®: High-Definition Procedures"

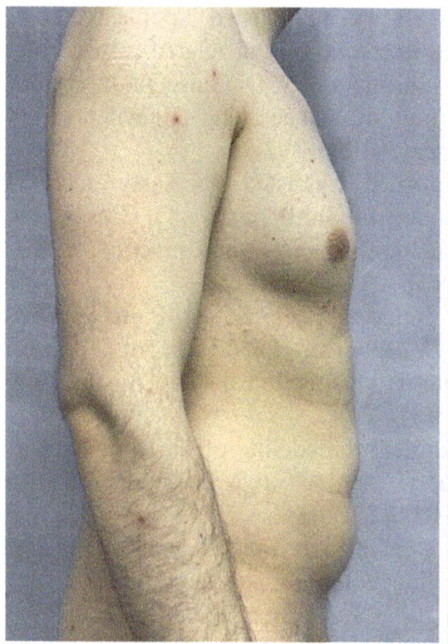
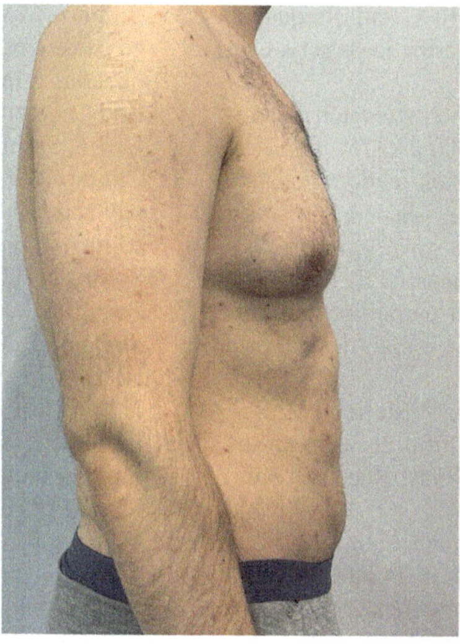
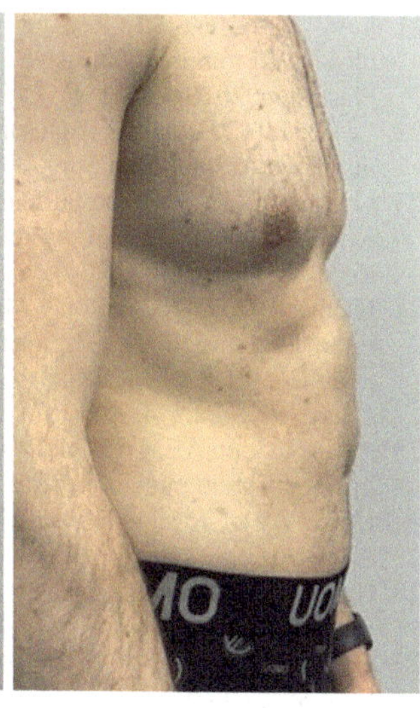

Fig. 30 Before, 3 months after and 1 year after ultrasound liposuction with abdominoplasty—4D abdominoplasty. The used parameters of the ultrasound device are illustrated in Table 1 of Chapter "Minimally Invasive Ultrasound-Based Procedures: VASERlipo®: High-Definition Procedures"

References

1. Matarasso A, Aly A, Hurwitz DJ, Lockwood TE. Body contouring after massive weight loss. Aesthet Surg J. 2004;24:452.
2. Knoetgen J III, Petty PM, Johnson CH. Plastic surgery after bariatric surgery and massive weight loss. Mayo Clin Proc. 2005;80:136.
3. Giordano S, Victorzon M, Stormi T. Suominen E desire for body contouring surgery after bariatric surgery: do body mass index and weight loss matter? Aesthet Surg J. 2014;34(1):96–105.
4. Paul MA, Opyrchal J, Knakiewicz M, Jaremkow P, Duda-Barcik L, Ibrahim AMS, Lin SJ. The long-term effect of body contouring procedures on the quality of life in morbidly obese patients after bariatric surgery. PLoS One. 2020;15(2):e0229138.
5. Wiser I, Heller L, Spector C, Fliss E, Friedman T. Body contouring procedures in three or more anatomical areas are associated with long-term body mass index decrease in massive weight loss patients: A retrospective cohort study. J Plastic Reconstruct Aesthet Surg. 2017;70(9):1181–5.
6. Zook EG. Abdominoplasty following gastrointestinal bypass surgery. Plast Reconstr Surg. 1983;71(4):500–7.
7. Pitanguy I. Evaluation of body contouring surgery today: a 30-year perspective. Plast Reconstr Surg. 2000;105:1499.
8. Kamper MJ, Galloway DV, Ashley F. Abdominal panniculectomy after massive weight loss. Plast Reconstr Surg. 1972;50:441.
9. Ogawa T, Hattori R, Yamamoto T, Gotoh M. Safe use of ultrasonically activated devices based on current studies. Expert Rev Med Devices. 2011;8(3):319–24.
10. Hunstad JP, Remus R. Atlas of abdominoplasty. Amsterdam: Elsevier; 2009.
11. Al-Basti HB, El-Khatib HA, Taha A, Sattar HA, Bener A. Intraabdominal pressure after full abdominoplasty in obese multiparous patients. Plast Reconstr Surg. 2004;113:2145.
12. Aly AS. Body contouring after massive weight loss. St. Louis, MO: Quality Medical Publishing; 2006. p. 400.
13. Illouz Y, DeVillers Y. Body sculpturing by lipoplasty. 1st ed. Edinburgh: Churchill Livingstone; 1989.
14. Bolton MA, Pruzinsky T, Cash TF, Persing JA. Measuring outcomes in plastic surgery: body image and quality of life in abdominoplasty patients. Plast Reconstr Surg. 2003;112:619.
15. Heddens CJ. Body contouring after massive weight loss. Plast Surg Nurs. 2004;24:107.
16. Hoyos AE, Prendergast PM. High definition body sculpting. Berlin: Springer; 2014. p. 73–80.
17. Mulholland RS. The BodyTite Book, vol. 261. 2nd ed; 2021. p. 734–50.
18. Dayan E, Burns AJ, Rohrich RJ, Theodorou S. The use of radiofrequency in aesthetic surgery. Plast Reconstr Surg Glob Open. 2020;8(8):e2861.
19. Theodorou SJ, Del Vecchio D, Chia CT. Soft tissue contraction in body contouring with radiofrequency-assisted liposuction: a treatment gap solution. Aesthet Surg J. 2018;38:S74–83.
20. Mulholland RS. Radiofrequency energy for non-invasive and minimally invasive skin tightening. Clin Plast Surg. 2011;38:437–48.

21. Levy AS, Grant RT, Rothaus KO. Radiofrequency physics for minimally invasive aesthetic surgery. Clin Plast Surg. 2016;43:551–6.
22. Le Louarn C, Pascal JF. High superior tension abdominoplasty. Aesthet Plast Surg. 2000;24:375.
23. Lockwood T. High-lateral-tension abdominoplasty with superficial fascial system suspension. Plast Reconstr Surg. 1995;96:603.
24. Fuente del Campo A, Rojas Allegretti E, Fernandez Filho JA, Gordon CB. Regional dermolipectomy as treatment for sequelae of massive weight loss. World J Surg. 1998;22:974.
25. Aly AS, Cram AE, Chao M, Pang J, McKeon M. Belt lipectomy for circumferential truncal excess: the University of Iowa experience. Plast Reconstr Surg. 2003;111:398.
26. Hoyos AE, Prendergast PM. High definition body sculpting. Berlin: Springer; 2014. p. 147–69.
27. Dellon AL. Fleur-de-lis abdominoplasty. Aesthet Plast Surg. 1985;9:27.
28. Cimino WW. History of ultrasound-assisted lipoplasty. In: Shiffman MA, Di Giuseppe A, editors. Body contouring: art, science, and clinical practice. Berlin: Springer; 2010. p. 399.
29. Cimino WW. The physics of soft tissue fragmentation using ultrasonic frequency vibrations of metal probes. Clin Plast Surg. 1999;26:447–61.
30. Scuderi N, Devita R, D'Andrea F, Vonella M. Nuove prospettive nella liposuzione la lipoemulsificazone. Giorn Chir Plast Ricostr ed Estetica. 1987;2(1):33–9.
31. Zocchi ML. Clinical aspects of ultrasonic liposculpture. Perspect Plast Surg. 1993;7:153–74.
32. Zocchi ML. Ultrasonic assisted lipoplasty. Clin Plast Surg. 1996;23(4):575–98.
33. Troilius C. Ultrasound-assisted lipoplasty: is it really safe? Aesthet Plast Surg. 1999;23(5):307–11.
34. Baxter RA. Histologic effects of ultrasound-assisted lipoplasty. Aesthet Surg J. 1999;19:109–14.
35. Cimino WW. Ultrasonic surgery: power quantification and efficiency optimization. Aesthet Surg J. 2001;21(3):233–40.
36. Cimino WW. Ultrasound-assisted lipoplasty: basic physics, tissue interactions, and related results/complications. In: Shiffman MA, Di Giuseppe A, editors. Body contouring: art, science, and clinical practice. Berlin: Springer; 2010. p. 392.
37. Cimino WW. VASER-assisted lipoplasty: technology and technique. In: Shiffman MA, Di Giuseppe A, editors. Liposuction principles and practice. Berlin: Springer; 2006. p. 239–44.
38. Jewell ML, Fodor PB, de Souza Pinto EB, Al Shammari MA. Clinical application of VASER–assisted lipoplasty: a pilot clinical study. Aesthet Surg J. 2002;22(2):131–46.
39. Illouz YG. Surgical remodeling of the silhouette by aspiration lipolysis or selective lipectomy. Aesthet Plast Surg. 1985;9(1):7–21.
40. Villegas FJ. A novel approach to abdominoplasty: TULUA modifications (transverse plication, no undermining, full liposuction, Neoumbilicoplasty, and low transverse abdominal scar). Aesthet Plast Surg. 2014;38:511–20.
41. Hoyos A, Perez M. Dynamic-definition male pectoral reshaping and enhancement in slim, athletic, obese, and gynecomastic patients through selective fat removal and grafting. Aesthet Plast Surg. 2012;36(5):1066–77.
42. Hoyos AE. High definition liposculpture. Bucaramanga: XIII International Course of Plastic Surgery; 2003.
43. Ersek RA, Salisbury AV. Abdominal etching. Aesthet Plast Surg. 1997;21(5):328–31.
44. Hoyos AE, Perez ME, Domínguez-Millán R. Variable sculpting in dynamic definition body contouring: procedure selection and management algorithm. Aesthet Surg J. 2021;41(3):318–32.
45. Hoyos AE, Millard JA. VASER-assisted high-definition liposculpture. Aesthet Surg J. 2007;27(6):594–604.

Gluteoplasty in Combination with Radiofrequency and Ultrasound Procedures

Introduction

The etiological factors determining the patient's need and desire for correction in the area of the buttock are as follows [1, 2]:

- Patients with massive weight loss
- Lipodystrophy
- Patients with skin elasticity loss due to ageing processes
- Genetic predisposition
- Postoperative deformities
- Postmenopausal changes
- Aesthetic noxa

For the first time in 1964, Pitanguy proposed a buttock lifting technique, which included: an incision along the gluteal fold, continuing along the medial surface of the thigh with subsequent excision at the expense of lifting the ptosis buttocks. The technique so described often leads to an unsatisfactory result—a flat contour of the buttocks, smoothing of the lordosis in the lumbar spine, visible scars, accentuation of the supratrochanteric depression. Millard first emphasized the importance of the aesthetic units and the normal anatomical proportions in this area, while Lockwood contributed with an emphasis on the fascial suspension. The so-called Brazilian butt lift is increasingly applied in our days. Introduced by Pitanguy in 1990, this technique is based on buttock lifting using lipotransfer and/or silicone implants. The shape of the buttocks is determined by the gluteal muscles—mainly m.gluteus maximus et medius; the bony pelvic component; the distribution of adipose tissue—with the greatest effect regarding the contour of the area; the skin elasticity in the area.

Preoperatively, each half of the buttocks is subdivided into four quadrants, and the ideal buttocks should have the same volume ratio in relation to the lateral and medial parts, as well as in relation to the cranial and caudal parts. The accurate assessment is based on the assessment of the volume excess or deficit in each of these parts compared to the other three.

In terms of aesthetics, the so-called V-shape zone—upper inner gluteal-sacral junction is of primary importance. Ideally, the superior-medial insertion of the gluteal muscles is well defined and has a semicircular course in the cranial direction. The peak of this contour is 3–4 cm above the beginning of the intergluteal cleft. Any incisions below the level of this contour lead to deformities of the area. When the area is not well defined due to the lack of muscle tone and/or the excess of adipose tissue, the buttocks look unattractive and flattened, especially in the lateral aspect [3].

In terms of aesthetics another key component is the so-called Diamond-shape zone—lower

Supplementary Information The online version contains supplementary material available at https://doi.org/10.1007/978-3-031-33350-7_8. The videos can be accessed individually by clicking the DOI link in the accompanying figure caption or by scanning this link with the SN More Media App.

E. Sharkov, *Body Contouring Surgery*, https://doi.org/10.1007/978-3-031-33350-7_8

inner gluteal fold-leg junction. When evaluating this area, the intergluteal cleft is taken as the midline. The upper end of the cleft is easily differentiated, while the lower end is taken to be the point where the buttocks begin to diverge to the left and right. Ideally, this point of separation begins in the lower 2/3–3/4 of the musculature and the area has the shape of a diamond [3]. In this case, the infragluteal fold in its medial part runs along a line that forms an angle of 45° with the vertical bisector of the diamond. With the smoothing of the area, the line becomes horizontal, and in case of excess fat in the area, it is oriented in the cranial direction.

The presacral area begins at the level of L5 and reaches the beginning of the intergluteal cleft; it should be shorter than the latter, ideally being 1/2–1/4 of its length. If the presacral area is twice as long as the intergluteal cleft, the illusion of buttocks that are short, flattened, caudally disposed and underdeveloped is created. If the presacral area is shorter than 1/4 of the length of the intergluteal cleft and there is excess fat in the lower-medial gluteal area, the illusion of an elongated and straight intergluteal cleft is created [3].

An important aesthetic criterion is the absence of depressions along the lateral contour of the buttocks. Proportionally, the ideal lateral contour is characterized by the following ratio: the presacral area, which is delicately concave, forming an 'S' shape together with the buttock; the gluteal volume is most pronounced in the middle third of the buttocks, as the volume cranial to the middle third is equal to that caudal to it, forming a 'C' shape; the peak of the central accumulation corresponds to the level of the pubis bone. Determining the level of the largest volume is the basis of the choice of surgical technique [4].

The ideal length of the intergluteal cleft is 1/2 of the length of m.gluteus maximus, as it is centred relative to it, so that 1/4–1/3 of the gluteal volume is cranial to the beginning of the cleft and 1/4–1/3 of it is caudal to the end of the cleft.

Accurate preoperative marking is the basis of the precise surgical intervention. The positioning of the postoperative cicatrix is considered. The scar should be positioned along the course of the postoperative line that marks the upper border of the buttocks cranially. To identify this line, it is necessary to palpate the insertion of m.gluteus maximus from medial to lateral—it presents from the angle of the V-zone to spina iliaca posterior-superior, then follows the labia externa of crista iliaca, not crista iliaca itself. It is necessary to identify the most superior point of the muscle insertion along the midline of the gluteal region. Intraoperatively, the level of the caudal incision is also determined on the surgical table by pulling the soft-tissue excess to the most cranial point of the insertion. Positioning the scar lower will result in a 'division' of the gluteal unit, while positioning it higher will result in an 'elongated' appearance of the buttocks.

Precise surgical execution is based on a good knowledge of the topographic-anatomical and aesthetic proportions in this area. Differentiation of the aesthetic proportions could be a serious challenge in patients after massive weight loss.

Techniques

Lipofilling

Lipofilling is a surgical intervention that involves taking adipose tissue (harvesting) from a relevant area of the body, purification of the adipose tissue by centrifugation or sedimentation and infiltration of the purified adipose tissue (supernatant) into the treated area. In lipofilling of the buttocks, the preferred donor areas are the inner and outer thighs, abdomen and back, armpits [5, 6]. Purification could be done both by centrifugation and sedimentation, and the subsequent infiltration is carried out strictly subcutaneously. Lipofilling is performed using a 3 mm Mercedes cannula manually (Figs. 1, 2 and 3 of Chapter "Vibrational Type of Liposuction").

Dermal Flaps

Superiorly Based Gluteal Flap

A technique that provides filling of the upper and middle floors of the buttocks.

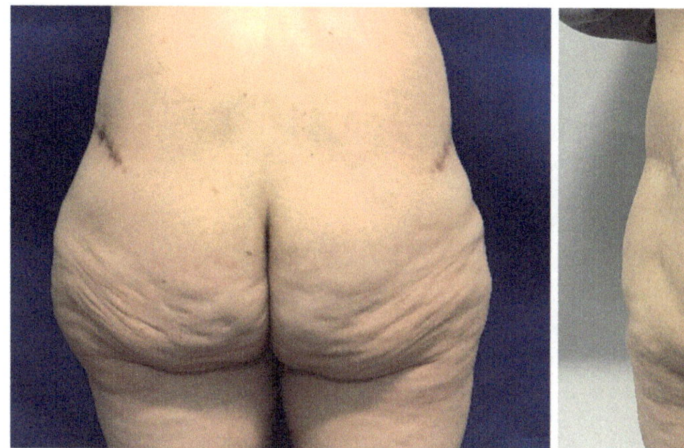
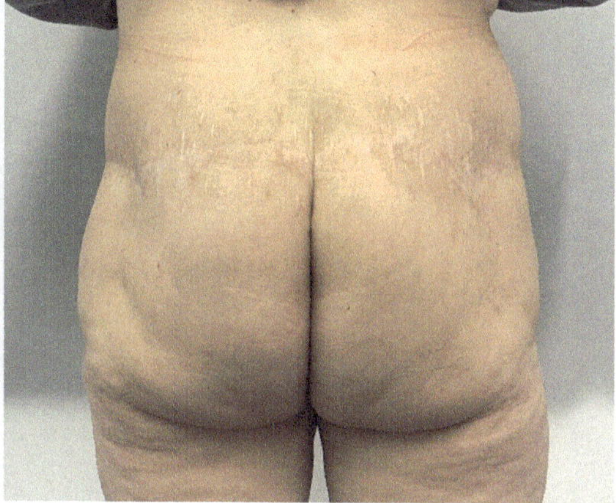

Fig. 1 A massive weight loss patient with a previously performed Fleur de Lis Abdominoplasty. Outcome 2 years after a medially based flap for lifting and buttock augmentation

In the past, dissection stopped at the level of the distal third of the muscle, where in the late postoperative period, after the swelling had subsided, a visible 'step-like' transition was obtained in the contour between the medial and distal third. In the present, precisely for this reason, it is believed that dissection should reach the level of the infragluteal fold. The flap should be fixed as low as possible to the muscle fascia. A disadvantage is that the lower floor of the buttocks often remains 'emptied', while good vascularization can be cited as an advantage.

Medially Based Rotation Gluteal Flap

This flap, first described by Young and Centeno, allows filling of the medial and lower third, but predilectionally fullness is achieved in the upper and middle third of the buttocks (Figs. 1 and 2). An advantage of this technique is that it allows for more even filling of the floors, while the main disadvantage is the limited arch of rotation of the flap—if the preoperative assessment is not good, a bulge deformity can be caused cranially by the rotation/in case of excessive pulling, the postoperative cicatrix may descend lower on the buttocks/the incidence of dehiscence is greater for the same reason (according to same authors, undermining and creating a pocket under the muscle fascia to the infragluteal fold reduces this risk).

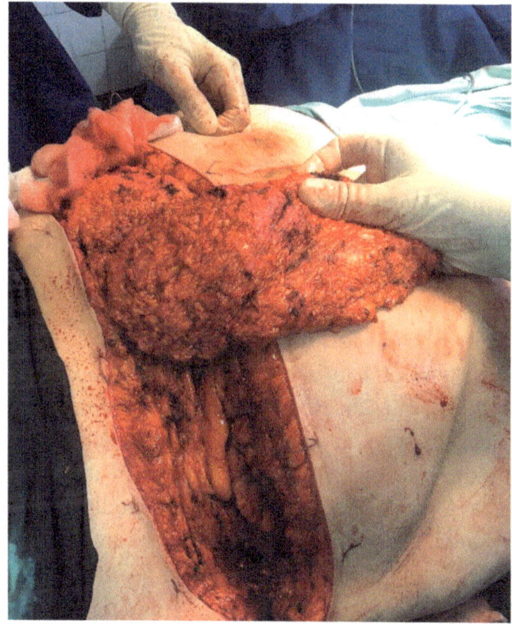

Fig. 2 Intraoperative presentation of a medially based flap in buttock augmentation

It is considered safe to lift the flap medially to 6–7 cm from the midline.

Centrally Based Gluteal Flap

With this type of technique, the flap advancement caudally is often insufficient and the inferior part of the buttocks remains 'empty'. This can be compensated by a lower design of the flap, but it

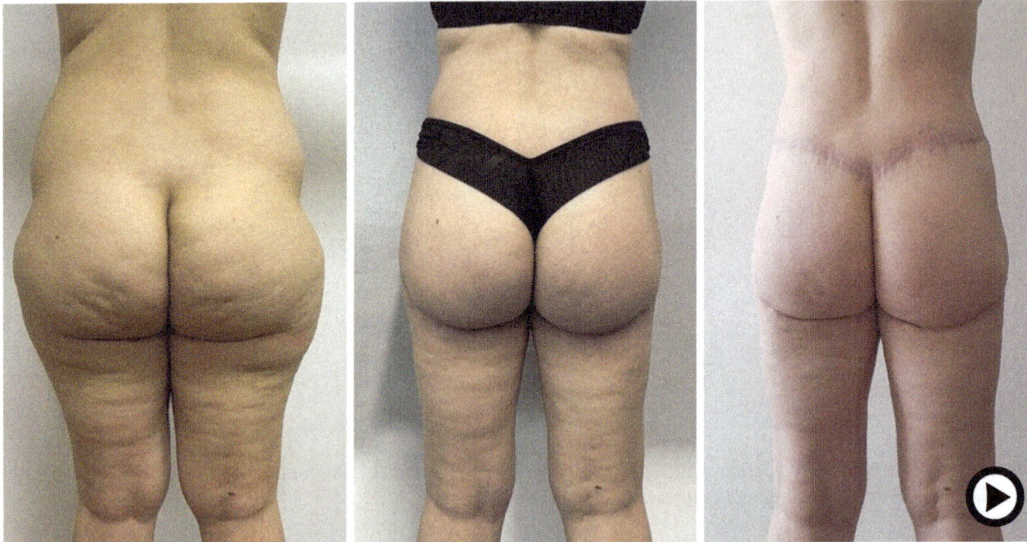

Fig. 3 Before 6 months and 1 year after BodyTite™ radiofrequency lipolysis and vibration assisted liposuction of the flanks and hips with N3 and N4 long curved cannula of Mercedes type + **gluteoplasty with** centrally based flap in combination with lipectomy in the area of "banana roll". Intraoperative demonstration of a centrally based pedicle (▶ https://doi.org/10.1007/000-b0e)

will be at the expense of dislocating the scar inferiorly on the buttocks, not following the aesthetic areas [7] (Figs. 3) (Video 1).

Inferiorly Based Gluteal Flap

This type of flap is an appropriate technique in patients with skin excess inferiorly, including infragluteally, who are characterized at the same time by the lack of soft-tissue projection in the same area. A good filling of the lower and middle floor is ensured, considering the possibility of an implant-based filling of the upper floor after 5–7 months.

Purse-String Gluteoplasty

With this technique, elliptical areas in the upper part of the buttocks are bilaterally deepithelialized, which are modelled using a purse-string that also passes through the fascia for the purpose of fixation. Tightening it increases the projection.

Implant-Based Augmentation

When performing this type of contouring in the area, the preoperative assessment of the height-to-width ratio of the muscle (not of the buttocks) in posterior and lateral aspect is of primary importance, i.e. an assessment of where the volume is concentrated.

- Assessment in posterior aspect
  - Short muscle—round implant;
  - high muscle—anatomical implant;
  - border muscle—any type of implant could be used depending on the desired result.
- Assessment in lateral aspect:
  - when the volume is concentrated inferiorly—a round implant because it will give volume in the medial and superior floors, making the volumes equal.
  - When the volume is concentrated in the medial floor—an anatomical implant, but actually any type would be suitable depending on the desired effect.
  - When the volume is concentrated superiorly—an anatomical implant because it will give volume in the middle and inferior floors, making the volumes equal.
- In preoperative terms, the following should also be taken into consideration:
- Selection of incision site

- Central median sacral incision—it is believed that it is associated with a greater risk of dehiscence and exposure of the implant, especially with larger volume
- Bilateral intergluteal incision—the incision remains hidden in the fold and at the same time the less vascularized sacral area is avoided
- Implant position
- Subcutaneous—prohibited due to the insufficient soft-tissue cover and the high complication rate; subfascial; intramuscular; submuscular [8–12] (Fig. 4a)

Combined Technique of Skin Excision and Insertion of Implants Fig. 4b

The performance of this type of combined technique aims to achieve the best possible result in contouring the area not only in terms of volume, but also in terms of degree of loose skin. The procedure is based on excision of the cutaneous–subcutaneous excess in a cranial direction and implantation of the gluteal prostheses intramuscularly through the already created surgical incision [8–12].

Application of Non-invasive and Minimally Invasive Techniques in Gluteoplasty Procedures

(a) Intraoperatively
- **Radiofrequency procedures:**
  - **BodyTite™:** The author recommends radiofrequency in adjacent areas—flanks, inner and outer thighs, 'banana roll', back area, lower back area. The radiofrequency is performed after lipoaspiration in cases of BBL, due to otherwise compromising the fat viability. The parameters are: 20 W cannula with one sensor/40 power/40 ext. cut off. The purpose is to achieve 8–10 kJ of energy per 10 cm^2 of treated area on 2 cm depth [13, 14]. The author does not recommend using a radiofrequency procedure in the buttock area in cases of autoaugmentation and combined excision-implant-based techniques, due to a possible compromise in the blood supply of the flap; in cases of BBL, due to the heating effect on the tissues with a possible reduction in the survival of the transferred adipose tissue. In cases of augmentation gluteoplasty by means of implants, the BodyTite procedure could be applied to achieve additional tightening and lifting in the same area, as the parameters do not differ from the above in cases of treatment of adjacent areas.
  - **Morpheus8 Body™:** At the end of the surgery radiofrequency microneedling procedure could be applied in order to improve the elasticity of the surrounding and covering skin (in cases of implant-based augmentation) and only of the surrounding skin away of the lipotransfer and/or the incision site (in cases of BBL, flap-based autoaugmentation, combined excision-implant based procedures) [15, 16]. The procedure parameters are as follows:

    7-5-3 mm burst mode depth with 30 kJ, 3 stacks per place, and the procedure can be repeated in the late postoperative period, on the 45th postoperative day, after which a third one can be performed for optimal effect, again in 45 days.
- **Ultrasound procedures**
  - **Vaserlipo®:** Ultrasound treatment is possible in all of the neighbouring areas [17].
  - **The most important factor when doing BBL is to stay at 70 °C as the highest possible parameter on VASER different modes (the author recommends 60 °C); the lipoaspiration should be around 18 mmHG and not higher; otherwise we could compromise the vitality of the fat that will be transferred.**
- **Vibration-assisted liposuction**
  - Vibration assisted liposuction is used for the purpose of harvesting adipose

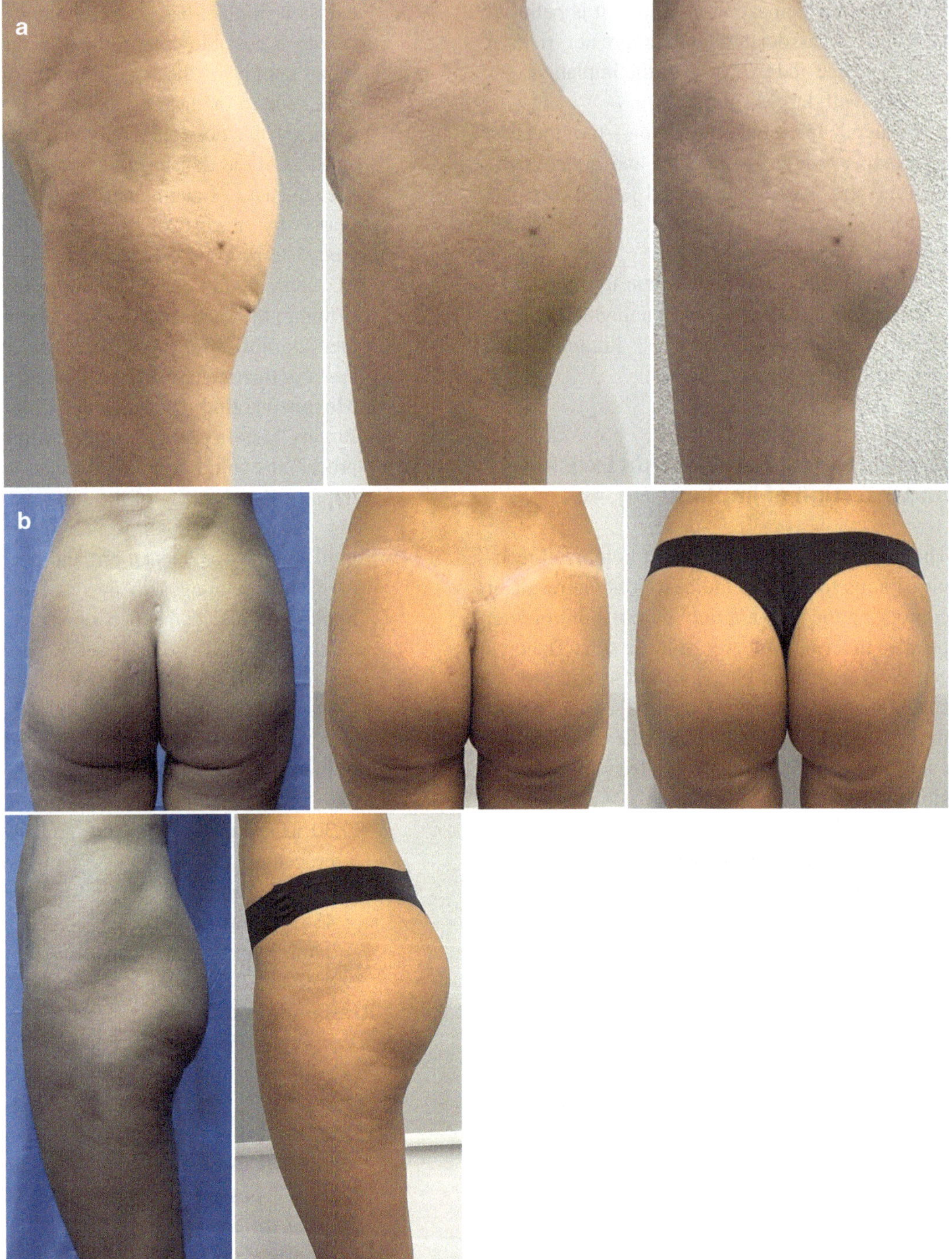

Fig. 4 (**a**) Before and after submuscular augmentation with 225 cc round implants—before 1 month and 6 months post op. (**b**) Before and 6 months after skin excision and intramuscular implantation of 225cc round implants in the buttock. BodyTite in combination with vibration assisted liposuction performed in neighbouring areas—outer thighs; FaceTite in the area of the "banana" roll. Vibration assisted liposuction in the area of the flanks

tissue, but also for the purpose of achieving a 360° definition involving the abdomen, flanks, thighs, buttocks and the area of the so-called banana roll. The author recommends using the following cannulas—Mercedes type N3 and 4, long and short curved and bent types [17–26].

- **Radiofrequency procedures in combination with ultrasound procedures and vibration-assisted liposuction for gluteoplasty procedures**
  - 1 The area of the flanks, inner and outer thighs, 'banana roll' area—VASERlipo® with two-ring probe (first VASER mode on 60% superficially and then continuous C mode on 60% deep). This is followed by **vibration-assisted liposuction** using Mercedes type cannulas N3 and N4 long and short, bent and curved. **Morpheus8 Body** 7-5-3 mm Burst Mode depth with 30-45 kJ, 3 stacks per place and 20–30% overlapping.
  - 2 The area of the flanks, inner and outer thighs, "banana roll" area—vibration assisted liposuction using Mercedes type cannulas N3 and N4 long and short, bent and curved. The treatment of the mentioned areas ends with BodyTite 20 W cannula/40 power/40 ext. cut off/8–10 energy per 10 cm² of treated area. ± Morpheus8 Body 7-5-3 mm burst mode depth with 30–45 kJ, 3 stacks per place and 20–30% overlapping.
  - In cases of implant-based techniques, the same parameters can be used in the buttock area with an additional lifting effect. The author does not recommend using a radiofrequency procedure in the buttock area in cases of: augmentation and combined excision-implant based techniques, due to a possible compromise in the blood supply of the flap; in cases of BBL, due to the heating effect on the tissues with a possible reduction in the survival of the transferred adipose tissue.
  - **Extremely contributory is the effect of additional tightening of the skin in the area of the so-called banana roll, where the FaceTite™ cannula can be used. In the area that is otherwise difficult to tighten and lift, the radiofrequency tightening of the skin finds a very positive application** (Fig. 5).
  - 3A Lipofilling using a 3 mm Mercedes type Basket cannula manually (Fig. 6, 7, 8 and 9).
  - 3B Auto-augmentation using a soft-tissue flap.
  - 3C Implant-based augmentation procedures
  - 3D Combined technique of skin excision and implants based augmentation.

(b) Secondary procedures

- **Radiofrequency procedures:**
  - **BodyTite™, FaceTite™, AccuTite™** are used to correct contour irregularities and/or additional skin tightening. The goal is to reach parameters as follows: 70 °C for destruction of subcutaneous fat accumulation and 40 °C for additional tightening of the skin, and in each case the goal is to achieve 8–10 kJ of energy per 10 cm² of treated area [27]. Wait sixth months to optimally assess the contour deformity after the surgical intervention.
  - **Morpheus8 Body™:** The parameters of the procedure are: 7-5-3 mm burst mode depth with 30 kJ, 3 stacks per place. On the 45th day, after which a third one can be performed for optimal effect, again in 45 days.
  - **EVOLVE X™: The procedure is applied to each of the adjacent areas, but not to the buttock area when lipofilling has been performed.** The procedure requires a cycle of several sessions and the expected

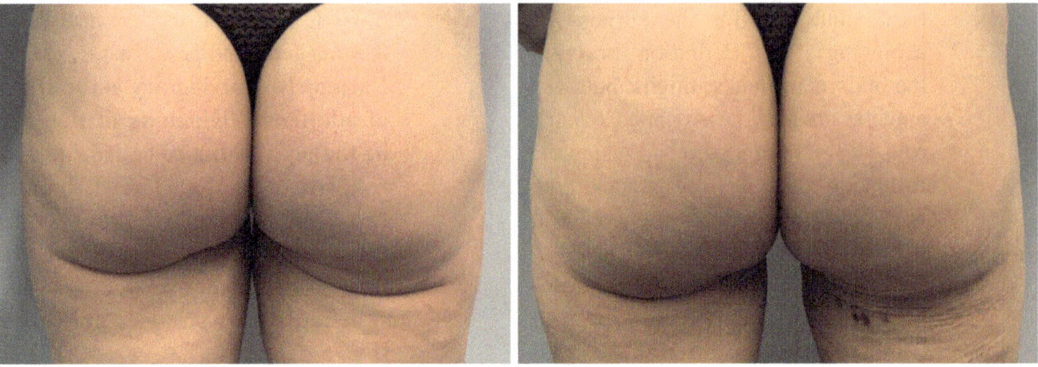

Fig. 5 Before and correction of asymmetry from previous liposuction in the banana roll area, using FaceTite. Eight Kilojoule on the right side of the patient have been done

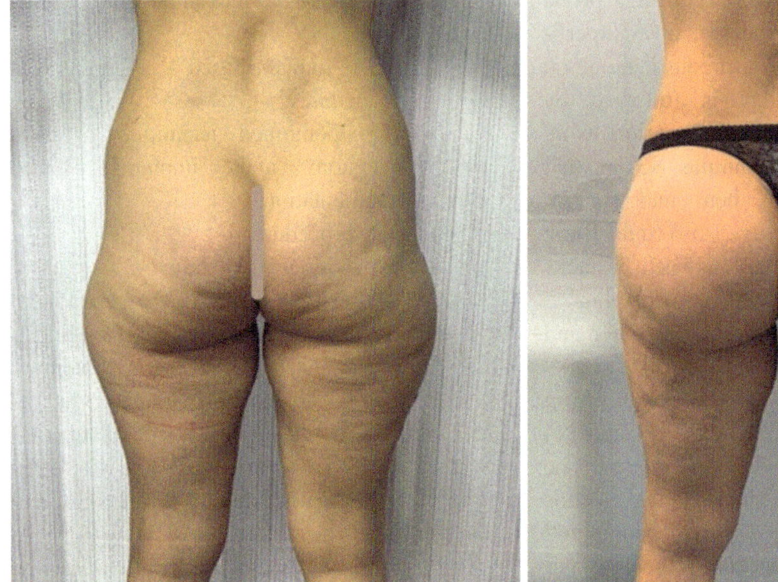

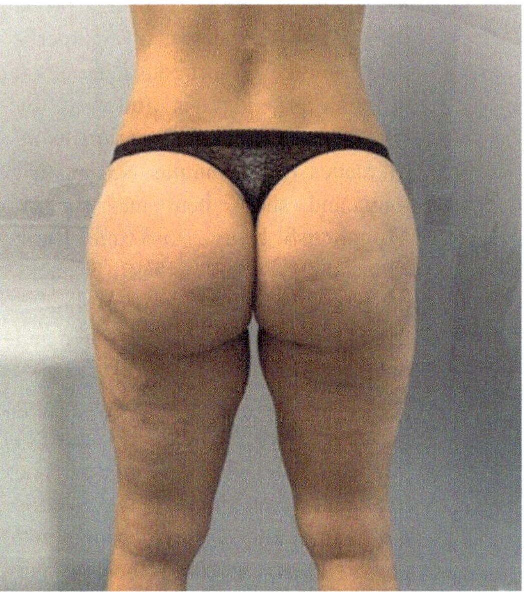

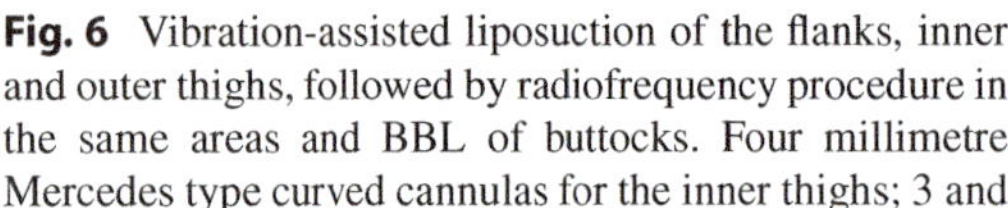

Fig. 6 Vibration-assisted liposuction of the flanks, inner and outer thighs, followed by radiofrequency procedure in the same areas and BBL of buttocks. Four millimetre Mercedes type curved cannulas for the inner thighs; 3 and 4 mm Mercedes type curved cannulas for the outer thighs. Infiltration of 300 cc per side, using 3 mm basket cannula. Purification of the fat was done by sedimentation. Early postoperative result—1 month after the procedure

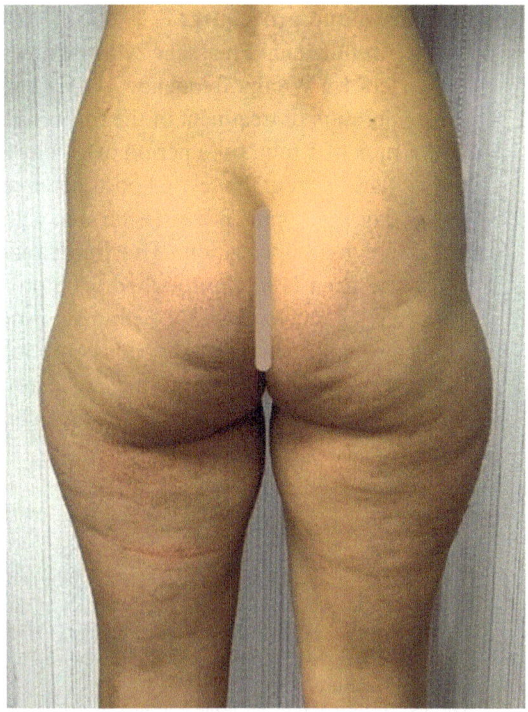

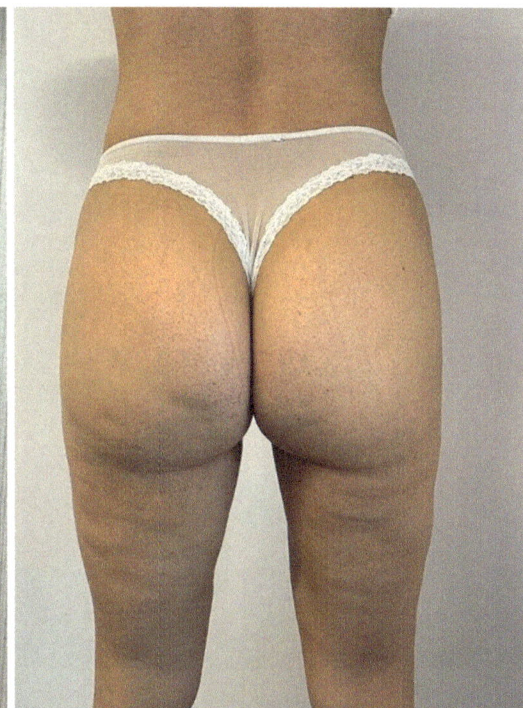

Fig. 7 Vibration-assisted liposuction of the flanks, inner and outer thighs, followed by radiofrequency procedure in the same areas and BBL of buttocks. Four millimetre Mercedes type curved cannulas for the inner thighs; 3 and 4 mm Mercedes type curved cannulas for the outer thighs. Infiltration of 300 cc per side, using 3 mm basket cannula. Purification of the fat was done by sedimentation. 1 year after the procedure. Early results of the same patient are shown in Fig. 6

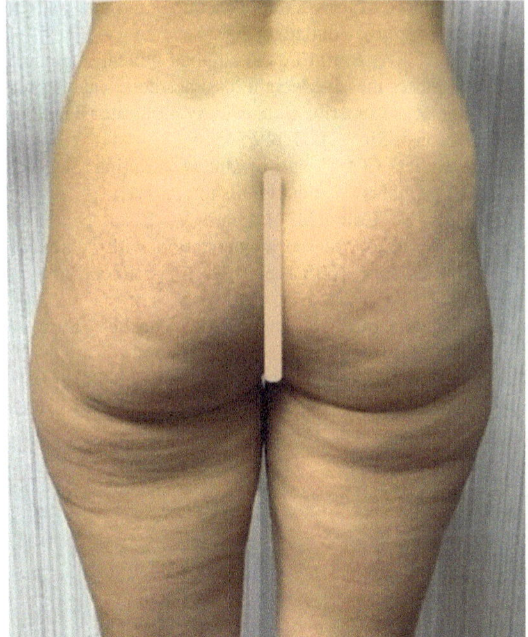

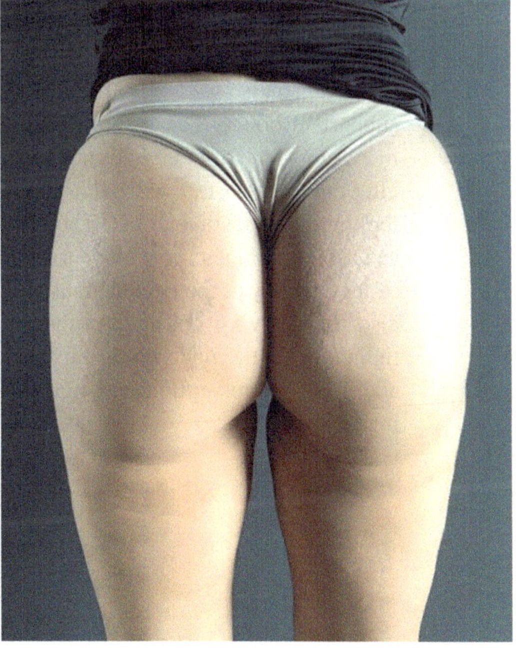

Fig. 8 Vibration-assisted liposuction of the flanks, inner and outer thighs, followed by radiofrequency procedure in the same areas and BBL of buttocks. Four millimetre Mercedes type curved cannulas for the inner thighs; 3 and 4 mm Mercedes type curved cannulas for the outer thighs. Infiltration of 250 cc per side, using 3 mm basket cannula. Purification of the fat was done by sedimentation. The result is 1 year after the procedure

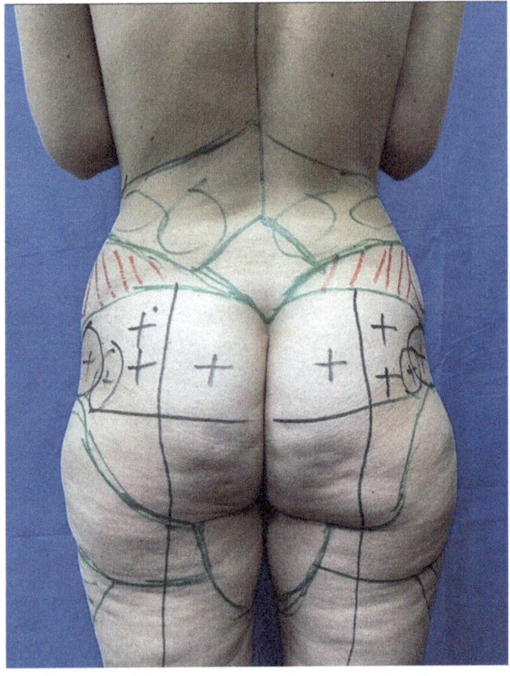

Fig. 9 Preoperative marking—the areas in green and red are subject of vibration assisted liposuction using Mercedes type cannulas N3 and N4 long and short bent and curved. The treatment of the mentioned areas ends with BodyTite 20 W cannula/40 power/40 ext. cut off/8–10 energy per 10 cm^2 of treated area. In the areas marked in black colour, lipofilling will be performed using a 3 mm Mercedes type cannula

improvement is 15–20% with a mostly supportive effect. The author recommends this type of intervention to start after the tenth postoperative day when looking for a positive effect. The procedure contributes not only to the faster recovery of the treated areas, but also to achieving optimal results by tightening of the underlying muscles, additional fat resorption and tightening of the skin.

- **Ultrasound procedures**
  - An ultrasound massage with parameters 1.5 W/cm^2, frequency 3 MHz and duration of treatment of the respective area of 5 min, for a period of 10 days, starting from the second postoperative day, is recommended in each area with previous liposuction. **The lipotransfer area is left untouched.** The process accelerates the drainage of oedema and improves venous outflow, thereby accelerating the recovery period and improving the final results.

References

1. Gonzalez UM. A review of the present status of the correction for sad buttocks. Mexico: IV Congress of the International Society of Aesthetic Plastic Surgery; 1977.
2. Gonzalez Ulloa M. Gluteoplasty: a ten-year report. Aesthet Plast Surg. 1991;15:85.
3. Aly AS. Body contouring after massive weight loss. St Louis, MO: Quality Medical Publishing; 2006. p. 237–301.
4. Lack EB. Contouring the female buttocks: Liposculpting the buttocks. Dermatol Clin. 1999;17:815.
5. Coleman SR. Structural fat grafting. St. Louis, Missouri: Quality Medical Publishing; 2004.
6. Rhoda S. Narins safe liposuction and fat transfer. Oxfordshire: Routledge; 2003.
7. Colwell A, Borud L. Autologous gluteal augmentation after massive weight loss: aesthetic analysis and role of the superior gluteal artery perforator flap. Plast Reconstr Surg. 2007;119:345–56.
8. Mendieta CG. The art of gluteal sculpting. St Louis, MO: Quality Medical Publishing; 2011.
9. Petit F, Colli M, Badiali V, Ebaa S, Salval A. Buttocks volume augmentation with submuscular implants: 100 cases series. Plast Reconstr Surg. 2022;149(3):615–22.
10. Mendieta CG. Gluteoplasty. Aesthet Surg J. 2003;23(6):441–55.
11. Robles JM, Tagliapertra JC, MA YG. Gluteoplastia de aumento: implante submuscular. Cir Plast Iberolatinoamer. 1984;10:365–75.

12. Vergara R, Marcos M. Intramuscular gluteal implants. Aesthet Plast Surg. 1996;20:259.
13. Dayan E, Burns AJ, Rohrich RJ, Theodorou S. The use of radiofrequency in aesthetic surgery. Plast Reconstr Surg Glob Open. 2020;8(8):e2861.
14. Theodorou SJ, Del Vecchio D, Chia CT. Soft tissue contraction in body contouring with radiofrequency-assisted liposuction: a treatment gap solution. Aesthet Surg J. 2018;38:S74–83.
15. Mulholland RS. Radiofrequency energy for non-invasive and minimally invasive skin tightening. Clin Plast Surg. 2011;38:437–48.
16. Levy AS, Grant RT, Rothaus KO. Radiofrequency physics for minimally invasive aesthetic surgery. Clin Plast Surg. 2016;43:551–6.
17. Hoyos AE, Prendergast PM. High definition body sculpting. Berlin: Springer; 2014. p. 73–80.
18. Cimino WW. The physics of soft tissue fragmentation using ultrasonic frequency vibrations of metal probes. Clin Plast Surg. 1999;26:447–61.
19. Ogawa T, Hattori R, Yamamoto T, Gotoh M. Safe use of ultrasonically activated devices based on current studies. Expert Rev Med Devices. 2011;8(3):319–24.
20. Zocchi ML. Clinical aspects of ultrasonic liposculpture. Perspect Plast Surg. 1993;7:153–74.
21. Zocchi ML. Ultrasonic assisted lipoplasty. Clin Plast Surg. 1996;23(4):575–98.
22. Troilius C. Ultrasound-assisted lipoplasty: is it really safe? Aesthet Plast Surg. 1999;23(5):307–11.
23. Baxter RA. Histologic effects of ultrasound-assisted lipoplasty. Aesthet Surg J. 1999;19:109–14.
24. Illouz YG. Surgical remodeling of the silhouette by aspiration lipolysis or selective lipectomy. Aesthet Plast Surg. 1985;9(1):7–21.
25. Hoyos AE, Prendergast PM. High definition body sculpting, vol. 95-117. Berlin: Springer; 2014. p. 147–64.
26. Hoyos AE, Millard JA. VASER-assisted high-definition liposculpture. Aesthet Surg J. 2007;27(6):594–604.
27. Mulholland RS. The bodytite book, vol. 261. 2nd ed. Rijeka: IntechOpen; 2021. p. 734–50.

Thigh Lift in Combination with Radiofrequency

Introduction

The procedure is used:

- in patients after massive weight loss. Often, the intervention is performed after a previous correction of an adjacent area, due to the fact that, when performing a previous abdominoplasty and especially belt lipectomy, deformities in the thigh area would be positively influenced to a greater or lesser extent.
- in obese patients, the area could be subjected to liposuction, which, depending on the degree of fat deposits and the qualitative of the skin, could be combined with or followed by excisional procedure.
- in patients after massive weight loss, deformities in this area most often have a horizontal and vertical component, which requires performing a vertical thigh lift or transverse or circumferential thigh lift.
- in the presence of an isolated horizontal excess in the medial area, it can be proceeded to an inner thigh lift. Here it is mostly about patients with skin excess in the area because of frequent weight variations and/or age changes. In terms of aetiology, the cause of the available skin excess could also be iatrogenic noxa—previous liposuction in the area.

Historically, for the first time in 1964, Pitanguy performed the so-called thigh/ buttock lift, which was an excision along the course of the gluteal fold continuing horizontally along the medial surface of the thigh. The approach was based on an excision of the ptosed tissues gluteally (lifting them is the basis of modern trends). The outcome was smoothing of the gluteal contour, obliteration of the lordosis in the lumbar region and accentuation of the trochanteric depression—signs of ageing, not of youth. Tissue suspension in the thigh area involved only a skin suture—the outcome was a visible and wide scar caudally dislocated over time, vulvo-vaginal deformities and dysfunctions.

For the first time in 1987, Al Aly proposed a technique with Colles' fascia suspension, which resulted in long-lasting results with no extension and no caudal dislocation of the scar. Fixation of the elevated cutaneous–subcutaneous flap to Colles' fascia is a key point in the medial thigh lift procedures in order to achieve long-lasting results with a well-positioned postoperative scar.

Excisional and/or liposuction techniques in the thigh area must always be performed in accordance with the topographic-anatomical specificity of the thighs.

Liposuction techniques must be performed in accordance with the so-called zones of adhesions, which in the thigh area are, respectively, the medial 1/3 on the inner surface, the distal 1/3 on the lateral surface, the distal 1/3 on the posterior surface.

The type and degree of excess in the area are essential. The presence of cutaneous–subcutaneous excess with a predominant skin component

E. Sharkov, *Body Contouring Surgery*, https://doi.org/10.1007/978-3-031-33350-7_9

suggests massive weight loss and/ or age-related changes in the area, which requires performing excisional techniques ± liposuction procedures. With an accompanying fat component and preserved skin elasticity, the procedures can be limited to the area of non- and/or minimally invasive techniques. In the presence of a fatty component and compromised skin elasticity, the following options exist as a surgical plan: lipoaspiration techniques in combination with radiofrequency procedures intra- and postoperatively with the option for an excisional procedure at the second stage in case of insufficiently satisfactory result regarding skin retraction; lipoaspiration techniques in combination with excisional techniques in one surgical procedure; lipoaspiration techniques in combination with excisional techniques and radiofrequency techniques—Morpheus 8 Body in order to improve the quality of the skin in the area.

Techniques

Inner Thigh Lift (Medial Thigh Lift)

Preoperatively, the inguinal fold is marked—posteriorly the marking continues just before becoming visible when viewed from behind; anteriorly it continues just to the level of tuberculum pubicum. Using a pinch test, the excision volume is determined as a width—no more than 4–6 cm are recommended.

The patient is in gynaecological position.

Depending on the local status, the procedure could be preceded by a liposuction technique in the area.

A skin incision is made along the superior marking, and dissection to the level of the superficial fascia, after which the dissection is continued in caudal direction in order to intraoperatively assess the width of the planned excision. Posteriorly, the incision should not be continued along the gluteal fold.

If it is considered appropriate, additional dissection can be made in inferior direction. Some authors use a cannula for liposuction, and with this additional separation even reach the level of the knee, if necessary.

Accurate identification of tuberculum pubicum, ramus ischiopubicum and Cooper's ligament. Anterior from tuberculum pubicum (the area of attachment of m.adductor longus), the soft tissues in the area between mons pubis and trigonum femorale must be left intact—only superficial dissection is allowed, leaving the subdermal fat intact—this provides preservation of the lymphatic network and a. et vv. pudendae ext. and reduces the risk of complications related to lymphatic drainage [1].

Fascial suspension—it is started posteriorly by pulling the inferior flap in antero-cranial direction in order to prevent dog-ears posteriorly (without excessive tension and without vulvo-vaginal deformities). Anteriorly, the suspension will be between the SFS and ramus ischiopubicum, tuberculum pubicum and Cooper's ligament [1–3] (Fig. 1).

Vertical Thigh Lift

Preoperative marking is performed as follows: cranially it is started from the area of insertion of m.gracillis and the most distal point of the cutaneous–subcutaneous excess is reached caudally, in some cases below the knee level (Figs. 2, 3a, b and 4). Using a pinch test, the excision volume is determined without excessive tension circumferentially, applying a 'double ellipse' technique analogous to that used in a brachioplasty procedure. Transverse markings connect the ellipse (respectively inner ellipse) postero-anteriorly and help for a better and accurate intraoperative orientation [1–5].

The patient is in gynaecological position. Depending on the local status, the procedure could be preceded by liposuction of the area. According to some authors, the procedure begins with liposuction due to the fact that the available subcutaneous fat would limit an adequate excision without excessive tension in the subsequent closure of the defect. After the liposuction is performed, the transverse antero-posterior markings are stitched by reference sutures in order to re-evaluate the excision. The skin excision itself is made from caudal to cranial direction on the principle of 'segmental resection closure'—a tech-

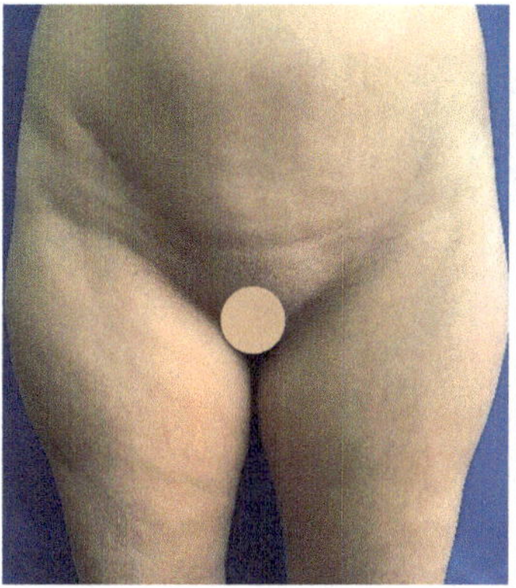
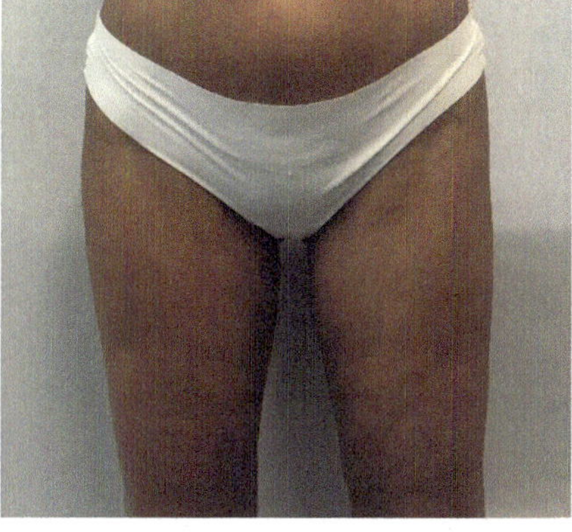
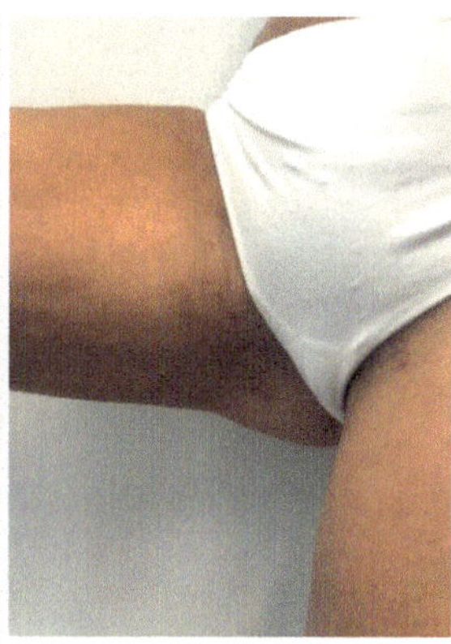

Fig. 1 Inner thigh lift—Vibration-assisted liposuction in combination with medial thigh lift. With this degree of fat accumulation in a middle-aged patient and acceptable skin elasticity, a possible technique is the combination of vibration-assisted liposuction and BodyTite™ radiofrequency technique in order to 'spare' the need for excision and, accordingly, postoperative cicatrix. The result is 1 year after the procedure

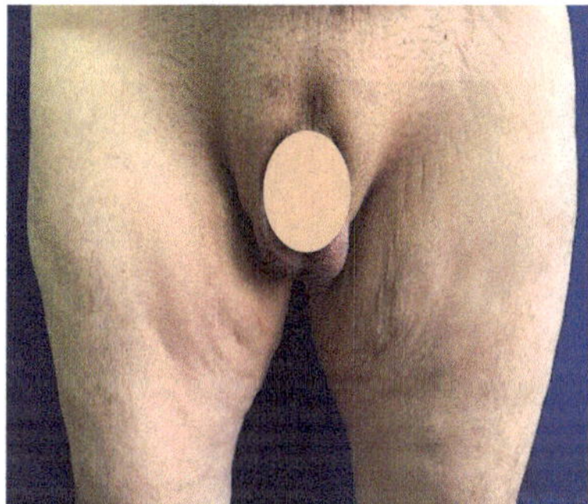
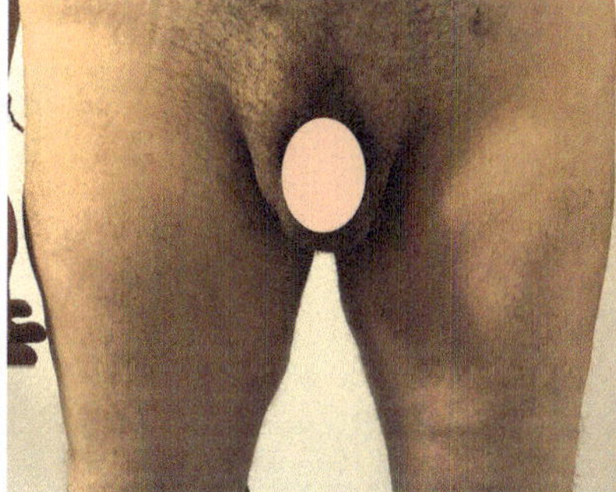
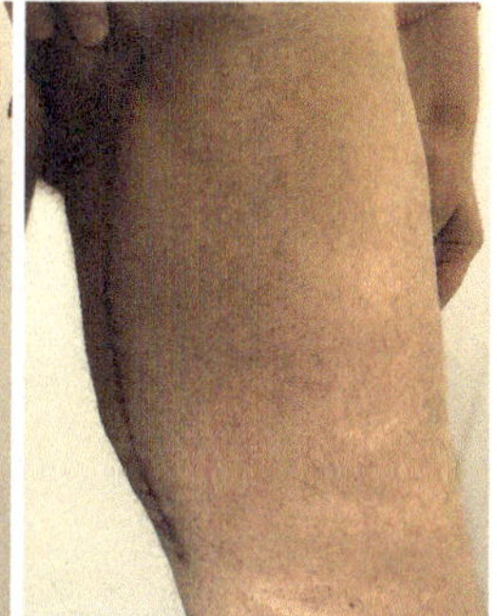

Fig. 2 Vertical thigh lift—result 1 year after the procedure in a patient after massive weight loss. The procedure was performed as a second stage in the overall surgical plan for body contouring. Six months before the lifting, a belt lipectomy was performed. The postoperative cicatrix in the area of the thigh is illustrated

nique that ensures the prevention of intraoperative soft-tissue oedema [1–5]. During the excision, the aim is to preserve the subcutaneous fat in order to preserve the lymphatic and venous drainage of the lower limbs. Thorough haemostasis. Redon drains. Fascial suspension, layered suture.

Application of Non-invasive and Minimally Invasive Techniques in Thigh Lift Procedures

(a) Intraoperatively

- **Radiofrequency procedures:**
  - **BodyTite™**: BodyTite is performed in the following areas—inner thighs, outer thighs, 'banana roll'. The parameters used are as follows: 20 W cannula/70 int cut off/40 ext. cut off/—the purpose is to achieve 8–10 kJ energy per 10 cm^2 of treated area, and depending on the preoperative pinch test, it is worked at 2 or 3 cm. The working techniques are, respectively, 'stamping' (melting the fat cells by reaching 70 °C int cut off) and lining (tightening the skin by reaching 40 °C ext. cut off) [6, 7]. The author does not recommend using BodyTite in the inner thighs in cases of excisional and/or combined lipoaspiration excisional techniques, due to the possible risk of compromising the blood supply as a result of the ablative effect of the radiofrequency.
  - **Morpheus8 Body™:** At the end of the surgery radiofrequency microneedling

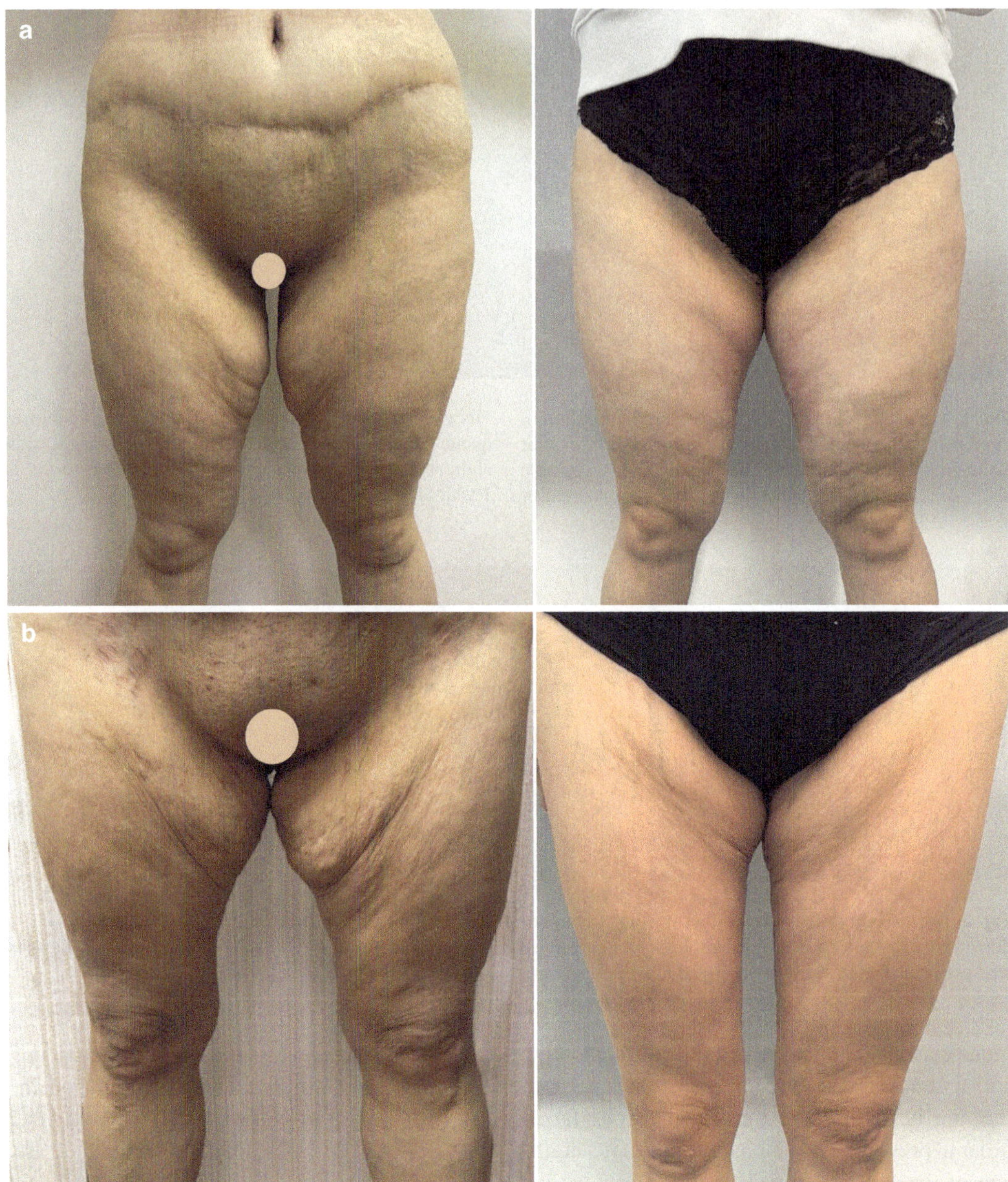

Fig.3 (**a**) Vertical thigh lift in combination with vibration-assisted liposuction—6 month after the procedure in a patient after massive weight loss. The procedure was performed as a second stage in the overall surgical plan for body contouring. Six months before the lifting, a belt lipectomy was performed. (**b**) Vertical thigh lift in combination with vibration-assisted liposuction—6 month after the procedure in a patient after massive weight loss. The procedure was performed as a second stage in the overall surgical plan for body contouring. Six months before the lifting, Fleur De Lis abdominoplasty was performed. In both cases (**a**) and (**b**) there is still soft tissue excess in the upper inner part of the thigh, suggesting Transverse thigh lift would have been better choice as possible procedure (Fig. 4)

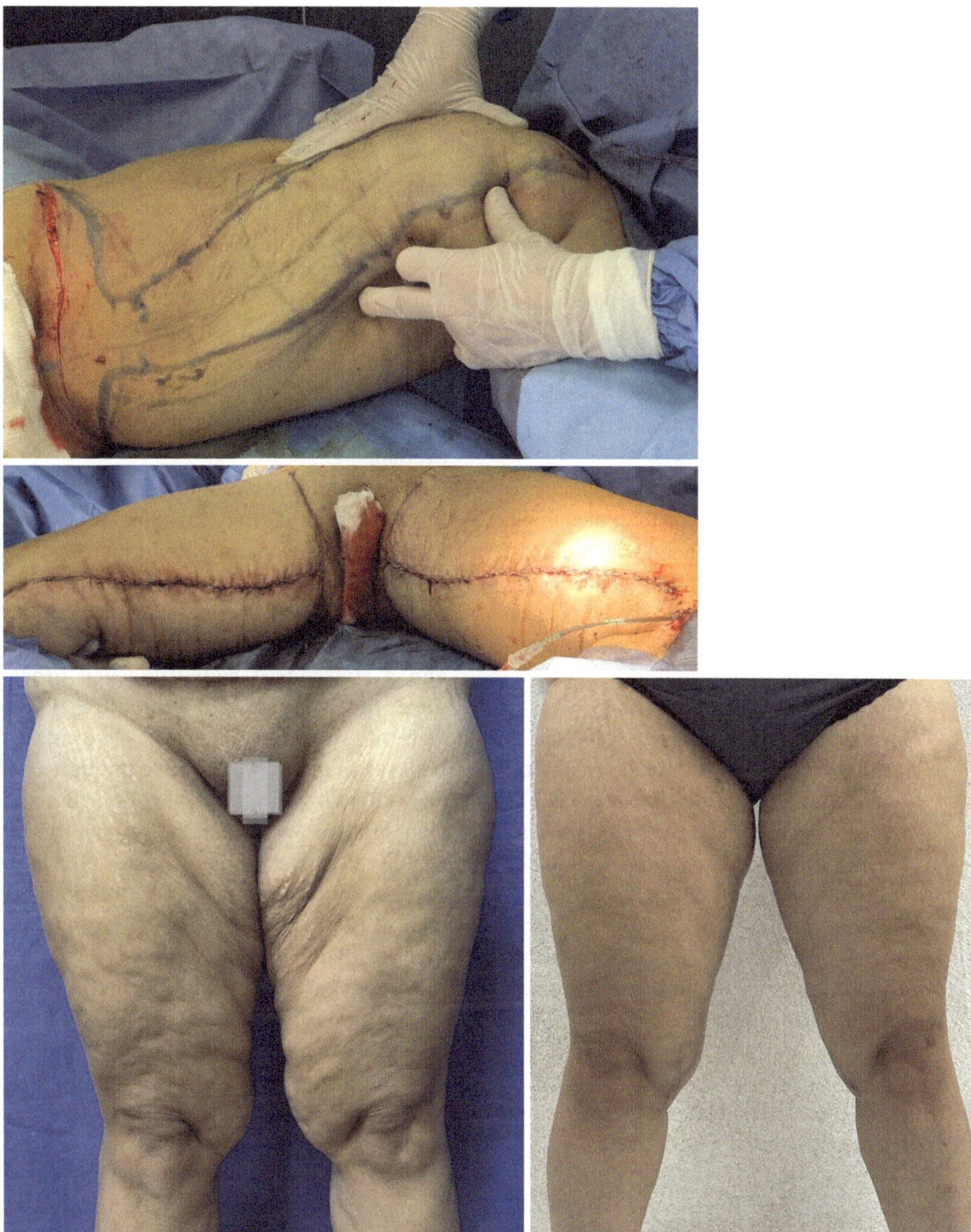

Fig. 4 Combination of vertical and inner medial thigh lift (Transverse thigh lift) with vibration-assisted liposuction. Demonstration of the preoperative markings and wound closure immediately after the procedure. Six months before the thigh lift, abdominoplasty has been performed in other clinic. Before and 6 months after

could be applied. The goal is to improve the elasticity of the surrounding and covering skin and only of the surrounding skin away of the incision side (in cases of surgical excision). The procedure parameters are as follows:

7–5-3 burst mode depth with 30 kJ, 3 stacks per place, (30–40% overlapping when without excision of skin & no overlapping when close to the excision side—stay at least 2 cm away) and microneedling can be repeated on the 45th postoperative day, again in 45 more days.

- **Ultrasound procedures**
  - **Vaserlipo®:** Ultrasound treatment is possible in the area of the inner thigh, but also in all of the neighbouring areas. VaserLipo and the subsequent vibration-assisted liposuction should precede possible radiofrequency procedure—Morpheus8 Body.
- **Vibration-assisted liposuction**
  - vibration-assisted liposuction is used to remove excess fat both in the area of the inner thighs and in all adjacent areas. The author recommends using the following cannulas: Mercedes type N3 and 4, long and short curved and bent types [8].
- **Radiofrequency procedures, ultrasound procedures, vibration-assisted liposuction for medial and vertical thigh lift procedures**

Minimally Invasive Techniques in Combination with Each Other

1 The inner and outer thigh areas, the 'banana roll' area, the knees—VASERlipo® with 2-ring probe (first VASER mode on 60% superficially and then continuous C mode on 60% deep) [8].

2 Vibration assisted liposuction using Mercedes type cannulas N3 и N4 long and short bent and curved [8].

3 The treatment of the said areas ends with:

3A To tighten the skin - BodyTite 20 W cannula with one sensor/20 power/40 ext. cut off/8–10 kJ energy per 10 cm^2 of treated area ± 7–5-3 mm burst mode depth with 30 kJ, 3 stacks per place—**when VASERlipo hasn't been done as part of the procedure**.

3B To tighten the skin and melt the fat—40 W cannula/70 int cut off/40 ext. cut off/: the purpose is to achieve 8–10 kJ energy per 10 cm^2 of treated area, as—depending on the preoperative pinch test—it is worked at 2 or 3 cm ± 7-5-3 mm Burst Mode depth with 30 kJ, 3 stacks per place—**when VASERlipo hasn't been done as part of the procedure.**

3C Morpheus8 Body™—7-5-3 mm depth burst mode with 30 kJ, 3 stacks per place, 30–40% overlapping.

The effect of additional tightening of the skin in the area of the 'banana roll' with FaceTite is extremely contributory.

The author recommends that in cases of treatment in the inner thigh area, with a combination of VASERlipo® with liposuction and a subsequent radiofrequency procedure, the latter should be limited to the level of Morpheus8 Body™. The author believes that this would have the best possible effect both in terms of contouring and skin quality, without bringing an unreasonably high risk of possible side effects.

The possible combinations for treating the area of the inner thighs, which are recommended by the author, are:

Option 1–1 **(for possible definition) + 2 (for lipoaspiration) + 3C (for tightening)—provides contouring and definition of the area and tightening of the skin;**

Option 2–2 **(for lipoaspiration) + 3A (for tightening) or 3B (tightening and fat destruction)—provides contouring of the area, tightening of the skin, lasting results regarding the reduction in fat deposits** (Fig. 5);

Option 3–3A (taking into consideration only the BodyTite™ parameters, excluding those specified for Morpheus8 Body™) + 3C**—provides optimal tightening of the skin and is a possible option to surgical excision in moderately loose skin (Fig. 6).**

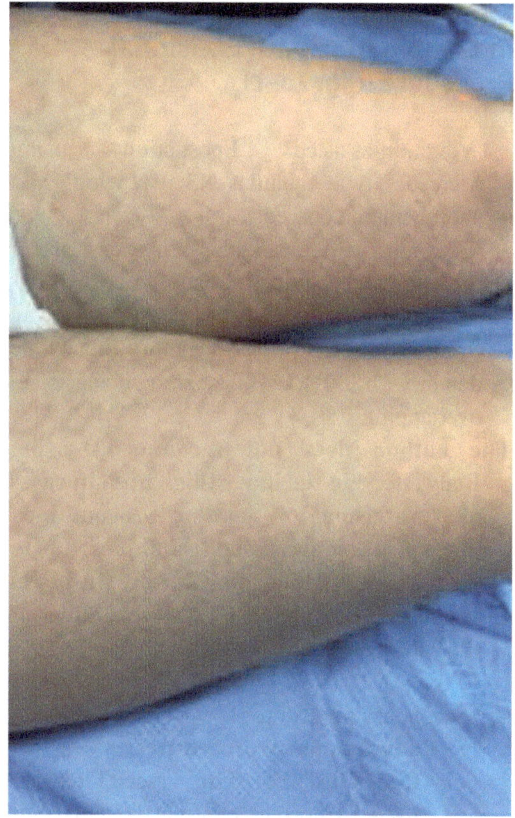

Fig. 5 Intraoperatively—Vibration-assisted liposuction with BodyTite™ of the inner thighs in combination with Morpheus8 Body™ of the thighs and knees—40 W cannula/70 int cut off/40 ext. cut off / The purpose is to achieve 8–10 kJ energy per 10 cm^2 of treated area, as—depending on the preoperative pinch test—it is worked at 2 or 3 cm ± 7-5-3 mm burst mode, 3 stacks per place, 30 kJ

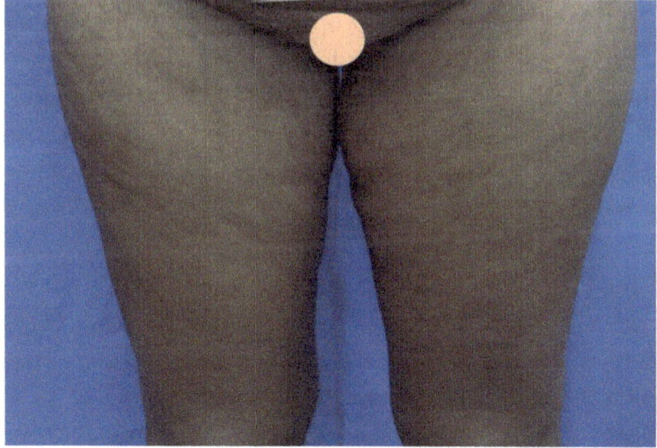

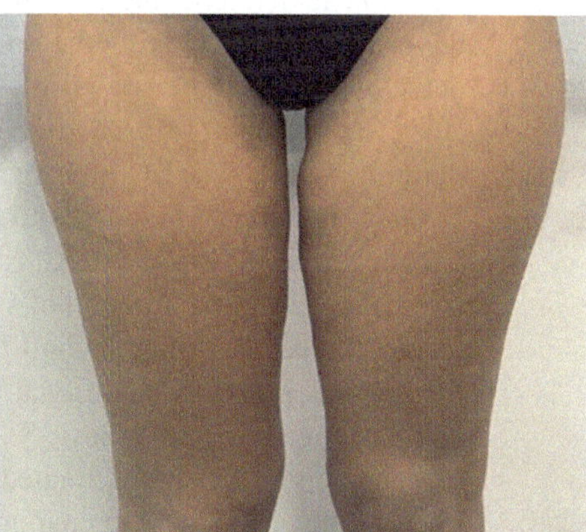

Fig. 6 Patient with previous liposuction performed in another clinic, loose skin and irregularities, who does not wish to have a postoperative scar. Six months after BodyTite 20 W cannula with one sensor/40 power/40 ext. cut off/8–10 kJ energy per 10 cm^2 of treated area + Morpheus8 Body™—7-5-3 mm Mode depth with 30 kJ, 30–40% overlapping, 3 stacks per place. One can notice the tightening effect on the skin and the still present unevenness from the previous procedure on the left. The patient is satisfied with the result, given her knowledge that it is impossible to correct the unevenness without excision

Minimally Invasive Techniques in Combination with Excisional Procedure (Fig. 7a–c)

1 Vibration-assisted liposuction using Mercedes type cannulas N3 и N4 long and short bent and curved.
2 Excision of the available skin excess using the surgical techniques already described.
3 Morpheus8 Body™—stay at least 2 cm away from the incision side; 7-5-3 mm Burst Mode depth with 30 kJ, 3 stacks per place no overlapping.

The author does not recommend using BodyTite™ in the inner thigh area in cases of excisional and/or combined lipoaspiration-excisional techniques, due to the possible risk of compromising the blood supply as a result of the ablative effect of the radiofrequency.

(b) Secondary procedures
- **Radiofrequency procedures:**
  - **BodyTite™, FaceTite™, AccuTite™** are used to correct contour irregularities and skin laxity. Use the specified tip depending on the area of the surgical defect. For large deformity—the BodyTite cannula is used and small deformity—the FaceTite and AccuTite cannulas are used. The goal is to reach parameters as follows: 70 °C for the internal probe for destruction of subcutaneous fat accumulation and 40 °C for the external probe for additional tightening of the skin, and deposit 8–10 kJ of energy per 10 cm^2 of treated area [8–10]. The goal is to reach parameters as follows: 70 °C for destruction of subcutaneous fat accumulation and 40 °C for additional tightening of the skin, and in each case the goal is to achieve 8–10 kJ of energy per 10 cm^2 of treated area. Wait sixth months to optimally assess the contour deformity.
  - **Morpheus8 Body™** (Fig. 8): 7-5-3 mm burst mode depth with 30 kJ, 3 stacks per place, and the procedure is performed in the late postoperative period, on the 45th day, after which a third one can be performed for optimal effect, again in 45 days.
  - **EVOLVE X™:** The author recommends the procedure as part of the postoperative management of each of his patients who underwent the said procedures for minimally invasive contouring of the body. The procedure requires a cycle of several sessions, and the expected improvement is 15–20% with a mostly supportive effect. The author recommends this type of interventions to start after the tenth postoperative day when looking for a positive effect. The procedure contributes not only to the faster recovery of the treated areas, but also to achieving optimal results by tightening of the underlying muscles, additional fat resorption and tightening of the skin.
- **Ultrasound procedures**
  - An ultrasound massage with parameters 1.5 W/cm^2, frequency 3 MHz and duration of treatment of the respective area of 5 min, for a period of 10 days, starting from the second postoperative day, is recommended in each area with previous liposuction. The process accelerates the drainage of oedema and improves venous outflow, thereby accelerating the recovery period and improving the final results.

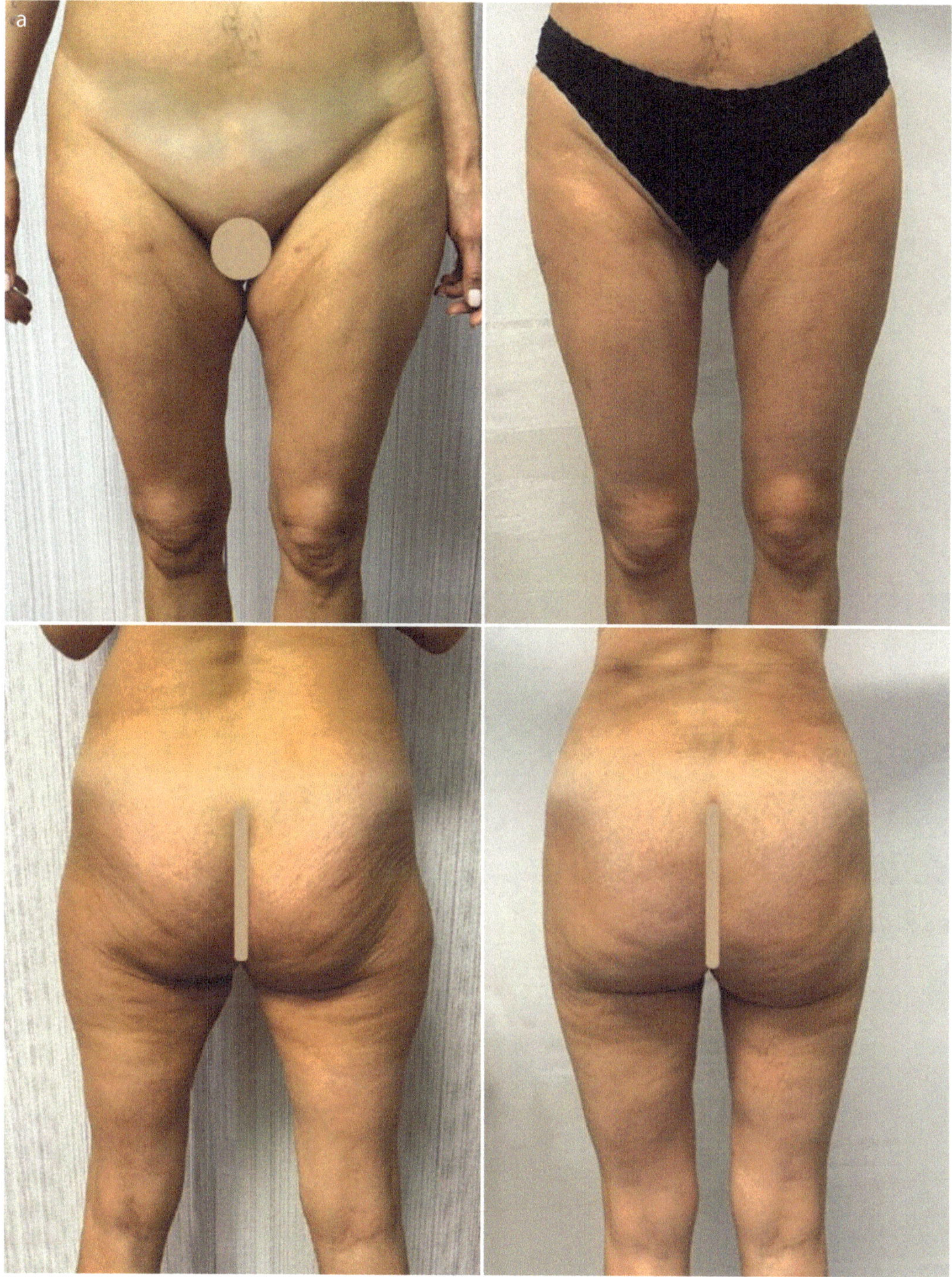

Fig. 7 (**a**) 1 year after vibration-assisted liposuction in combination with medial thigh lift + vibration assisted liposuction and BodyTite™ of the outer thighs. (**b**) Before and 6 months after. Thirty eight-year-old female patient with massive weight loss, who underwent medial thigh lift in combination with Morpheus8 Body™. (**c**) Before and 6 months after. Thirty eight-year-old female patient with massive weight loss, who underwent medial thigh lift in combination with Morpheus8 Body™

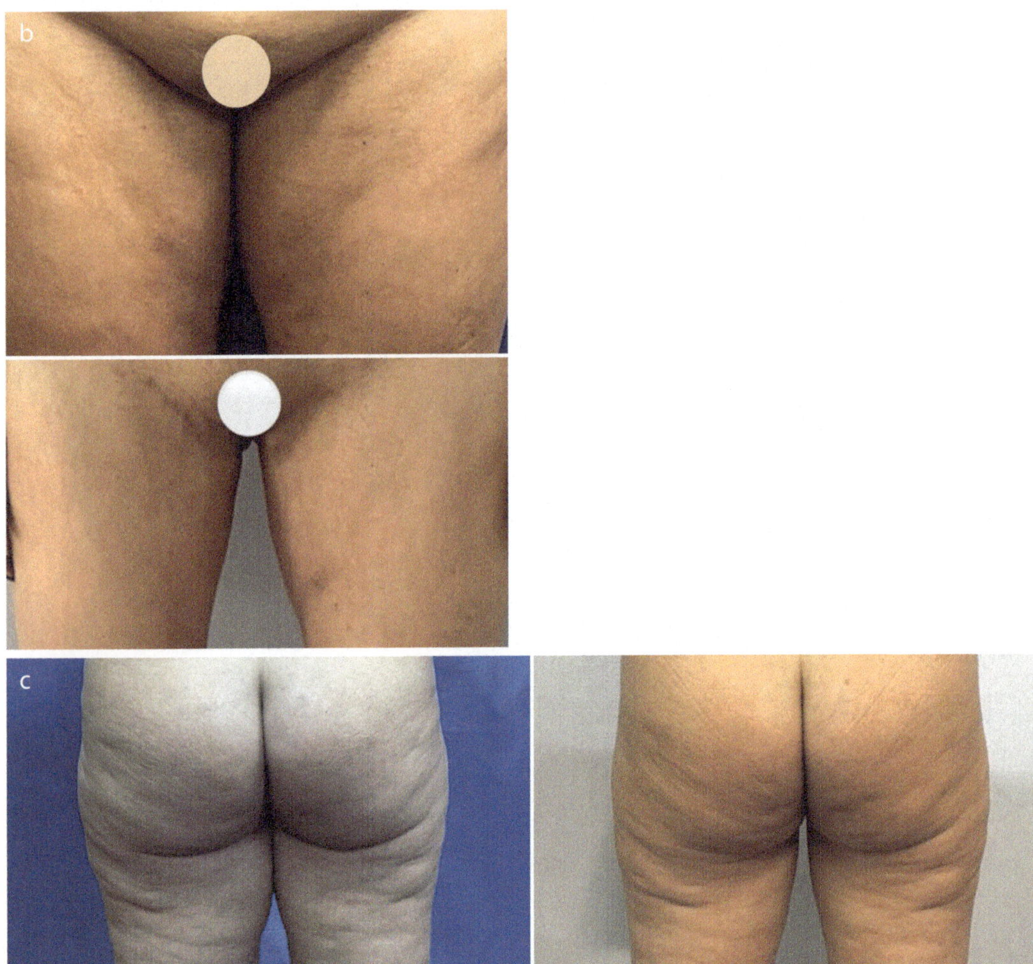

Fig. 7 (continued)

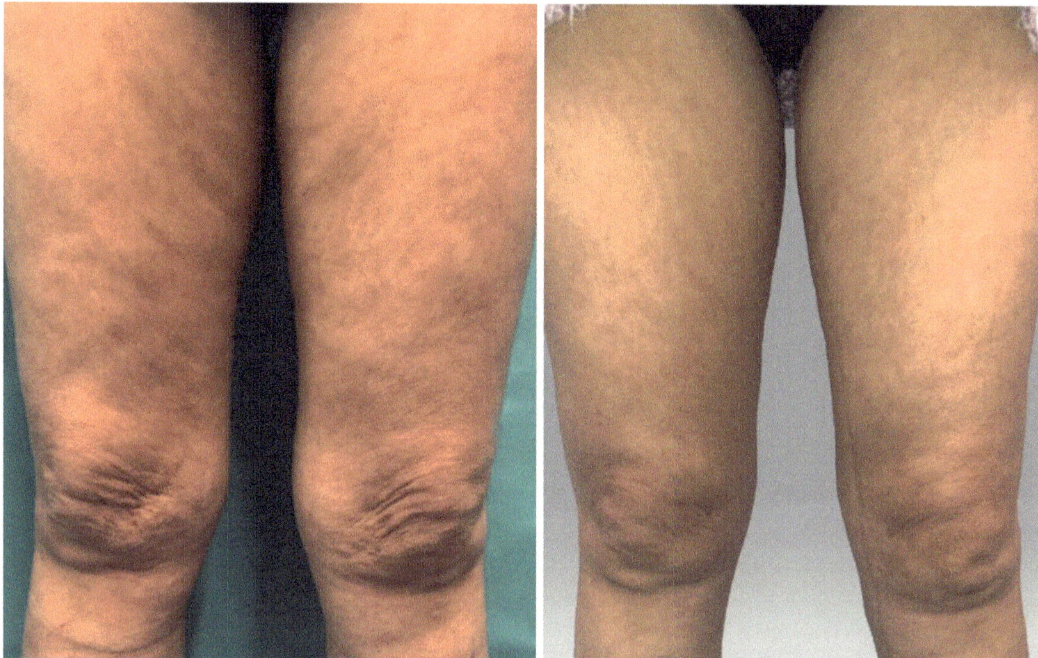

Fig. 8 Three months after one Morpheus8 Body™ procedure—The procedure parameters are as follows: 7-5-3 mm burst mode, 30–40% overlapping, 30 kJ, 3 stacks per place

References

1. Aly AS. Body contouring after massive weight loss. St Louis, MO: Quality Medical Publishing; 2006. p. 213–36.
2. Lockwood TE. Fascial anchoring technique in medial thigh lifts. Plast Reconstr Surg. 1988;82:299.
3. Lockwood TE. Lower body lift with superficial fascial system suspension. Plast Reconstr Surg. 1993;92:1112.
4. Hurwitz DJ. Approach to the medial thigh lift after weight loss. In: Rubin PJ, Matarraso A, editors. Aesthetic surgery after weight loss. Philadelphia: Saunders Elsevier; 2007. p. 113–30.
5. Rubin P, Jellew ML, Richter DF, Uebel CO. Body contouring and liposuction. Philadelphia: Saunders Elsevier; 2013. p. 353–74.
6. Mulholland RS. The BodyTite book. 2nd ed. Rijeka: IntechOpen; 2021. p. 801–2.
7. Mulholland RS. Radiofrequency energy for non-invasive and minimally invasive skin tightening. Clin Plast Surg. 2011;38:437–48.
8. Hoyos AE, Prendergast PM. High definition body sculpting, vol. 137–143. Berlin: Springer; 2014. p. 193–204.
9. Theodorou SJ, Del Vecchio D, Chia CT. Soft tissue contraction in body contouring with radiofrequency-assisted liposuction: a treatment gap solution. Aesthet Surg J. 2018;38:S74–83.
10. Levy AS, Grant RT, Rothaus KO. Radiofrequency physics for minimally invasive aesthetic surgery. Clin Plast Surg. 2016;43:551–6.

Lower Body Lift Procedures in Combination with Minimally Invasive and Non-invasive Techniques

Introduction

For the first time in 1987, Al Aly proposed a technique with Colles' fascia suspension, which resulted in long-lasting results with no expansion and no caudal dislocation of the scar. Fixation of the elevated cutaneous–subcutaneous flap to Colles' fascia is a key point, but in cases of circumferential thigh lift, fixation to additional immobile structures cranially is also essential in order to prevent the expansion of the scar and the re-ptosis of the tissues—fixation to the inguinal ligament and periosteum of spina iliaca anterior superior. The author used 2/0 Ethibond when placing these anchoring sutures.

In an anatomical aspect, respect and non-invasion in the area of trigonum femorale are extremely important, which could lead to serious complications, including lymphocele when the lymphatic basin in the area is compromised.

The performance of an excisional and/or lipoaspiration technique in the thigh area must always be in accordance with the topographic-anatomical specificity of the thighs.

The performance of lipoaspiration techniques must be in accordance with the so-called zones of adhesions, which in the thigh region are, respectively, the medial 1/3 on the inner surface, the distal 1/3 on the lateral surface, the distal 1/3 on the posterior surface.

Techniques

A key point is the accurate preoperative marking, which includes markings for Vertical Thigh Lift + marking on the lateral surface of the thigh and posteriorly in the buttock area. Cranially, it is started from the zone of insertion of m.gracillis and the most distal point of the cutaneous–subcutaneous excess is reach caudally, in some cases below the level of the knee. Using the pinch test, the volume of the excision is determined, without excessive tension circumferentially, as the 'double ellipse' technique is applied. Transverse markings connect postero-anteriorly the ellipse (respectively the inner ellipse) and help for a better and accurate intraoperative orientation. Laterally from the cranial part of the vertical marking, a horizontal line is marked along the course of the inguinal ligament; anterior superior iliac spine; crista iliaca posterior and sacrum. Caudally from this line, using the pinch test, the volume of the excision is determined, respectively, the line serves as a cranial marking of the future excision [1–4] (Fig. 1a, b, video to Fig. 1b).

The intervention begins with the patient in supine position. Depending on the local status, the procedure could be preceded by liposuction of the area. After the liposuction is performed,

Supplementary Information The online version contains supplementary material available at https://doi.org/10.1007/978-3-031-33350-7_10. The videos can be accessed individually by clicking the DOI link in the accompanying figure caption or by scanning this link with the SN More Media App.

E. Sharkov, *Body Contouring Surgery*, https://doi.org/10.1007/978-3-031-33350-7_10

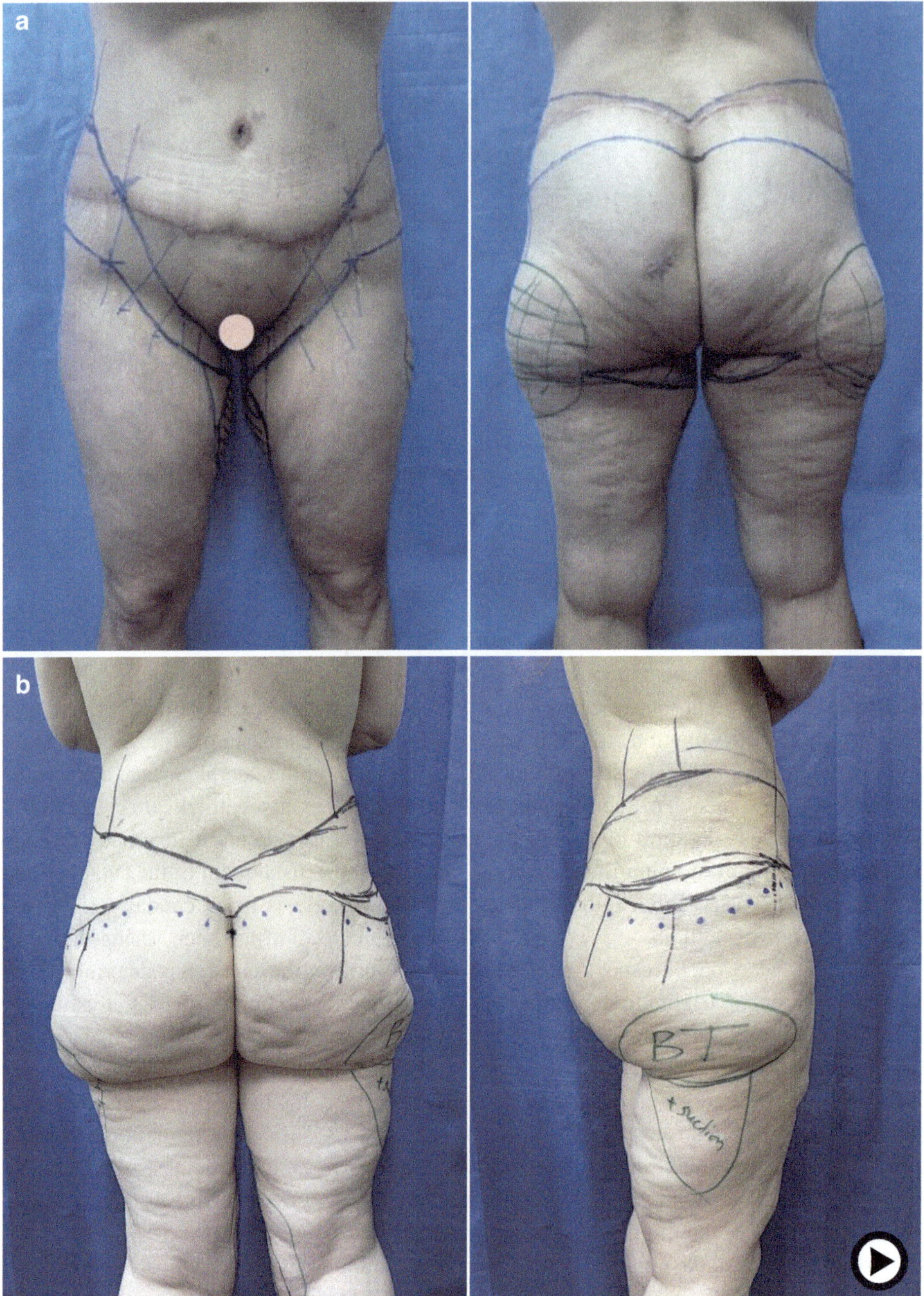

Fig. 1 (**a**) A 45-year-old female patient with massive weight loss and belt lipectomy performed 1 year ago. Preoperative marking of spiral thigh lift continued caudally as vertical thigh lift. BodyTite™ in combination with vibration-assisted liposuction in the outer thigh area—optimization of the final aesthetics with less tension during the wound closure. (**b**) A 55-year-old female patient with massive weight loss, abdominoplasty and vertical thigh lift done in another clinic 1 year ago. Preoperative marking of spiral thigh lift in combination with BodyTite™ with vibration-assisted liposuction in the outer thigh area. The blue markings are those that the author would prefer as excisional limits in conditions of isolated excisional procedure. The black markings are those that the author will follow when combining the excisional procedure with BodyTite™ of the outer thigh area. Overall, the BodyTite™ of the neighbouring area in those cases of spiral thigh lift provides as with the possibility to reduce the volume of the excision without diminishing the final outcome. Demonstration of BodyTite on the outer thigh area in combination with spiral thigh lift (▶ https://doi.org/10.1007/000-b0f)

the transverse antero-posterior markings are stitched by reference sutures in order to re-evaluate the excision. The skin excision itself is made from caudal to cranial direction on the principle of 'segmental resection closure'—a technique that ensures the prevention of intraoperative soft-tissue oedema [1–4]. During the excision, the aim is to preserve the subcutaneous fat in order to preserve the lymphatic and venous drainage of the lower limbs. Thorough haemostasis. Redon drains. Fascial suspension, wound closure. An excision of the antero-lateral part of the marked horizontal excess is made along the line of the inguinal ligament and spina iliaca anterior superior. Caudally, the tissues are dissected in order to prevent tension during closure and dilatation of the postoperative scar. 2/0 Ethibond anchoring sutures are placed in the already described areas, and the surgical wound is closed layer by layer [1–6]. At this stage, the author suggests rotating the patient in a prone position and a similar approach to the area posteriorly.

Application of Non-invasive and Minimally Invasive Techniques in Lower Body Lift Procedures

Intraoperatively (Figs. 2 and 3)

1. Vibration-assisted liposuction using Mercedes type cannulas N3 and N4 long and short bent and curved along the medial surface of the thigh—the author believes that liposuction prior to excision gives an advantage in terms of achieving an accurate volume of the excision and provides additional separation of the surrounding tissues, which in turn facilitates the closure of the operative defect and prevents the expansion of the postoperative scar.
2. Excision of the available skin excess by the surgical techniques already described.
3. The author recommends using BodyTite™ on the outer thigh area [7, 8]. The parameters used are as follows: 20 W cannula with one sensor/40 power/40 ext. cut off/—the purpose is to achieve 8–10 kJ energy per 10 cm^2 of treated area, as it is worked at 2 cm depth. The work technique is "lining" (tightening the skin by reaching 40 °C ext. cut off).
4. Morpheus8 Body™—7-5-3 mm Burst Mode with 30 kJ, 3 stacks per place no overlapping for diminishing the injury of the skin already treated with the BodyTite™. Stay at least 1. 5 cm away from the incision sides. The procedure can be repeated in the late postoperative period, on the 45th postoperative day, after which a third one can be performed for optimal effect, again in 45 days.

The author recommends the combination thus described in order to optimize the results achieved. The use of vibration-assisted liposuction allows for an optimal excision volume, reduces the tension in the closure of the surgical wound and prevents the expansion of the postoperative scar. The BodyTite™ on the outer thigh area of the thighs optimizes the tightening effect and improves the overall appearance of the area, reduces the volume of the excision in the lower back area without diminishing the final results. Finishing the procedure with an application of Morpheus8 Body™ has an additional tightening effect, improves the quality of the skin, and has beneficial impact on the cellulite changes in the area.

2. Secondary procedures

(a) Radiofrequency procedures:

- **BodyTite™, FaceTite™, AccuTite™** are used to correct contour irregularities and skin laxity. Use the specified tip depending on the area of the surgical defect. For large deformity—the BodyTite cannula is used and small deformity—the FaceTite and AccuTite cannulas are used. The goal is to reach parameters as follows: 70 °C for the internal probe for destruction of subcutaneous fat accumulation and 40 °C for the external probe for additional tightening of the skin, and deposit 8–10 kJ of energy per 10 cm^2 of treated area [9, 10]. Wait sixth month to optimally assess the contour deformity.

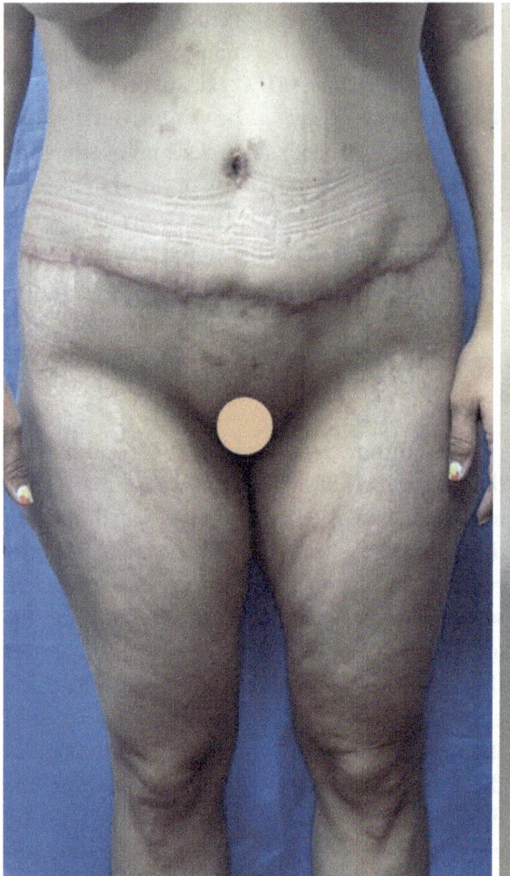

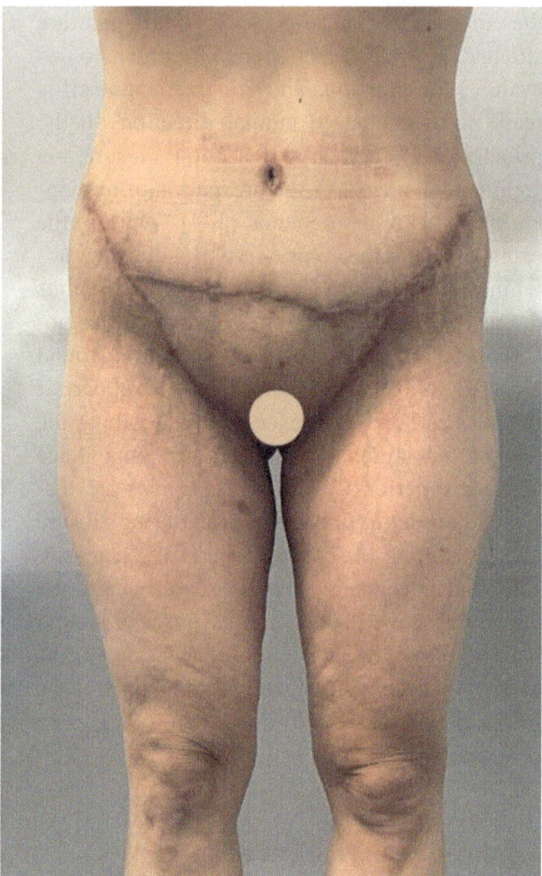

Fig. 2 45-year-old female patient with massive weight loss and belt lipectomy performed 1 year ago. Early postoperative period—sixth postoperative month—spiral thigh lift with continuation caudally as vertical thigh lift and BodyTite™ in combination with vibration-assisted liposuction in the outer thighs

- **Morpheus8 Body™**: 7-5-3 mm burst mode depth with 30 kJ, 3 stacks per place, and the procedure is performed in the late postoperative period, on the 45th day, after which a third one can be performed for optimal effect, again in 45 days.
- **EVOLVE X™:** The author recommends the procedure as part of the postoperative management of each of his patients who underwent the said procedures for minimally invasive contouring of the body. The procedure requires a cycle of several sessions and the expected improvement is 15–20% with a mostly supportive effect. The author recommends this type of interventions to start after the tenth postoperative day when looking for a positive effect. The procedure contributes not only to the faster recovery of the treated areas, but also to achieving optimal results by tightening of the underlying muscles, additional fat resorption and tightening of the skin.

(b) Ultrasound procedures

- An ultrasound massage with parameters 1.5 W/cm^2, frequency 3 MHz and duration of treatment of the respective area of 5 min, for a period of 10 days, starting from the second postoperative day, is recommended in each area with previous liposuction. The process accelerates the drainage of oedema and improves venous outflow, thereby accelerating the recovery period and improving the final results.

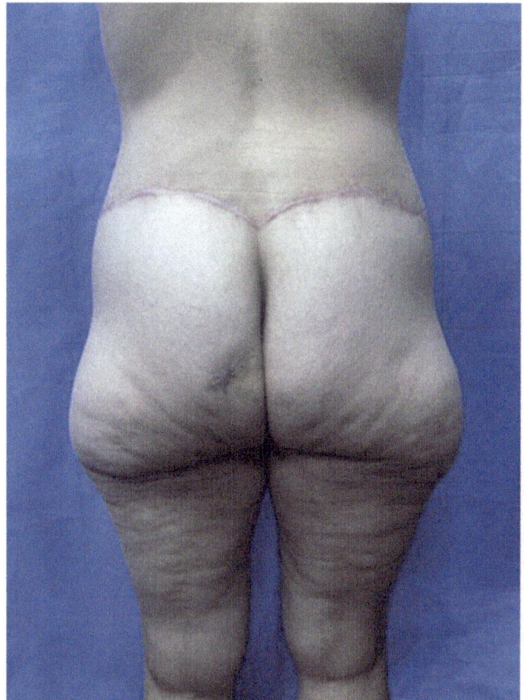

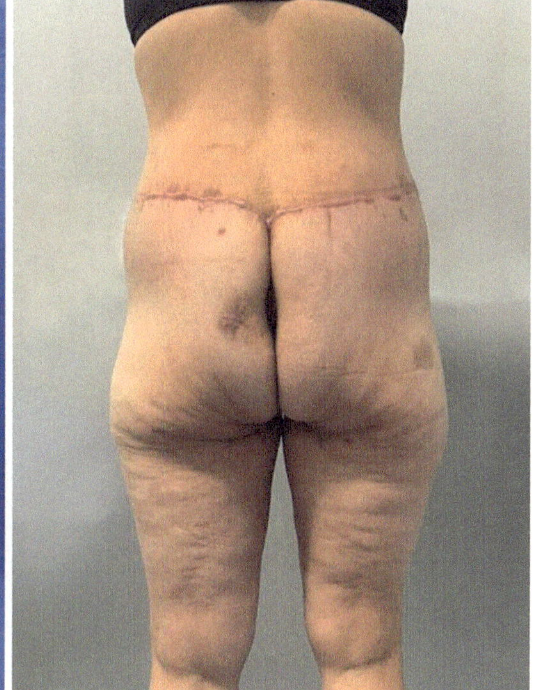

Fig. 3 A 45-year-old female patient with massive weight loss and belt lipectomy performed 1 year ago. Early postoperative period—sixth postoperative month—spiral thigh lift with continuation caudally as vertical thigh lift and BodyTite™ in combination with vibration-assisted liposuction in the outer thighs

References

1. Hurwitz DJ. Comprehensive body contouring. Theory and practice. New York: Springer; 2016. p. 81–104.
2. Kim SW, Han HH, Seo JW, Lee JH, Oh DY, Ahn ST, Rhie JW. Two cases of lower body contouring with a spiral and vertical medial thigh lift. Arch Plast Surg. 2012;39(1):67–70.
3. Sozer SO, Agullo FJ, Palladino H. Spiral lift: medial and lateral thigh lift with buttock lift and augmentation. Aesthet Plast Surg. 2008;32:120–5.
4. Kolker AR, Xipoleas GD. The circumferential thigh lift and vertical extension circumferential thigh lift: maximizing aesthetics and safety in lower extremity contouring. Ann Plast Surg. 2011;66:452–6.
5. Lockwood TE. Fascial anchoring technique in medial thigh lifts. Plast Reconstr Surg. 1988;82:299.
6. Lockwood TE. Lower body lift with superficial fascial system suspension. Plast Reconstr Surg. 1993;92:1112.
7. Mulholland RS. The BodyTite book. 2nd ed. Rijeka: IntechOpen; 2021. p. 801–2.
8. Mulholland RS. Radiofrequency energy for non-invasive and minimally invasive skin tightening. Clin Plast Surg. 2011;38:437–48.
9. Theodorou SJ, Del Vecchio D, Chia CT. Soft tissue contraction in body contouring with radiofrequency-assisted liposuction: a treatment gap solution. Aesthet Surg J. 2018;38:S74–83.
10. Levy AS, Grant RT, Rothaus KO. Radiofrequency physics for minimally invasive aesthetic surgery. Clin Plast Surg. 2016;43:551–6.

Mastopexy Techniques and Radiofrequency Procedures in Neighbouring Areas

Introduction

Depending on Regnault grade of ptosis, correction could be performed using different techniques of mastopexy:

- Inverted-T Technique: in Regnault grade III ptosis with significant skin excess both in vertical and horizontal aspect
- Circumareolar Techniques: in Regnault grade I and II ptosis—periareolar deepidermization technique according to Peixoto and periareolar round-block techniques according to Benelli
- Techniques of vertical mastopexy: in grade I and II ptosis, in which periareolar deepidermization is performed in combination with vertical incision and deepidermization, in some cases also lipoaspiration procedures
- Techniques of augmentation mastopexy: by means of pure augmentation techniques in case of minor ptosis; by means of periareolar or vertical or inverted-T deepidermization in combination with augmentation in case of depleted parenchyma and respectively Regnault grade I-II-III ptosis [1].

Supplementary Information The online version contains supplementary material available at https://doi.org/10.1007/978-3-031-33350-7_11. The videos can be accessed individually by clicking the DOI link in the accompanying figure caption or by scanning this link with the SN More Media App.

Historically, a number of eminent surgeons can be mentioned, whose discoveries contributed immeasurably to the development of mastopexy surgical techniques:

- Peixoto popularized the periareolar deepidermization, as in 1985 Peled [2, 3] described a purse-string suture technique for the first time, and in 1990 Spear [4] systematized rules for estimating the optimal diameter of the ring, subject to deepidermization
- The periareolar round-block mastopexy was introduced by Benelli [5]; an option of such technique is that of Goes, who uses a mesh that fixes to the breast wall
- In 1969, Claude Lassus introduced the vertical mastopexy technique in which he left the feeding of the nipple-areolar complex (NAC) on a superiorly based thick dermoglandular pedicle; no skin undermining is performed and en block resection of skin, fat and gland [6] is performed. In 1990, Lejour modified the described technique by including high undermining subcutaneously and adding a lipoaspiration technique in the lower poles of the breast [7];
- Hall-Findlay is an option of vertical mastopexy with preservation of the feeding of the nipple-areolar complex (NAC) on a superior-medial dermoglandular pedicle [8]
- In historical terms we can also mention the techniques of Hammond—Short Scar Periareolar Inferior Pedicle Reduction

E. Sharkov, *Body Contouring Surgery*, https://doi.org/10.1007/978-3-031-33350-7_11

Mammaplasty; the technique of Marchac as a modification of inverted-T mastopexy [9, 10]

Knowledge of the anatomical features of the area is of primary importance in performing this type of surgical interventions:

Blood supply to the breast is carried out by:

- A. thoracica interna—its perforators provide the dominant blood supply to the breast
- A. thoracica lateralis
- Intercostal perforators
- Perforators of a. thoracoacromialis
- Rr. anteriores et posteriors of aa. intercostales and mainly of fifth and sixth intercostal artery

Venous drainage—the superficial venous network may be very well developed in some patients, and it is important to try to preserve it as much as possible in order to reduce any possible postoperative venous congestion.

Lymphatic drainage—the breast has a superficial and a deep lymphatic plexus, with the lymph from the former going to the axillary lymph nodes and the lymph from the latter going to the lymph nodes under the pectoralis major muscle (Rotter's lymph nodes), and from there to the axillary lymph nodes – Grossman's lymphatic pathway. Some lymphatic vessels from the deep lymphatic plexus reach the mediastinal lymph nodes, and the lymphatic vessels from the lower-medial quadrants of the breasts drain to the hepatic and subdiaphragmatic lymph nodes—Gerota's lymphatic pathway.

Innervation—supraclavicular branches; lateral intercostal branches of the second to the sixth intercostal nerves; anterior intercostal branches of the second to the sixth intercostal nerves; the lateral branch of the fourth intercostal nerve is predominant for the formation of the subareolar plexus of the nipple-areolar complex (NAC).

Fascial strengthening apparatus—the gland is wrapped, located between lamina anterior et posterior of Scarpa's fascia. Lamina posterior separates the breast from the underlying m.pectoralis major. Between the two sheets of Scarpa's fascia, there are intraparenchymal fibrous septa (Cooper's ligaments), which are also part of the breast strengthening apparatus. There is also a horizontally oriented fibrous septum, which is at the level of the fourth to fifth rib and, roughly speaking, divides the breast into superior 2/3 and inferior 1/3. It starts from the pectoral fascia and is accompanied by a vascular arcade and nerve branches, and the said vascular and nerve branches are of particular importance in relation to the nipple-areolar complex (NAC). The septum in question is of significant importance in the formation of a feeding pedicle for the nipple-areolar complex (NAC)—for example, in the formation of a lower feeding pedicle; in order to preserve the blood supply to the nipple-areolar complex (NAC), it is good to shape the pedicle in such a way that the vessels located caudal to the septum remain preserved.

Mastopexy techniques are based on the removal of only skin and possibly a minimal amount of glandular parenchyma, which is the main difference with reduction mammoplasty techniques. Traditional mastopexy techniques are often insufficient to achieve adequate contouring in patients with significant reduction in body weight. This type of patient are a challenge to surgery due to the presence of significant cutaneous–subcutaneous excess and Regnault Grade III ptosis, accompanied by a lateral disposition of the available mammary gland, which is often found to be hypoplastic as well [11]. What has been said above determines the use of Inverted-T technique as a main method, with the appropriate choice of the type of feeding pedicle for the nipple-areolar complex (NAC). In men, the cases of hyperplasia of the gland, presented with available gynecomastia, which requires extirpation of the glandular tissue and excision of the available cutaneous–subcutaneous excess, prevail. In both men and women after massive weight loss, the transposition of NAC as a free nipple graft is widely used.

Inverted-T technique—a technique using the so-called Wise pattern of preoperative delineation is widely used in patients after massive weight loss [12].

The choice of feeding pedicle for NAC depends both on the patient's local status and on the surgeon's evaluation:

- Double-horizontal according to Strombeck [13]
- Double-vertical according to McKissock [14]
- Superiorly based feeding pedicle according to Wise [15]
- Inferiorly based feeding pedicle according to Ribeiro [16]—an option preferred by the author due to the good feeding of NAC and tissue suspension adequate in nature and duration in time
- Centrally based feeding pedicle—an option preferred by the author, which involves extensive subcutaneous undermining circumferentially around a centrally based feeding pedicle and fixation of a medial and lateral glandular flap to and superior to the feeding pedicle, resulting in maximal remodelling and centrocranial fixation of the glandular tissue [17, 18]
- Medial pedicle according to Strombeck [19]
- Superior-medial pedicle according to Hall-Findlay

The specificity of this type of patients suggests a 'continuation' of the Wise pattern lateral pedicle toward and even to the posterior axillary line. This would allow to simultaneously remove the skin excess on the lateral surface of the chest and use the underlying lipodermal flap for additional autologous augmentation of the breast.

In patients after massive weight loss, the so-called L-type of skin excision with a short arm pointing laterally toward the axilla is used. This technique is widely used especially in patients with significant soft-tissue excess on the lateral surface of the chest, where the short arm of the L-incision can be continued and even passed into skin incisions in other topographic-anatomical areas (L-type brachioplasty; back-bra-lift, etc.). In women, the short arm of the L-incision is limited to deepidermization with minimal or no underlying soft-tissue excision—the purpose is to use the lateral excess to further augment the lifted breast. In men, the short arm of the L-incision involves deepidermization with removal of excess subcutaneous soft tissue.

The free nipple graft technique is used in our practice—a technique in which the nipple-areolar complex (NAC) is transposed cranially on the already lifted breast, respectively, the contoured chest in men, in the form of a free autograft. NAC is taken and moved as a composite graft including skin, subcutaneous tissue and muscle fibres, in which only the fat and glandular tissue are removed. NAC is implanted on a deepidermized recipient site. Epidermolysis of the graft is usually observed in the early postoperative period, which fades away spontaneously over time. The accurate positioning of NAC both in terms of left and right symmetry and in terms of distance from the inframammary folds (IMF) is considered.

In male patients after massive weight loss, with significant skin excess and/ or severe gynecomastia (Simon or Rohrich Grade IV), the free nipple transfer technique is considered—a technique with/without extirpation of the underlying glandular tissue (depending on local status). Both Inverted-T with Wise pattern technique and L-type incision can be used, and if there is a need for contouring in the chest area and lifting and/or contouring of adjacent areas (abdomen, chest lateral surface), dermal flaps are used from caudal and lateral, which are transposed and fixed in a cranial direction.

Techniques

Breast Lift in Pseudoptosis and Regnault Grade I Ptosis, Author's Preferred Techniques

Augmentation Mastopexy with Periareolar Deepidermization

The author uses a periareolar approach with subsequent submuscular positioning of round ergonomic implants. Periareolar deepidermization with subsequent cerclage using 2/0 Ethibond is performed (Figs. 1 and 2).

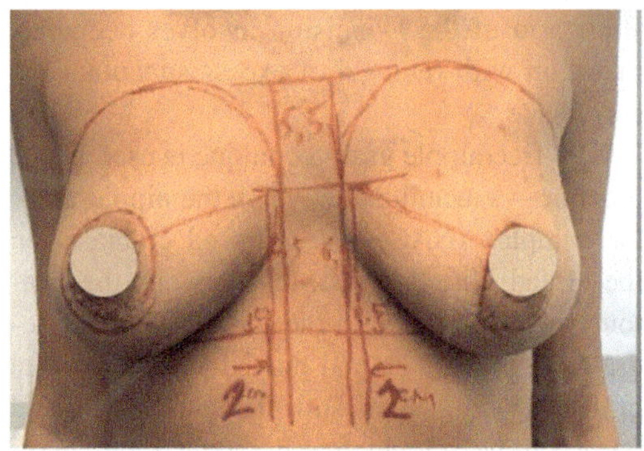

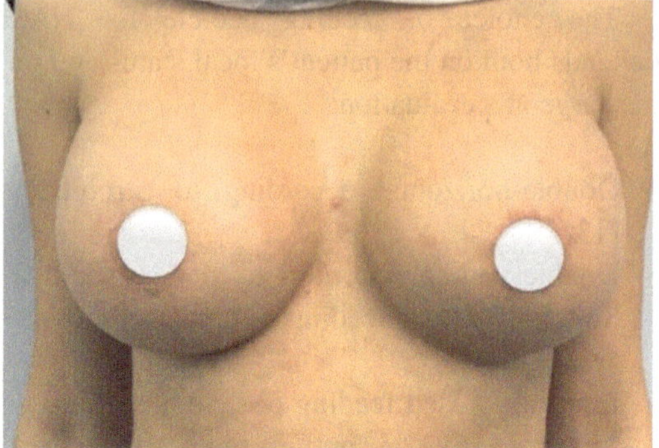

Fig. 1 Augmentation mastopexy with periareolar deepidermization. Before and 6 months after

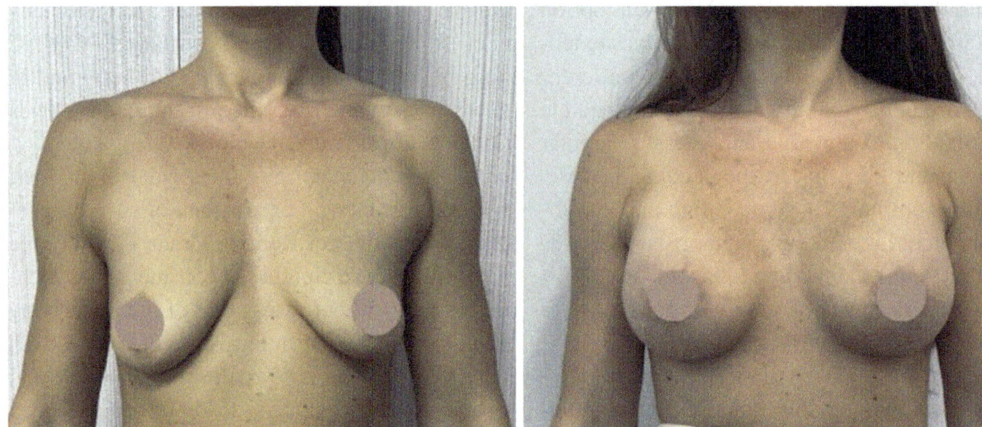

Fig. 2 Augmentation mastopexy with periareolar deepidermization and symmetrization of the breast. Before and 6 months after

Breast Lift in Regnault Grade II-III Ptosis, Author's Preferred Techniques

Inverted-T Mastopexy

Preoperative marking is made according to the so-called wise pattern. Inferior pedicle (Figs. 3, 4, 5 and 6) (with a width of at least 7 cm) or the centrally based feeding pedicle (Fig. 7, Video 1) (preferred options by the author) could be used. Incisions are shaped according to the type of 'inverted horseshoe', respectively, inverted-T. In patients without serious weight reduction and available glandular parenchyma, there is an option to minimally remove the glandular tissue in a superior and/ or medial and/or lateral aspect to the pedicle. In patients after massive weight loss due to depleted subcutaneous soft-tissue reserves and lack of volume, reduction techniques are rarely required and after fixation of the pedicle cranially to the second to third rib, the lateral and medial cutaneous–subcutaneous-glandular pillars are fixed by pulling in a medial direction on the inferior feeding pedicle or by fixation to the central feeding pedicle in a direction towards itself and cranially in order to shape the breast in the shape of a 'round implant' [20], and the defect is closed layer by layer.

The author uses a technique he calls a 'tissue bra', in which caudal portions of the medial and lateral soft-tissue pillars are fixed to the inferior feeding pedicle in order to further prevent subsequent ptosis. (Figs. 4 and 5; Video 2).

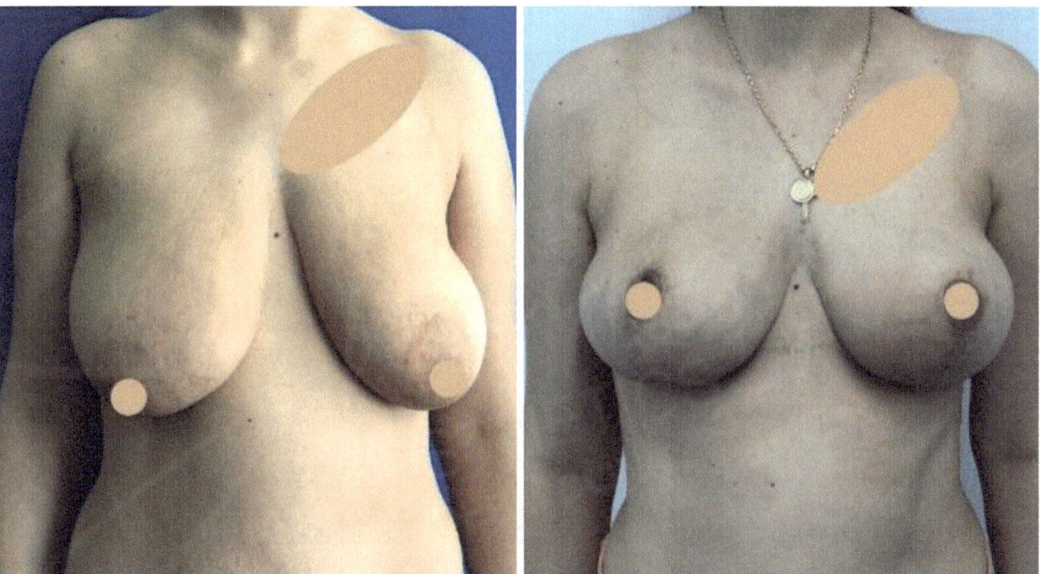

Fig. 3 Inverted-T mastopexy of inferior feeding pedicle. Before and 6 months after

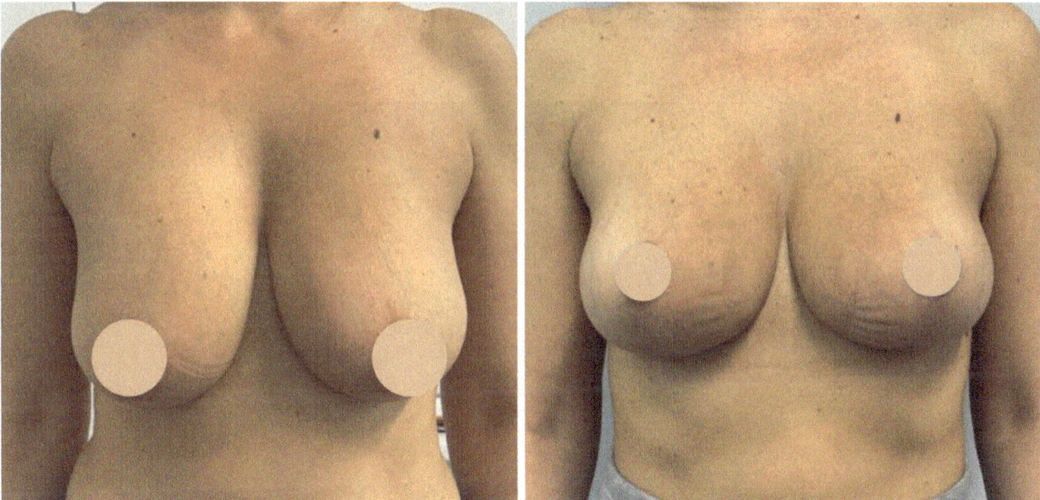

Fig. 4 Inverted-T mastopexy of inferior pedicle using the 'tissue bra' technique described by the author. Before and 1 year after

Inverted 'T' Mastopexy: Inverted-T Technique with Pedicled Flap of Subcutaneous Adipose Tissue from the Lateral Part of the Chest (Fig. 8)

Preoperative marking is carried out according to the so-called wise pattern, marking an elliptical skin island with soft-tissue excess present in the lateral part of the chest. Due to the depleted subcutaneous soft-tissue reserves and the lack of volume after fixation of the inferior pedicle in a cranial direction, deepidermization of the lateral skin island is performed, which is separated circumferentially and then pulled and transposed in a medial direction, passing over the inferior pedicle [21]. The lateral and medial cutaneous–

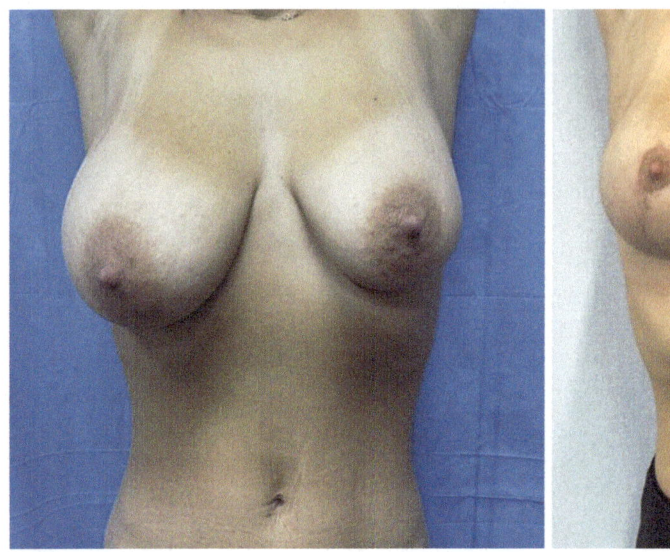

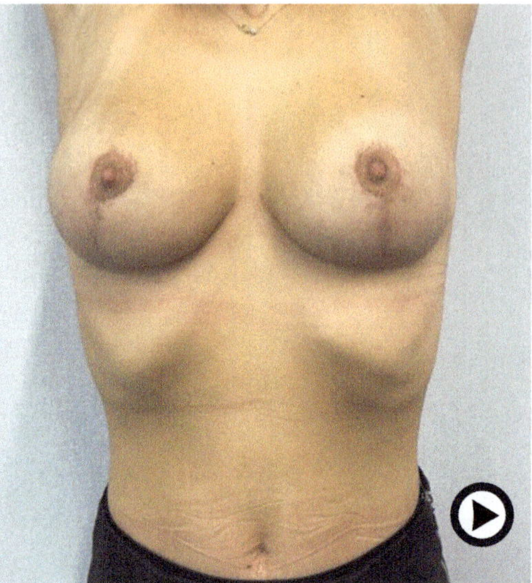

Fig. 5 Inverted-T mastopexy and breast symmetrization. The pexy was performed with an inferior pedicle using the 'tissue bra' technique described by the author. Before and 6 months after the procedure. Mastopexy with inferior pedicle using the 'tissue bra' technique described by the author, in which caudal portions of the medial and lateral soft-tissue pillars are fixed to the inferior feeding pedicle to further prevent subsequent ptosis (▶ https://doi.org/10.1007/000-b0h)

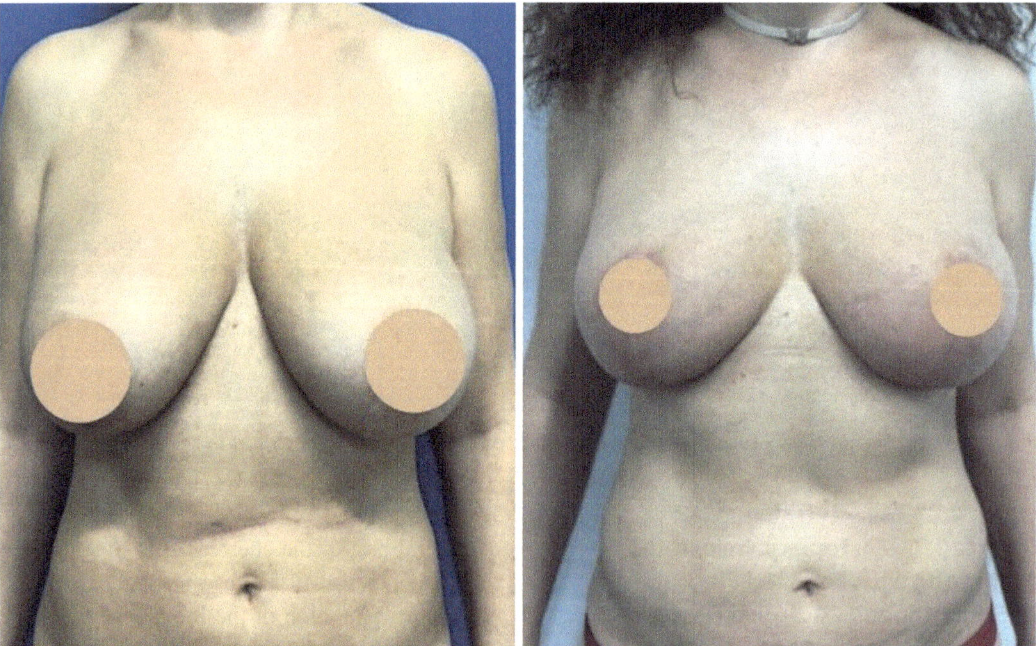

Fig. 6 Inverted-T mastopexy of inferior feeding pedicle. Before and 1 year after

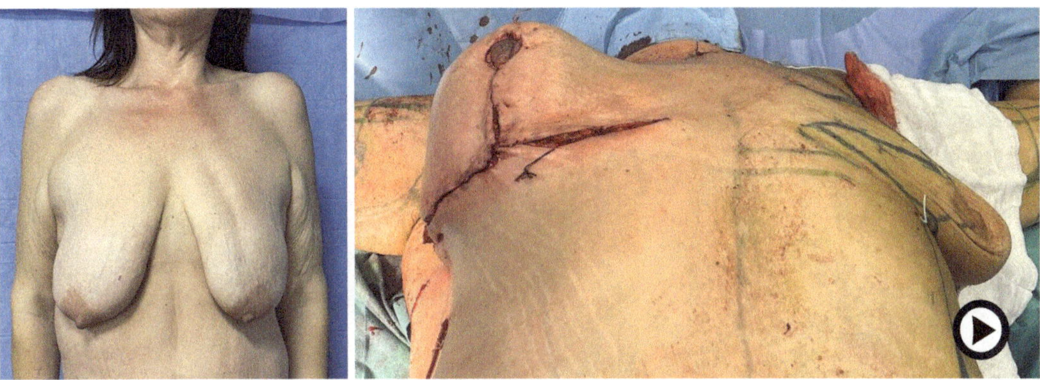

Fig. 7 A patient after massive weight loss—inverted-T mastopexy of centrally based pedicle. Intraoperative modelling of the pedicle with fixation of the lateral and medial pillars to the centrally-based pedicle (▶ https://doi.org/10.1007/000-b0g)

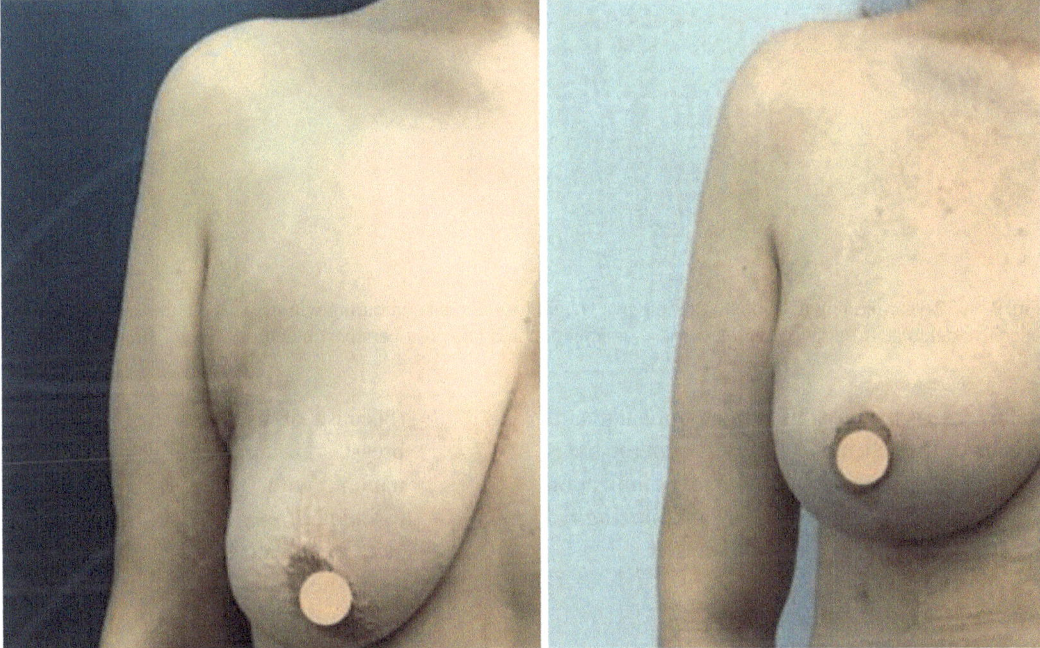

Fig. 8 Inverted-T mastopexy with inferior pedicle and soft-tissue from the lateral side of the chest. Before and 6 months after in patient after massive weight loss

subcutaneous-glandular pillars are fixed by pulling in the medial direction and the defect is closed layer by layer. Volume correction after removal of excesses could also be implant-based, but due to the specificity of the intervention and the associated intra- and postoperative risks in this type of patients, the author prefers volume replacement to be performed with adjacent own tissues, whenever possible. Implant-based techniques for the purpose of augmentation of the already lifted tissues, if necessary, are mainly used as a subsequent stage in a plan for contouring the area.

Breast Contouring with Free Nipple Transfer [22] (Fig. 9)

This type of surgical techniques is used when there is a significant degree of soft-tissue ptosis. The intervention enables precise positioning of NAC both in women and in men, as an advantage

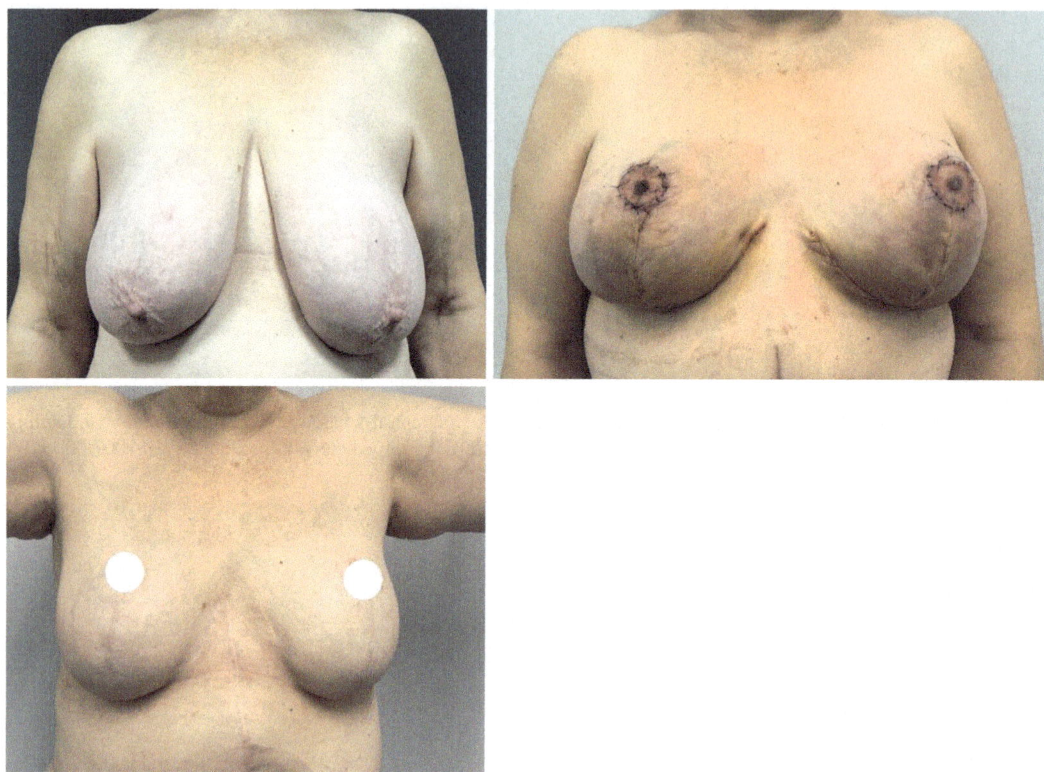

Fig. 9 A 72-year-old female patient after massive weight loss. Breast contouring with free nipple transfer. Early postoperative outcome—14 days after the surgical intervention and late postoperative outcome—2 years after surgery

in this case is the possibility of additional manipulation of the subcutaneous reserves in the breast area for the purpose of volume optimization. Precise execution is the basis of minimizing risk in terms of survival of the free transfer.

Application of Non-invasive and Minimally Invasive Techniques in Mastopexy Procedures

(a) Intraoperatively

- Radiofrequency procedures:
  - **BodyTite™:** The author recommends using isolated radiofrequency therapy for breast lift only in cases of minor and/or pseudoptosis [23]. BodyTite™ is performed in the following areas: breast area—the parameters are as follows: 20 W cannula with one sensor/40 power/40 ext. cut off/2 cm depth—the purpose is to achieve 8–10 kJ of energy per 10 cm² of treated area. The author does not recommend using BodyTite™ (because of its ablative effect) in the breast area intraoperatively in combination with any type of pexy technique.
  - **FaceTite™/AccuTite™** in the armpits [24]. The goal is to improve the appearance in the breast area (Fig. 10; Video 3). The parameters are: FaceTite handpiece/70 int cut off/40 ext. cut off/—the purpose is to achieve 6–8 kJ energy. The work techniques are respectively 'stamping' (melting the fat cells by reaching 70 °C int temperature) and 'lining' (tightening the skin by reaching 40 °C ext. temperature), as the skin tightening precedes the subcutaneous fat destruction. The procedure finishes with lipoaspiration of the liquefied fat.
  - **Morpheus8 Body™** and Morpheus8™: In the area of the armpits (in combination with FaceTite) and in the area of the cleavage—the purpose again is

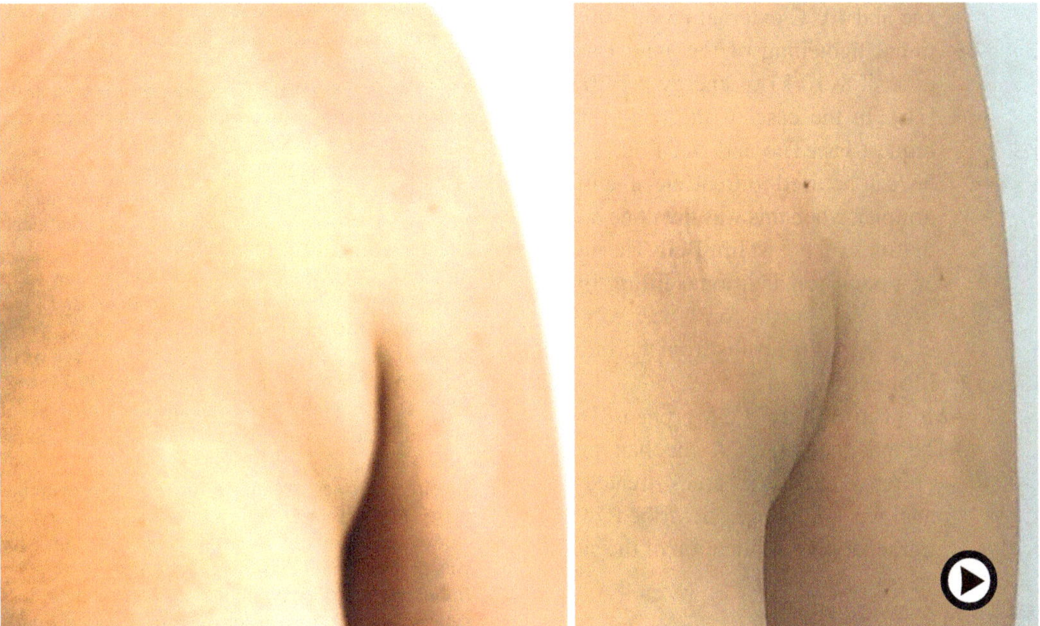

Fig. 10 AccuTite in the area of armpits before and 1 year after (▶ https://doi.org/10.1007/000-b0j)

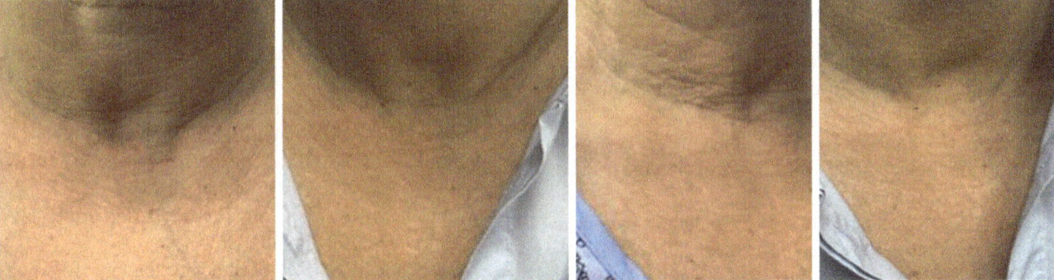

Fig. 11 **Morpheus8™**—45 days after one procedure with the following parameters—lower third of the neck and cleavage—4 mm/35 energy/3 stacks per place/50% overlapping/ fixed mode + neckline—3 mm/30 energy/2 stacks per place/30% overlapping/fixed mode + neckline 2 mm/15 energy/1 stack per place/cycle mode

not only to improve the appearance in the breast area using the mastopexy techniques above-described, but also to have an overall positive impact on the area on and around the breast [25]. The parameters are: **Morpheus8 Body™**—7-5-3 mm burst mode depth with 30 kJ, 3 stacks per place, and microneedling can be repeated on the 45th and 90th postoperative days. **Morpheus8™**—lower third of the neck and cleavage—4 mm/35 energy/3 stacks per place/50% overlapping/fixed mode + neckline 3 mm/30 energy/2 stacks per place/30% overlapping/fixed mode + neckline 2 mm/15 energy/1 stack per place/cycle mode (Fig. 11), and microneedling can be repeated on the 45th 90th postoperative days.

(b) Secondary procedures
- Radiofrequency procedures:
  - **BodyTite™, FaceTite™, AccuTite™** for contour irregularities and/ or additionally tightening of the skin. The goal is 70 °C internal probe for destruction of subcutaneous fat with sublethal damage to the connective tis-

sue and 40 °C external probe for additional tightening of the skin. Usually deposit 8–10 kJ of energy per 10 cm^2 [26]. In the case of mastopexy techniques, FaceTite and AccuTite cannulas can be used to treat the area of the armpits, when this was not done during the surgical breast lift. BodyTite can be an option for additional lifting in the breast area—wait for 1 year to properly assess the results from the surgical lifting.

- Morpheus8 Body™ § Morpheus8™:
- The parameters used, the handpieces preferred and the areas treated are analogous to those described in the intraoperative application of the same.

References

1. Romansky R, Tepavicharova P. Reconstructive and aesthetic surgery in women's breast Sofia, Bulgaria. 89–104.
2. Peled IJ, Zagher U, Wexler MR. Purse string suture for reduction and closure of skin defects. Ann Plast Surg. 1985;14:465.
3. Peled IJ, Zagher U. The concentric mastopexy and the purse string suture. Plast Reconstr Surg. 1991;87(2):385.
4. Spear SL, Kassan M, Little JW. Guidelines in concentric mastopexy. Plast Reconstr Surg. 2001;107:1294.
5. Benelli L. A new periareolar mammaplasty: the "round-block" technique. Aesthet Plast Surg. 1990;14:93.
6. Lassus C. New refinements in vertical mammaplasty. Chir Plast. 1981;6:81.
7. Lejour M. Vertical mammaplasty and liposuction of the breast. Plast Reconstr Surg. 1994;94:100.
8. Hall-Findlay EJ. Vertical breast reduction with a medially-based pedicle. Aesthet Surg J. 2002;22(2):185.
9. Hammond DC. Short scar periareolar inferior pedicle reduction (SPAIR) mammaplasty. Plast Reconstr Surg. 1999;103:890.
10. Marchac D, De Olarte G. Reduction mammaplasty and correction of ptosis with a short inframammary scar. Plast Reconstr Surg. 1982;69:45.
11. Hurwitz DJ. Comprehensive body contouring. Theory and practice. New York: Springer; 2016. p. 63–179.
12. Regnault P. Breast ptosis. Definition and treatment. Clin Plast Surg. 1976;130(4):779.
13. Stroembeck JO. Mammaplasty: report on a new technique based on the two-pedicle procedure. Br J Plast Surg. 1960;13:79.
14. McKissock PK. Reduction mammaplasty with a vertical dermal flap. Plast Reconstr Surg. 1972;49:245–52.
15. Wise RJ. A preliminary report on a method of planning the mammaplasty. Plast Reconstr Surg. 1956;17:17–367.
16. Ribeiro L. A new technique for reduction mammaplasty. Plast Reconstr Surg. 1975;55:330.
17. Hurwitz DJ, Golla D. Breast reshaping after massive weight loss. Semin Plast Surg. 2004;18:179–87.
18. Rubin JP. Mastopexy in the massive weight loss patient: dermal suspension and total parenchymal reshaping. Aesthet Surg J. 2006;26:214–22.
19. Stroembeck JO. Reduction mammaplasty: some observations and reflections. Aesthet Plast Surg. 1983;7:249.
20. Rubin P, Jellew ML, Richter DF, Uebel CO. Body contouring and liposuction. Philadelphia: Saunders Elsevier; 2013. p. 122–78.
21. Aly AS. Body contouring after massive weight loss. St Louis: Quality Medical Publishing; 2006. p. 361–77.
22. Thorek M. Possibilities in the reconstruction of the human form. NY Med J Rec. 1922;116:572.
23. Mulholland RS. The BodyTite book. 2nd ed. Rijeka: IntechOpen; 2021. p. 801–2.
24. Mulholland RS. Radiofrequency energy for non-invasive and minimally invasive skin tightening. Clin Plast Surg. 2011;38:437–48.
25. Theodorou SJ, Del Vecchio D, Chia CT. Soft tissue contraction in body contouring with radiofrequency-assisted liposuction: a treatment gap solution. Aesthet Surg J. 2018;38:S74–83.
26. Levy AS, Grant RT, Rothaus KO. Radiofrequency physics for minimally invasive aesthetic surgery. Clin Plast Surg. 2016;43:551–6.

Upper Body Lift Techniques in Combination with Minimally Invasive and Non-invasive Procedures

Introduction

Deformities in the upper torso are generally characterized by a vertical and horizontal component. The human body possesses areas of dense fascial connections between skin and the underlying musculoskeletal system, which in the thoracic region project anteriorly into the area of the sternum and posteriorly along the spine. During obesity, there will be no fat excess accumulation in these areas, and in subsequent weight loss, the adjacent areas will ptose around and caudal to them. This results in the so-called inverted-V deformity in the chest area anteriorly and in the subscapular area posteriorly. The lateral aspect of the inframammary fold (IMF) is also affected significantly, as the soft tissues in this area are equidistant both from the sternum and from the spine. Ptosis in this area can continue laterally and posteriorly and lead to the so-called lateral breast/upper back roll deformity [1].

Determining the position of the lateral part of the inframammary fold (IMF) is a key factor

- In the absence of caudal dislocation—isolated brachioplasty and breast lift/reduction procedures are the correct choice of surgical technique (Fig. 4)
- If it is inferiorly dispositioned—need for an upper body lift procedure (Fig. 3) [1]

Evaluation of available gynecomastia—the author uses two classification:

- Simon et al. classification—Grade I: Small enlargement without skin excess; Grade IIa: Moderate enlargement without skin excess; Grade IIb: Moderate enlargement with minor skin excess; Grade III: Marked enlargement with excess skin, mimicking female breast ptosis [2].
- Rohrich classification—Grade I: Minimal hypertrophy (<250 g) without ptosis; Grade II: Moderate hypertrophy (250–500 g) without ptosis. Grade III: Severe hypertrophy (>500 g) with grade I ptosis; Grade IV: Severe hypertrophy with grade II or grade III ptosis [3].

Techniques

Upper Body Lift

The author examines and describes the following techniques:

Supplementary Information The online version contains supplementary material available at https://doi.org/10.1007/978-3-031-33350-7_12. The videos can be accessed individually by clicking the DOI link in the accompanying figure caption or by scanning this link with the SN More Media App.

E. Sharkov, *Body Contouring Surgery*, https://doi.org/10.1007/978-3-031-33350-7_12

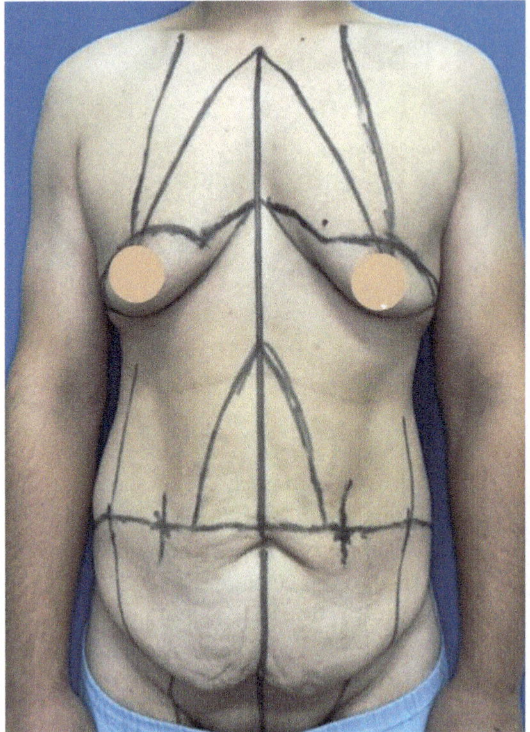

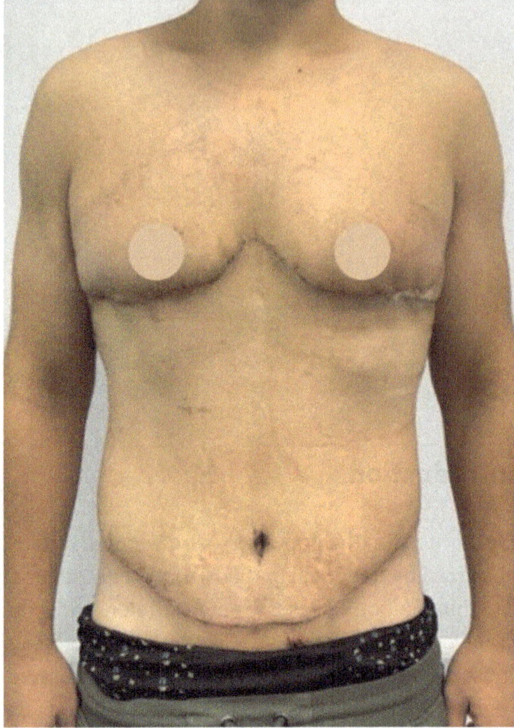

Fig. 1 Preoperative marking of upper body lift with free nipple transfer in a patient with massive weight loss. The marking also includes a one-stage Fleur De Lis abdominoplasty, and intraoperatively, after re-evaluation of the tissues, it is proceeded to extended abdominoplasty. The photo on the right shows an early postoperative outcome 14 days after the procedure

Isolated Lifting in the Pectoral Area in Male Patient After Massive Weight Loss

An elliptical excision of preoperatively marked cutaneous–subcutaneous excess in the pectoral area is performed (Fig. 1). Emphasis is placed on preserving the subcutaneous soft-tissue in the area onto the pectoral muscle in order to preserve the projection. Otherwise, the area is deprived of its masculine appearance associated with pronounced pectoral musculature. The author describes a technique with free nipple transfer (Fig. 2).

One-Stage Brachioplasty with Lateral Torso Contouring and Breast Lift in Female Patient After Massive Weight Loss

Brachioplasty is performed using techniques described in the brachioplasty section. In cases of L-brachioplasty with overlapping of the excision on the lateral surface of the chest with the lateral breast-back roll area, temporary closure of the short arm of the L-excision with staples is necessary for adequate assessment. It is proceeded to the lateral breast-back roll area—skin is excised and the cutaneous–subcutaneous flap is undermined caudally above the underlying muscle fascia. The flap is elevated cranially, the shoulder is pushed caudally, and the excess is excised. As a result, the vertical excess is eliminated, the lateral aspect of the inframammary fold (IMF) is elevated, and the lateral breast-back roll excess is excised [1]. A disadvantage is the possible presence of a dog-ear in the inferior-lateral aspect of the breast, which will be corrected later during the intervention on the breast. The surgical wound is closed layer by layer with an emphasis on Lockwood's fascia [4]. It is proceeded to the breast area, where the intervention will depend

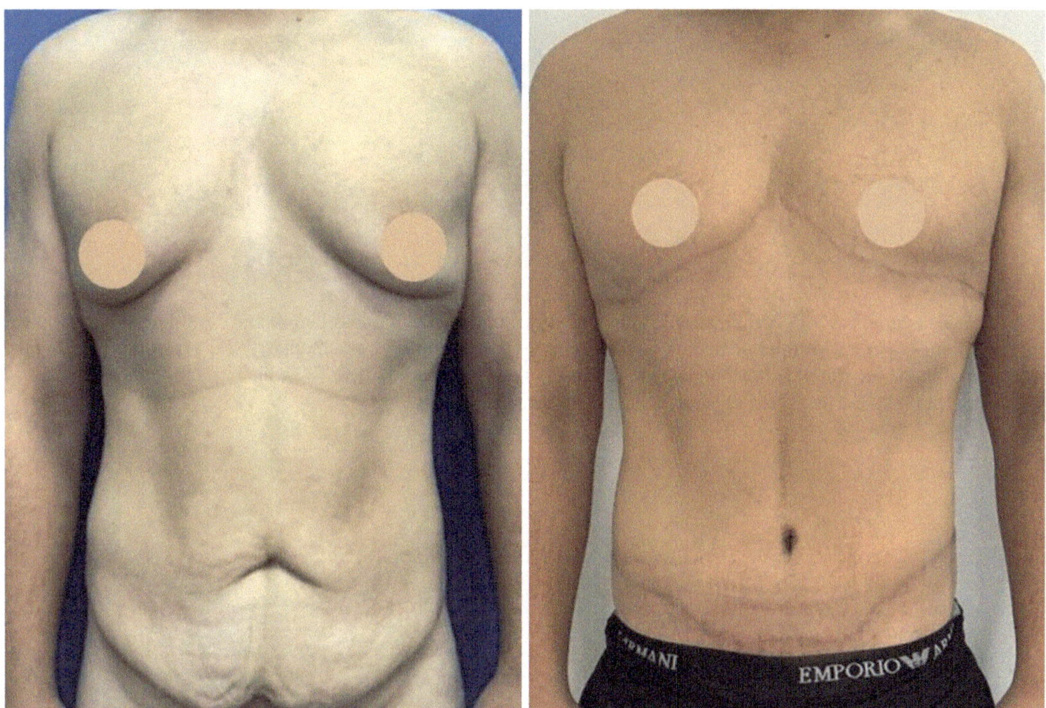

Fig. 2 Upper Body Lift with free nipple transfer in a patient with massive weight loss. One-stage extended abdominoplasty was also performed. The outcome is 1 year after the surgery

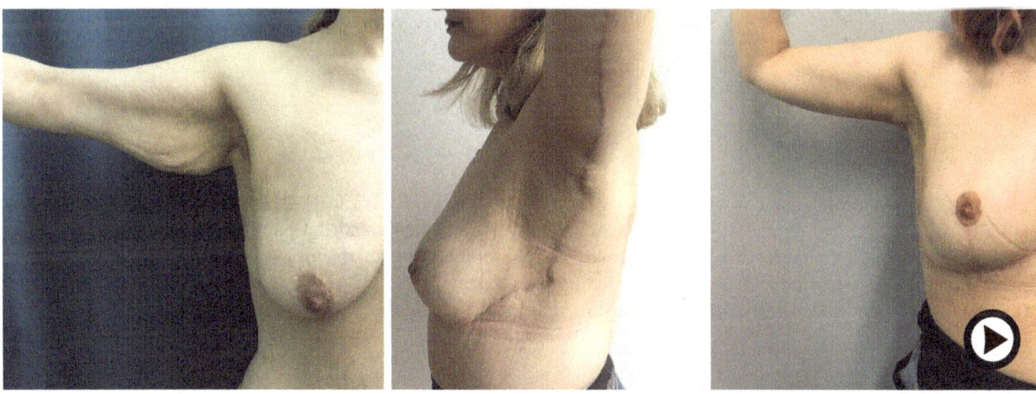

Fig. 3 One-time L-brachioplasty, with a scar positioned on the posterior surface of the upper arm, combined with inverted-T mastopexy with mobilization of the subcutaneous soft-tissue excess on the lateral surface of the chest for volume replacement in the breast area. NAC feeding is stored on an inferior pedicle by Ribeiro [5]. The photos illustrate a patient with massive weight loss—before and 1 year after the procedure. Mobilization of the subcutaneous soft-tissue excess on the lateral surface of the chest for volume replacement in the breast area (▶ https://doi.org/10.1007/000-b0m)

on the local status and gender—in men, reduction is most often required due to existing gynecomastia, while in women, reduction, pexy, augmentation or a combination is possible. In patients after massive weight loss, emphasis should be placed on fixing the inframammary fold (IMF) in a higher position (Figs. 3 and 4, Video 1).

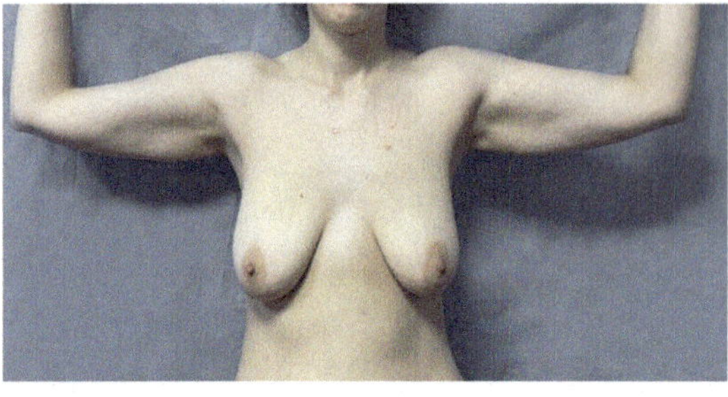

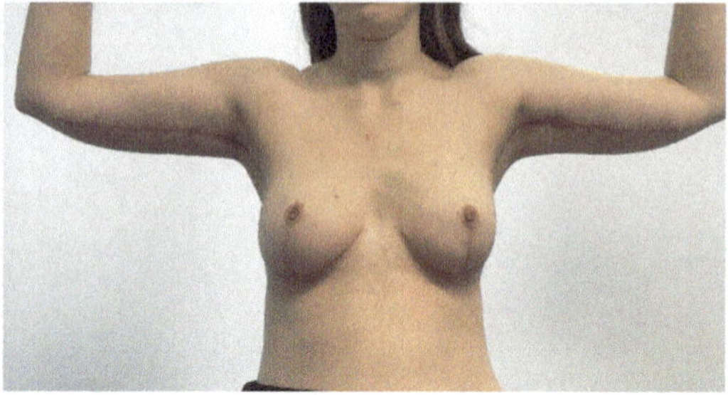

Fig. 4 L-Brachioplasty in combination with classic inverted-T mastopexy with inferior pedicle without continuation of the short arm of L-brachioplasty to the inframammary fold (IMF). The photos illustrate a patient after massive weight loss before and after the sixth postoperative month. The brachioplasty scar is positioned along the bicipital groove [6, 7], which is the author's preferred technique

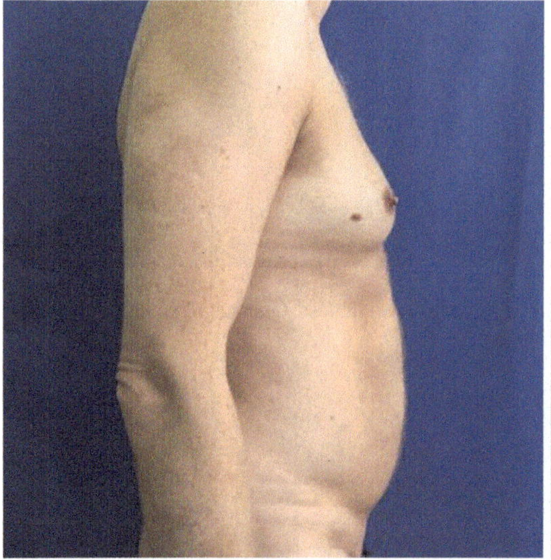

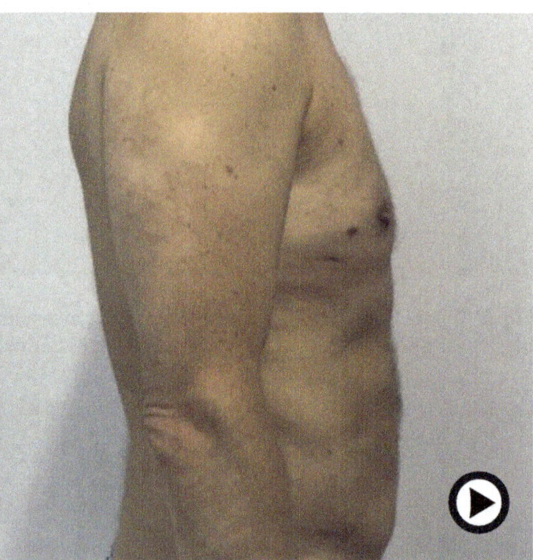

Fig. 5 A 60-year-old male patient with existing gynecomastia of mixed type, before and 1 year after vibration-assisted liposuction in the breast area, with extirpation of the glandular tissue using the above-described technique in combination with BodyTite™ radiofrequency in the same area. BodyTite™—the energy is delivered in subcutaneous plane, and the parameters are as follows 20 W cannula with one sensor/40 power/40 ext cut off/10 kJ energy per side, 2 cm depth (▶ https://doi.org/10.1007/000-b0k)

Treatment of Gynecomastia by Combination of Gland Extirpation and Radiofrequency Based Procedure

The author proposes a classic technique of gland extirpation through a semilunar incision. The procedure is preceded by vibration-assisted liposuction with an N3 Mercedes type long straight cannula in cases of mixed gynecomastia. The intervention ends with BodyTite—with an entry point in the deltopectoral groove, the application of energy is carried out strictly subcutaneously; the parameters used are—20 W cannula with one sensor/40 power/40 ext. cut off/; the goal is to achieve 8–10 kJ energy per 10 cm^2 of treated area, working at a depth of 2 cm [8]. The author does not recommend using BodyTite™ in the breast area intraoperatively in combination with any type of lifting technique. The purpose is to prevent possible skin sagging after extirpation of the gland (Fig. 5, Video 2).

Application of Non-invasive and Minimally Invasive Techniques in Upper Body Lift Procedures

A. **Intraoperatively**

- **Radiofrequency procedures**
  - **BodyTite™:** The author recommends the use of radiofrequency therapy for lifting and tightening the skin in the chest area. The procedure is performed with an inlet in the deltopectoral sulcus, the parameters used are as follow: 20 W cannula with one sensor/40 power/40 ext. cut off/—the purpose is to achieve 8–10 kJ energy per 10 cm^2 of treated area, working at a depth of 2 cm. **The author does not recommend using BodyTite™ in the breast area intraoperatively in combination with any type of lifting technique, due to the ablative effect of the procedure.**
  - **FaceTite™** is used in an **adjacent area (armpits)** for overall improvement of the appearance in the breast area in combination with isolated **Mastopexy** techniques and in surgical treatment of **Grade I, II, III gynecomastia**. The parameters used are as follow: FaceTite handpiece/70 int cut off/40 ext. cut off/—the purpose is to achieve 5–8 kJ energy. 'Stamping' (melting the fat cells by reaching 70 °C int cut off) and 'lining' (tightening the skin by reaching 40 °C ext. cut off), should be used. The skin tightening precedes the ablative effect on the subcutaneous adipose tissue [9–11]. The procedure finishes with lipoaspiration of the liquefied adipose tissue.
  - **Morpheus8 Body™ and Morpheus 8™:** In the area of the armpits (in combination with FaceTite™) and in the area of the cleavage—the purpose again is not only to improve the appearance in the breast area using the mastopexy techniques above-described, but also to have an overall positive impact on the area on and around the breast. The parameters are described in Chapter "Mastopexy Techniques and Radiofrequency Procedures in Neighboring Areas".
- **VASERlipo®:**
  - The author uses ultrasound treatment for definition in the breast area in mixed type of gynecomastia, pseudogynecomastia and obesity. The parameters are as follow: breast area, including the area lateral and caudal to the pectoral muscles: 2 ring people; first VASER mode on 80% superficially and then continuous mode C on 80% deep; 1 min per 100 mL of infiltrated solution [12].
- **Vibrational assisted liposuction:**
  - The author uses liposuction techniques in cases of mixed type of gynecomastia, in cases of pseudogynecomastia and obesity. In case of liposuction techniques in the breast area in male patients, the entry points hidden in the deltopectoral sulcus and immediately caudally to the nipple. Liposuction is performed using an N3 and N4 Mercedes type long straight cannula in the area caudal to the line that connects the deltopectoral sulcus with proc. xyphoideus (Fig. 6). Liposuction precedes the radiofrequency treatment of the area, and in cases where the aim is to achieve definition in the breast area, the vibration technique is preceded by ultrasound treatment of the area. In cases of definition in the breast area, liposuction is also performed on the lateral surface of the chest and in the area caudal to the pectoral muscle in order to 'empty' the fat deposits in these areas and define along the course of pectoralis major 'muscle' (Fig. 6) [12]. The procedure can be combined with intramuscular lipofilling for optimal definition, in which case radiofre-

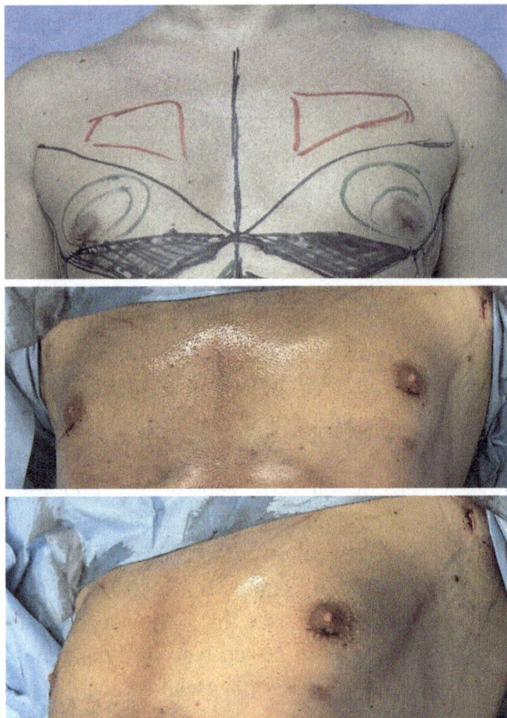

Fig. 6 Before and immediately after high-definition procedure in the chest area. The preoperative marking shows the liposuction area, marked in green, and the areas with maximum 'emptying' of the fat deposits, marked in black—'negative spaces', for the purpose of definition. The areas, marked in red, are for demonstration purposes—orientation in case of possible intramuscular lipotransfer under ultrasound guidance. Extirpation of glandular tissue was not required. No radiofrequency procedure was performed due to the patient's young age, preserved skin contractility, and absence of loose skin

quency treatment is avoided due to possible compromise of the lipotransfer survival.

- **Possible combinations depending on the patient's preoperative status:**
  A. **Male patients with massive weight loss**
     - **Upper Body Lift excisional procedure with free nipple transfer +/− treatment in the area of the armpits (FaceTite™, followed by vibration assisted liposuction, followed by Morpheus8 Body™) +/− treatment in the area of the arms (due to the etiological noxa, this type of patients are most often subject to excisional procedures in the area).**

  B. **Female patients**
     - **With massive weight loss: Inverted-T mastopexy in combination with L-Brachioplasty +/− Morpheus8™ in the area of the neckline. Again according to the author, treatment of the armpits area with radiofrequency does not find a one stage justified application.**
     - **Without massive weight loss: Inverted-T mastopexy in combination with radiofrequency procedures by neighbourhood—the possible combinations are described in Section Mastopexy.**

  C. **Patients with adipose tissue accumulation in the chest area and patients with gynecomastia**
     - **in isolated adipose tissue accumulation: VASERlipo® ultrasound treatment of the area + vibration assisted liposuction for definition +/− Morpheus8 Body™—(the parameters are 7–5–3 mm Burst Mode depth with 30 kJ, at 3 stacks. The procedure is performed 45, and possibly 90 days postop)**
     - **in patients with gynecomastia Grade I–IIa, IIb according to Rohrich: VASERlipo® ultrasound treatment of tissues + vibration-assisted liposuction for definition + extirpation of the gland without skin deepidermization + Morpheus 8 Body™ (the parameters are 7–5–3 mm Burst Mode depth with 30 kJ, at 3 stacks. The procedure is performed 45, and possibly 90 days postop)**
     - **in patients with gynecomastia Grade III according to Simon: the author recommends vibration-assisted liposuction + extirpation of the gland with skin deepidermization. If definition is desired, the author recommends that it be carried out at a second stage. One-time treatment of**

the area with BodyTite™ is not recommended, due to the ablative effect of the procedure.

B. **Secondary procedures:**
   - **Radiofrequency procedures**:
     - **BodyTite™, FaceTite™, AccuTite™** BodyTite™, FaceTite™, AccuTite™ for contour irregularities and/or additionally tightening of the skin. The goal is 70 °C internal probe for destruction of subcutaneous fat with sublethal damage to the connective tissue and 40 °C external probe for additional tightening of the skin. Usually deposit 8–10 kJ of energy per 10 cm^2 are required for optimal results. BodyTite can be an option for additional lifting in the area—wait for 1 year to properly assess the results from the surgical lifting.
     - **Morpheus8 Body™ and Morpheus8™**

   The parameters used, the handpieces preferred and the areas treated are analogous to those described for the intraoperative application of the same.
     - **Ultrasound procedures**

   In patients without skin excision—an ultrasound massage with parameters 1.5 W/cm^2, frequency 3 MHz and duration of treatment of the respective area of 5 min, for a period of 10 days, starting from the second postoperative day, is recommended in each area with previous liposuction. The lipotransfer area (if any) is left untouched. The process accelerates the drainage of oedema and improves venous outflow, thereby accelerating the recovery period and improving the final results.

References

1. Aly AS. Body contouring after massive weight loss. St Louis: Quality Medical Publishing; 2006. p. 59–83.
2. Simon BE, Hoffman S, Kahn S. Classification and surgical correction of gynecomastia. Plast Reconstr Surg. 1973;51:48–52.
3. Rohrich RJ, Ha RY, Kenkel JM, Adams WP Jr. Classification and management of gynecomastia: defining the role of ultrasound-assisted liposuction. Plast Reconstr Surg. 2003;111:909–23.
4. Lockwood TE. Superficial fascial system (SFS) of the trunk and extremities: a new concept. Plast Reconstr Surg. 1991;87(6):1009–18.
5. Ribeiro L. A new technique for reduction mammaplasty. Plast Reconstr Surg. 1975;55:330.
6. Hurwitz DJ. Comprehensive body contouring. Theory and practice. Berlin: Springer; 2016. p. 170–4.
7. Rubin P, Jellew ML, Richter DF, Uebel CO. Body contouring and liposuction. Philadelphia: Saunders Elsevier; 2013. p. 19–24.
8. Mulholland RS. The BodyTite book. 2nd ed. London: IntechOpen; 2021. p. 227–39.
9. Mulholland RS. Radiofrequency energy for non-invasive and minimally invasive skin tightening. Clin Plast Surg. 2011;38:437–48.
10. Theodorou SJ, Del Vecchio D, Chia CT. Soft tissue contraction in body contouring with radiofrequency-assisted liposuction: a treatment gap solution. Aesthet Surg J. 2018;38:S74–83.
11. Levy AS, Grant RT, Rothaus KO. Radiofrequency physics for minimally invasive aesthetic surgery. Clin Plast Surg. 2016;43:551–6.
12. Hoyos AE, Prendergast PM. High definition body sculpting. Berlin: Springer; 2014. p. 147–55.

Brachioplasty and Minimally Invasive Radiofrequency Procedures

Introduction

Different procedures of brachioplasty are used as follows

- in patients after massive weight loss
- in obese patients, the area can be subjected to liposuction with/without radiofrequency treatment with/without ultrasound definition, which can be combined with or followed by excision of the cutaneous–subcutaneous excess
- in patients after massive weight loss, deformities in this area most often continue with a present soft tissue excess with a predominant skin component on the lateral surface of the chest
- patients with lipodystrophy
- reduced skin elasticity and predominant skin excess as a result of natural ageing processes
- genetic predisposition

Historically, a number of eminent specialists in the field of plastic surgery can be listed

- Correa-Iturraspe et Fernandez—first aesthetic brachioplasty in 1954 [1]
- Pitanguy—in 1974 he was the first to regard the inner surface of the arm and the axilla as a common aesthetic unit; he was the first to describe a wavy line that extends along the inner surface of the biceps to the posterior axillary line and the inframammary fold with subcutaneous dissection in a posterior direction to form a posterior flap that is advanced forward—tension-free closure and satisfactory scar [2]
- Baroudi—tension-free closure with an incision of 2 cm above sulcus bicipitalis, the excision being elliptical [3]
- Lockwood—in 1995 he emphasized the importance of the superficial fascial system (SFS). Lockwood believed that the significant laxity of SFS resulted in predominant posterior positioning of the soft-tissue excess. SFS sutures—better contour effect and less tension during closure, better wound healing and better scar [4].

Anatomically, preservation of the venous vascular network is a key point in the prevention of undesirable excessive postoperative oedema of tissues in the area. Knowing the sensory innervation and preserving the relevant nerve branches is a key factor in maintaining normal sensation in the armpit and forearm area. It is essential to know the topographic-anatomical course of v. cephalica; v. basilica and v. thoracoepigastrica; n. intercostobrachialis; n. cutaneus antebrachia medialis; nn. cutanei brachii mediales; n. ulnaris et radialis. Identification of SFS (superficial fascial system) and its suspension during the closure of the postoperative defect is a key factor in the prevention of dilatation of the postoperative scar.

Supplementary InformationThe online version contains supplementary material available at https://doi.org/10.1007/978-3-031-33350-7_13. The videos can be accessed individually by clicking the DOI link in the accompanying figure caption or by scanning this link with the SN More Media App.

E. Sharkov, *Body Contouring Surgery*, https://doi.org/10.1007/978-3-031-33350-7_13

To make an accurate preoperative evaluation and refine the appropriate surgical approach, the **El-Khatib** classification [5] can be used:

- **Phase 1**—minimal amount of subcutaneous fat excess without ptosis—subject to circumferential liposuction
- **Phase 2—2a**—moderate amount of subcutaneous fat with I grade ptosis/up to 5 cm/—subject to staged liposuction
- **2b**—significant amount of fat with II grade ptosis/5–10 cm/—subject to excision with/without liposuction
- **Phase 3**—significant amount of subcutaneous fat with III grade ptosis/over 10 cm/—subject to excision with/without liposuction

Discussion regarding the position of the scar is essential—posterior (invisible to the patient, but visible to anyone else, especially when wearing short-sleeved clothes); medial in the bicipital sulcus (invisible to others and hidden to the patient when the arm is in neutral position—the author's preferred technique).

Techniques

Historically, variations of surgical techniques can be indicated both regarding the position of the scar, its length and the use of Z-plasty in the axilla and regarding the intraoperative technique (antero-posterior or distal-proximal approach in excision of the excess), as well as regarding its combination with minimally invasive procedures.

A. The length of the postoperative scar is predetermined by the volume of present excess
   - **Technique with short horizontal scar**—candidates are patients with excess mainly in the proximal 1/2–1/3 of the upper arm
   - **Technique with short horizontal scar in combination with vertical axillary excision**—N.B. the distal portion of the vertical excision should be shorter than the proximal one; thus, when closing the incision, the posterior edge of the axilla is shortened and this ensures adequate correction of the loose axillary skin
   - **Technique with isolated vertical excision in the axilla**—in rare cases of excess mainly in the proximal third of the upper arm and axilla. The technique is not preferred by the author due to the insufficiently satisfactory result in terms of present excess and its optimal removal
   - **Technique with long horizontal scar**—when the excess is along the entire upper arm, the excision will extend from the elbow to the axilla
   - **Technique with long horizontal scar in combination with vertical axillary excision**—when the excess is along the entire upper arm and axilla
   - **L-brachioplasty**—when the excess is along the entire upper arm, axilla and lateral surface of the chest
   - **Fish incision brachioplasty**—an option in bat-wing—a significant cutaneous–subcutaneous excess in the area between the olecranon and the axilla. The excision 'tail' is at the level of the axillary fold, along the line connecting the lateral edge of m. pectoralis major with the front edge of m. latissimus dorsi, and this line crosses the axilla and is denoted by 'T'. Angles of 45° are made from the posterior and anterior points, and a line that is 2/3 of the T is drawn anteriorly and a line that is 1/3 of the T is drawn posteriorly.

B. The position of the postoperative scar is determined after accurately informing the patient about the advantages and disadvantages of the posterior and medial positions of the cicatrix
   - **Posteriorly positioned scar**—the scar is invisible to the patient, but visible to everyone else when viewed posteriorly and when wearing short-sleeved clothes (Figs. 1 and 2).

     Preoperative marking—with arms brought to the shoulder at 90°, supination in the forearm and 90° elbow flexion: first, a mid-lateral line is drawn—a line in the

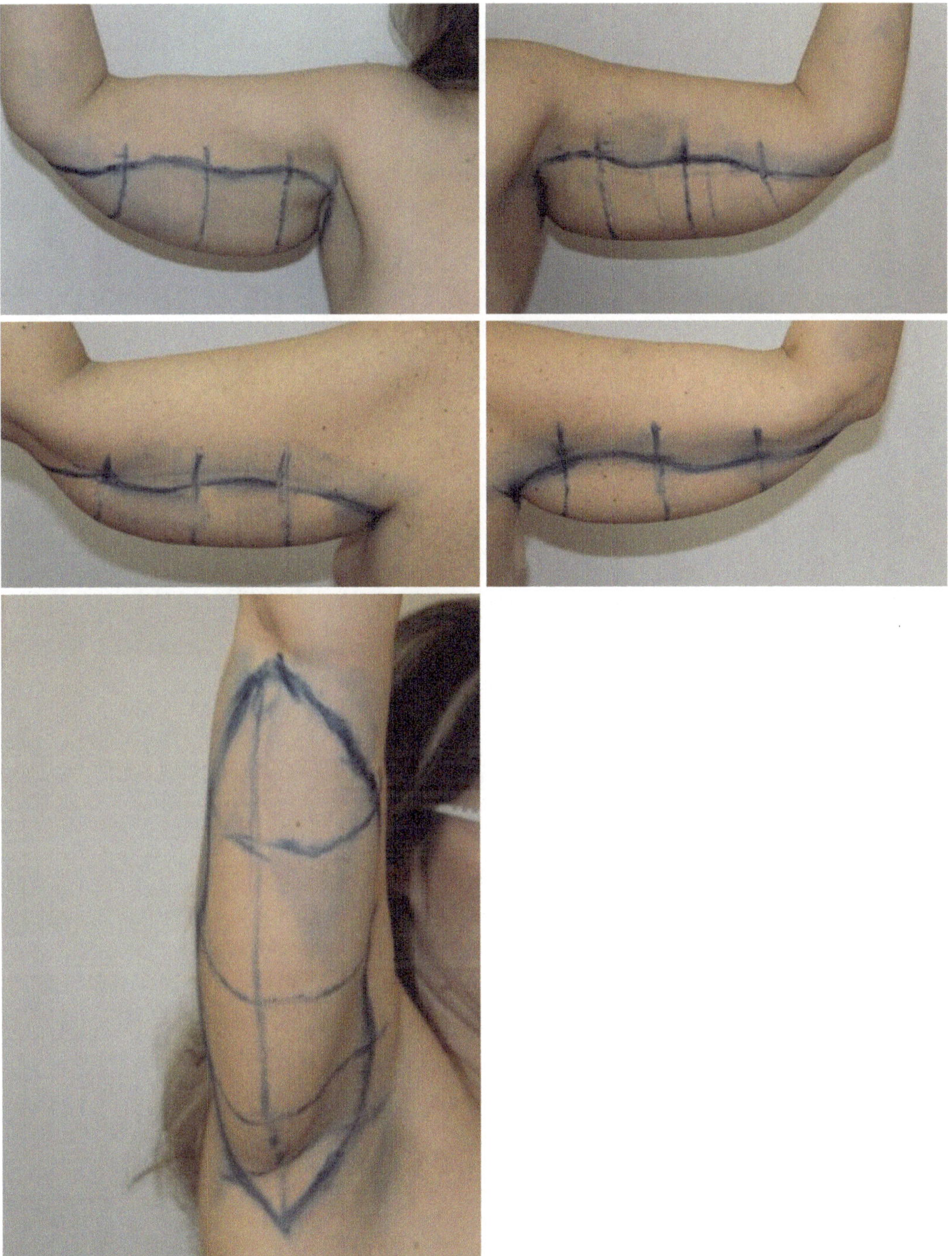

Fig. 1 Preoperative marking in posterior positioning of the scar

middle of the lateral surface of the armpit that connects the deltoid tubercle with the lateral tubercle of the elbow; second, the longitudinal axis of the ellipse is marked, which will be final position of the scar—it should go postero-medially and more pre-

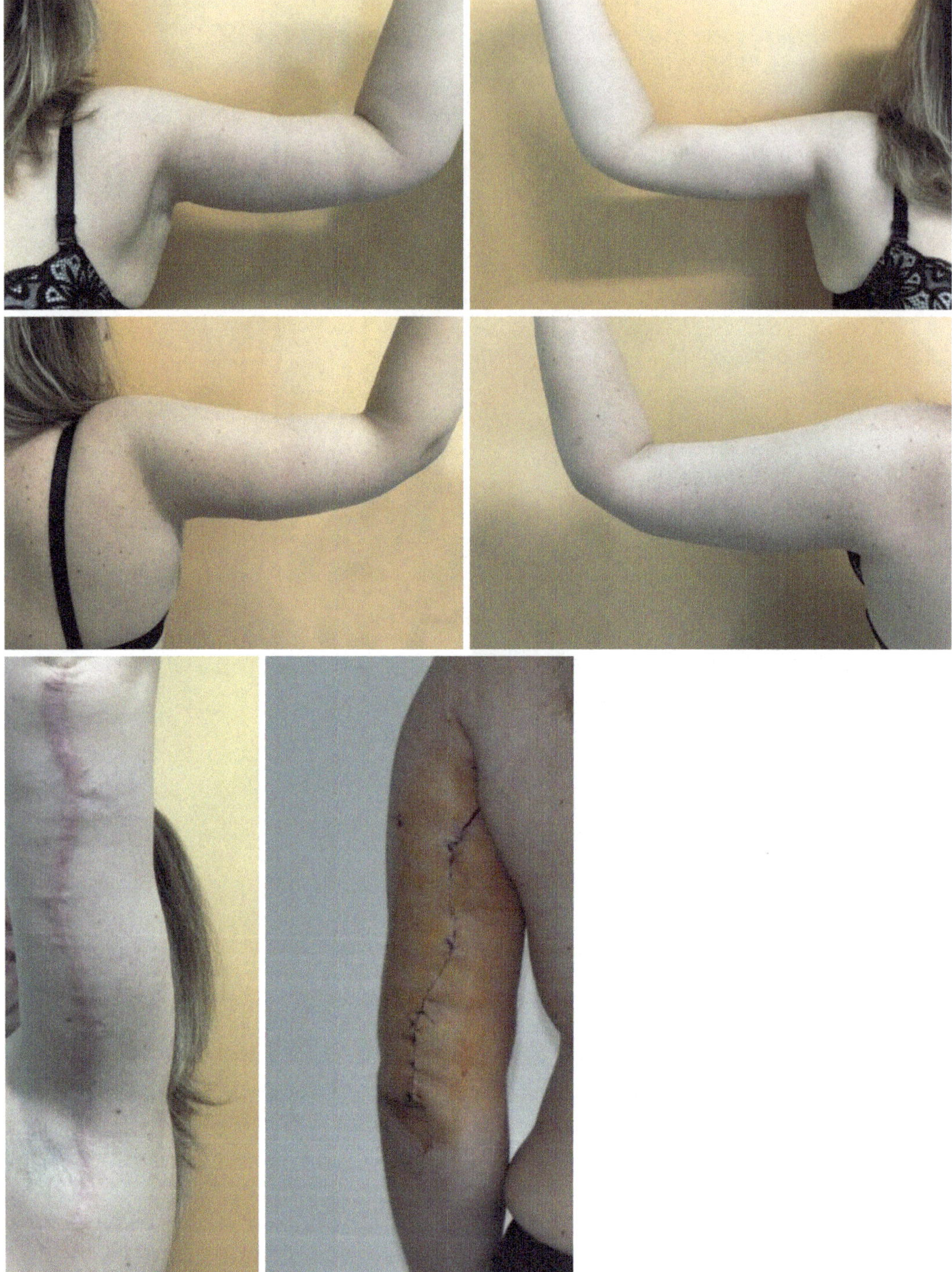

Fig. 2 18 months after brachioplasty with a posteriorly positioned scar and early postoperative outcome, visualizing the future position of the scar—invisible to the patient, but visible to everyone else

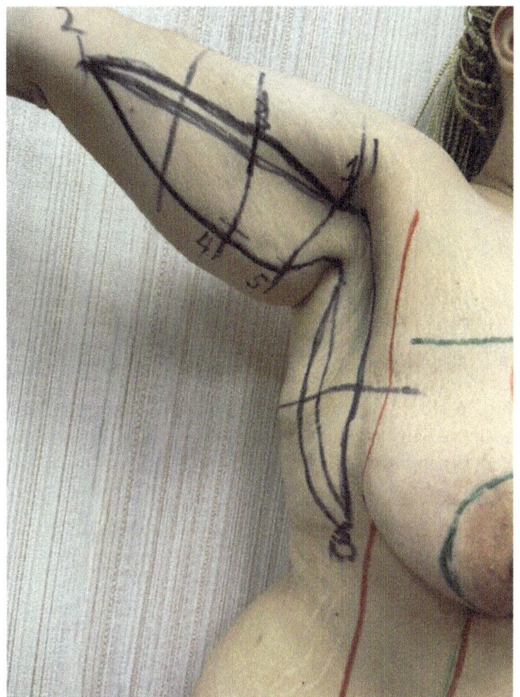

Fig. 3 Preoperative marking in medial positioning of the scar. In the specified case, an L-type Brachioplasty [8, 9] was performed, as the 'arm' on the lateral surface was marked in such a way that the anterior incision is 1.5 cm posterior to the lateral edge of pectoralis major sulcus, which makes this part of scar also 'invisible' when viewed in neutral arm position

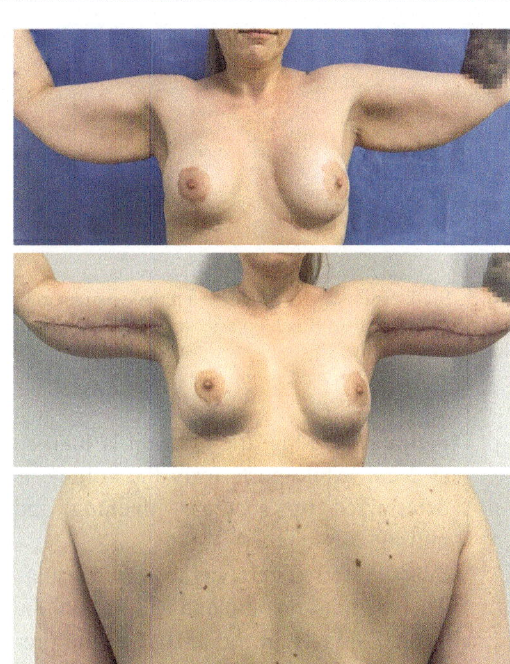

Fig. 4 Third postoperative month with medially positioned scar, 'invisible' posteriorly and in neutral position of the arm. Brachioplasty with vibrational type of liposuction superficially in the area to be excised. Liposuction has been done to provide wider excision and tension free closure. Vibration-assisted liposuction superficially in the area to be excised using a 4 mm long curved Mercedes type cannula. First stage in the performance of excisional brachioplasty in combination with vibration-assisted liposuction and radiofrequency techniques in the area of the upper arm and neighbouring areas—armpits and elbows (▶ https://doi.org/10.1007/000-b0q)

cisely posteriorly to the sulcus bicipitalis and more precisely between the biceps and triceps. This longitudinal axis is determined as follows: first, the circumference of the armpit is measured at its widest part at 90° abduction at the shoulder, then a point is plotted at a distance of 2/3 of the circumference anterior from the mid-lateral line and the line will go along this point—it should be 3–4 cm posterior from the bicipital sulcus [6].

- **Medially positioned scar (author's preferred technique)**—the scar remains hidden in the area between the arm and the lateral surface of the chest in neutral position of the upper limb. Preoperative marking (Figs. 3 and 4)—with arms brought to the shoulder at 90°, supination in the forearm and 90° elbow flexion: first, the bicipital sulcus is marked, then the deltopectoral sulcus in its cranial part is marked—point 1 [7]. Pulling the posterior flap at point 5 with a projection antero-medially and fixation to point 1 of the anterior flap results in neutralization of the need to use Z-plasty in the axilla. Superiorly from the

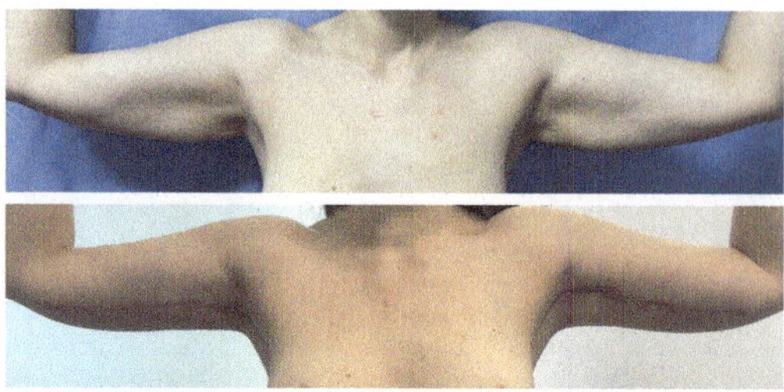

Fig. 5 Sixth postoperative month in a female patient after massive weight loss. Brachioplasty with medially positioned postoperative scar

bicipital marking, the incision is marked at 2 cm, while posteriorly the volume is determined by accurate pinching and pulling of tissues.

C. Author's preferred intraoperative technique

The author recommends a technique **without Z-plasty** in the axilla, as the prevention of contracture in the area is achieved by the above-described pulling and fixating of the posterior flap antero-medially in the area of the deltopectoral sulcus. The author uses **double ellipse technique**—an ellipse is drawn, the excision along which would probably result in the impossibility of closing the defect; therefore, a second ellipse is drawn inside the first one (using a pinch test, the degree of the excision is determined as X. The distance X would not allow us to adequately close the defect, due to which the level of the excision is reduced by ½ X both anteriorly and posteriorly). Intraoperatively, the approach is a **segmental-resection-closure** technique—the excision starts from the elbow to the axilla and when a marker is reached, a temporary stapler is placed [6]. The author believes that the use of the 'double-marked ellipse' technique enables an approach from the elbow to the axilla without the risk of probable inability to close the defect due to excessively wide excision. **Undermining the posterior flap** and advancing it anteriorly. After removal of the excess, deep fascial sutures are used and the surgical wound is closed in layers (Figs. 5, 6 and 7).

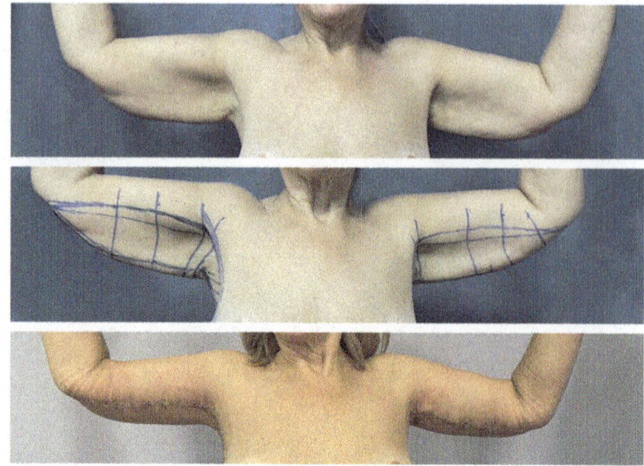

Fig. 6 Early postoperative results in L-brachioplasty with medially positioned postoperative scar and without Z-plasty in the axilla

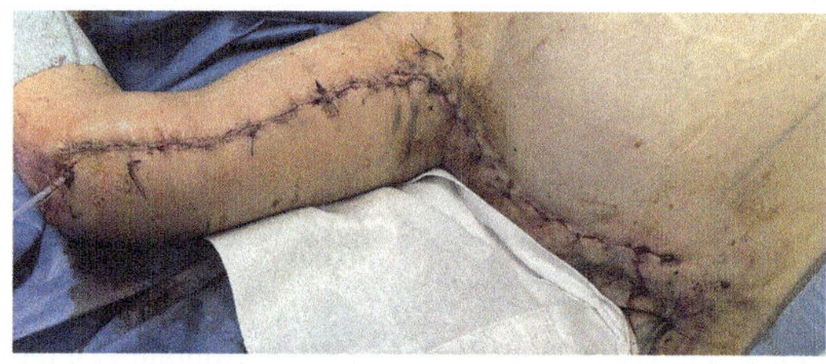

Fig. 7 Intraoperative view—L-brachioplasty with medially positioned scar, anteriorly advanced posterior flap, without the need for Z-plasty in the axilla, vertical scar on the lateral surface of the chest, positioned posterior to the lateral edge of the pectoralis major muscle

D. Application of non-invasive and minimally invasive techniques in brachioplasty procedures

(a) Intraoperatively

- **Radiofrequency procedures:**
  - **BodyTite™:** Use radiofrequency therapy +/− in combination with lipoaspiration of the upper arms and in neighbouring areas to achieve a single-stage overall contouring of the upper limb [10]. The procedure ablates subcutaneous fat and tightens the skin. The parameters are as follow: 20 W cannula/70 int cut off/40 ext. cut off for 8–10 kJ energy per 10 cm^2 and a depth of 2 or 3 cm (Fig. 8). The techniques are respectively 'stamping'

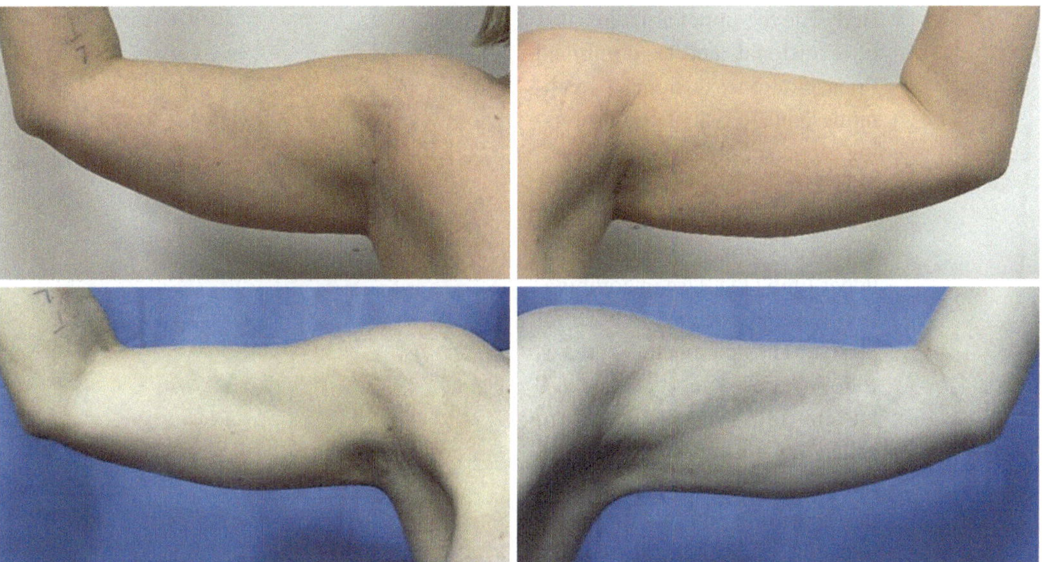

Fig. 8 Before and 6 months after BodyTite™ with vibration-based liposuction—20 W cannula/70 int cut off/40 ext. cut off/10 kJ energy per side at 2 cm depth. The working techniques are 'lining' (tightening the skin by reaching 40 °C ext. cut off) and 'stamping' (melting the fat cells by reaching 70 °C int cut off). The procedure ended with lipoaspiration of liquefied subcutaneous fat using a 4 mm long curved cannula −120 mL lipoaspirate per side

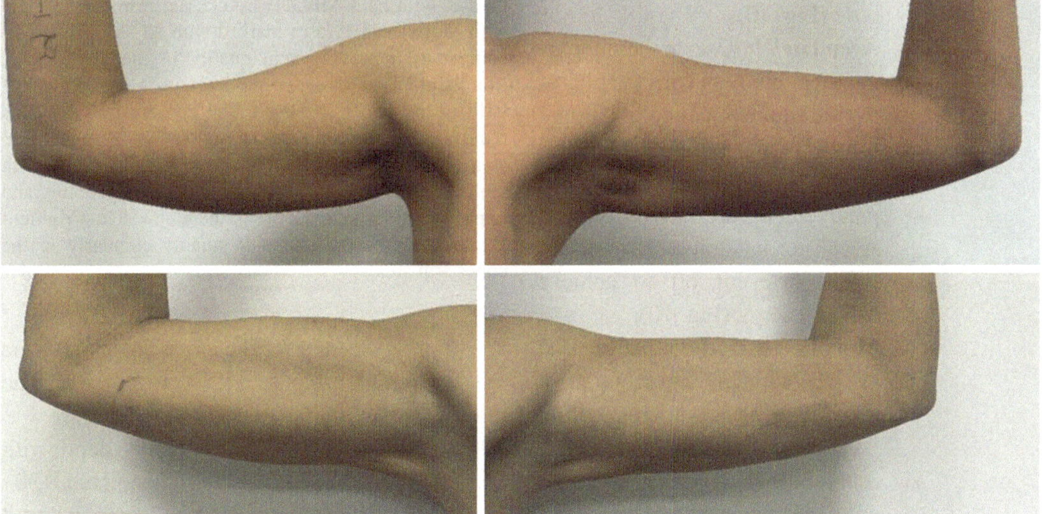

Fig. 9 Before and 6 months after BodyTite ™—20 W cannula with one sensor/40 power/40 ext. cut/10 kJ energy per side, working at a depth of 2 cm. The working technique is 'lining' (tightening the skin by reaching 40 °C ext. cut off)

(melting the fat cells by reaching 70 °C int cut off) and 'lining' (tightening the skin by reaching 40 °C ext. cut off). To tighten the skin, the parameters are as follows: 20 W cannula with one sensor/40 power/40 ext. cut off to achieve 8–10 kJ energy per 10 cm^2 of treated area, working at a depth of 2 cm (Fig. 9). Do not

BodyTite the upper arms in cases of excisional and/or combined lipoaspiration-excisional techniques, due to risk of compromising blood supply.

- **FaceTite™:** Use in neighbouring area (armpits) for overall improved appearance of the upper limb [11]. Use in combination with all options of brachioplasty. The parameters are as follows: FaceTite handpiece/70 int cut off/40 ext. cut off to achieve 6–8 kJ energy. The techniques are respectively 'stamping' (melting the fat cells by reaching 70 °C int cut off) and lining (tightening the skin by reaching 40 °C ext. cut off), as tightening the skin precedes the ablative effect on subcutaneous adipose. The procedure ends with lipoaspiration of liquefied adipose (Fig. 10).
- **AccuTite™:** Use in neighbouring area (elbows) with the aim of overall improvement of the upper limb. Use in combination with all options of brachioplasty. The parameters are as follows: AccuTite handpiece/70 int cut off/40 ext. cut off to achieve 6–8 kJ energy (Fig. 10);
- **Morpheus8 Body™:** At the end of the surgical intervention a radiofrequency microneedling improves elasticity of the surrounding and covering skin and only of the surrounding skin away of the incision side (in cases of surgical excision). The procedure could be applied not only for the arms, but also for the armpits [12] (Fig. 10). The parameters are as follows:
- 7–5–3 mm burst mode depth with 30 kJ, 3 stacks per place, (30–40% overlapping when without excision of skin and no overlapping when close to the excision side—stay at least 2.0 cm away.

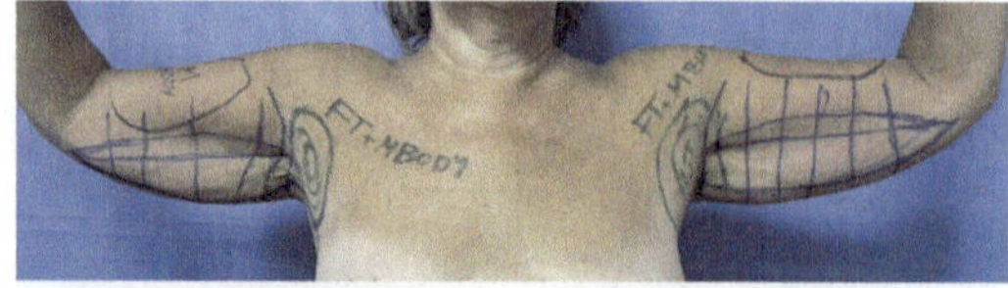

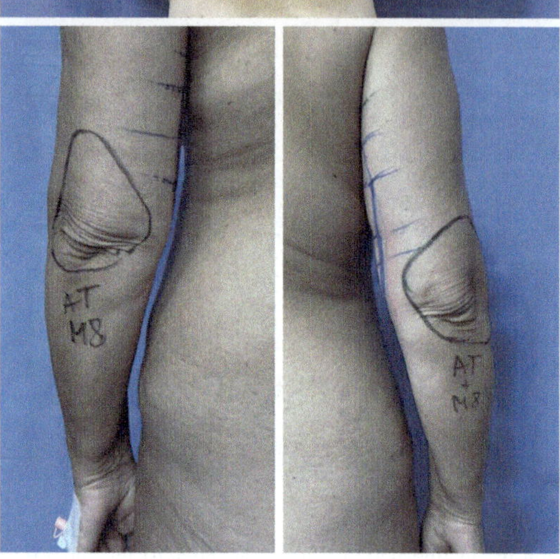

Fig. 10 Preoperative marking in a patient with brachioplasty in combination with vibration-assisted liposuction in the upper arm area; FaceTite™ with Vibration-Assisted Liposuction and Morpheus8 Body™ in the armpitS (area marked with FT + MBODY); AccuTite™ in combination with Morpheus8™ (area marked with AT+M8) for tightening and improving skin quality in the elbow area; Morpheus8 Body™ (area marked with MBODY) circularly in the upper arm area. The combination provides removal of excess skin and fat deposits in the upper arm area + tightening and improvement of skin quality with removal of excess fat in the armpit area + tightening and improvement of skin quality in the elbow area + tightening and improvement of skin quality circularly in the upper arm area

The procedure can be repeated on the 45th postoperative day, after which a third one can be performed for optimal effect, again in 45 days

- **Morpheus8™:** At the end of the surgical intervention radiofrequency microneedling could be applied to improve skin elasticity in the area of the elbows (Fig. 10). The parameters are as follows: 3 mm depth with 30–35 kJ, 3 stacks per place, 30–40% overlapping, Fixed Mode, 1 PPS + 2 mm depth with 15–20 kJ, 2 stacks per place, 20–30% overlapping, Cycle mode. The procedure can be repeated on the 45th postoperative day, after which a third one can be performed for optimal effect, again in 45 days.

- **Vibration-assisted liposuction**
  - Vibration liposuction is used to remove fat excess both in the area of the arms and in the area of the armpits. The following cannulas are used: Mercedes type N3 and 4, long and short curved and bent types [13]. Liposuction in combination with an excisional technique should be performed precisely and primarily in the area to be excised, with prevention of the subcutaneous fat component at the periphery of the marked excisional area (Fig. 10).
- **Radiofrequency procedures in combination with vibration-assisted liposuction and surgical excision of the skin excess—the author's approach.**

A. Combination of radiofrequency technique with vibration-assisted liposuction

Normal weight patients, but with fat deposits of the upper arm and without skin excess or with minimal skin excess and with potential for good skin contraction (Fig. 8).

1. Infiltration of Klein solution followed by a BodyTite™ procedure with the parameters described above
2. BodyTite™ is followed by vibration-assisted liposuction technique with the parameters described above
3. The procedure can be combined and completed with Morpheus8 Body™ in Burst Mode and with the parameters described above
4. Finally, neighbouring areas can also be treated: armpits with FaceTite and Morpheus8 Body™ and elbows with AccuTite™ and Morpheus8™, respectively

The above-described steps from 1 to 4 are performed in the indicated sequence.

B. Excisional technique in combination with vibration-assisted liposuction and radiofrequency treatment both in the area of the upper arm and neighbouring areas (Figs. 10, 11, 12, 13 and 14; Videos 1, 2, 3, 4 and 5)

1. Infiltration of Klein solution followed by superficial vibration-assisted liposuction in the area marked as the future excision
2. Excision of the cutaneous–subcutaneous excess of the type of segmental-closure skin excision from distal to caudal. The excision is made along the preoperatively marked internal ellipse. Undermining the posterior flap and advancing it anteriorly with subsequent fixation of Lockwood's fascia and layered closure of the surgical wound
3. FaceTite™ with vibration-assisted liposuction, followed by Morpheus8 Body™ in the area of the armpits, with the parameters described above
4. AccuTite™ followed by Morpheus8™ in the elbow area, with the parameters described above
5. Morpheus8 Body™ in the area of the upper arm circularly, but at a distance of at least 1.5–2 cm from the area of the postoperative scar. Burst mode is used according to the approach described above in terms of parameters.

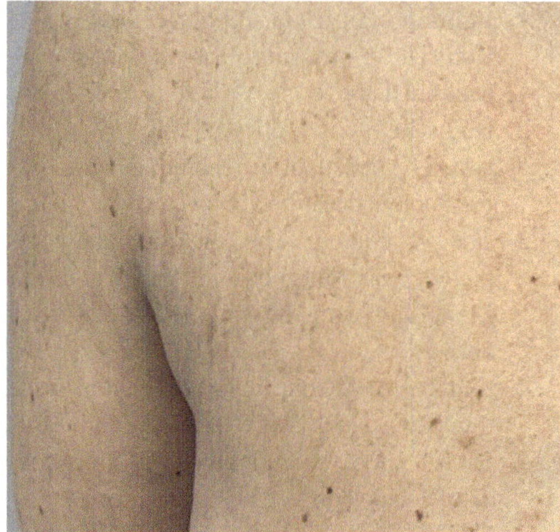

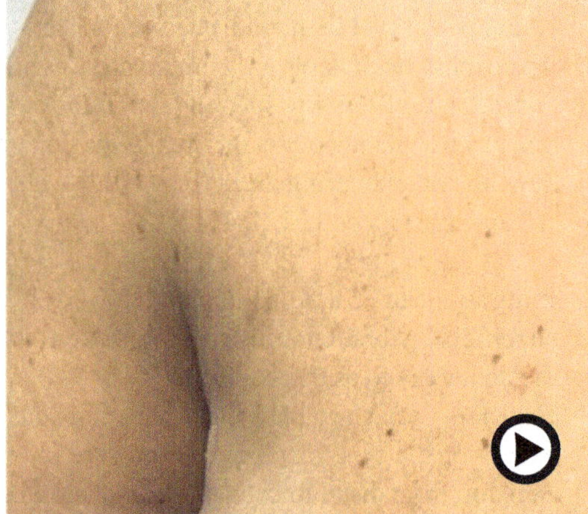

Fig. 11 6 months after brachioplasty in combination with vibration-assisted liposuction in the upper arms and FaceTite ™ with vibration-assisted liposuction and Morpheus8 Body™ in the armpit area. FaceTite™ followed by vibration-assisted liposuction using a short-angled Mercedes type cannula and Morpheus8 Body™. Third stage in the performance of excisional brachioplasty in combination with vibration-assisted liposuction and radiofrequency techniques in the upper arms and neighbouringareas—armpits(▶https://doi.org/10.1007/000-b0p)

The above-described steps from 1 to 5 are performed in the indicated sequence.

(b) Secondary procedures
  - **Radiofrequency procedures:**
- **BodyTite™, FaceTite™, AccuTite™** are used to correct contour irregularities and/ or additionally tighten the skin.
  - **Radiofrequency procedures:**
    - **BodyTite™, FaceTite™, AccuTite™** for contour irregularities and/or additional tightening of the skin. The goal is to reach the following parameters: 70 °C for destruction of subcutaneous fat deposits and 40 °C for additional tightening of the skin, and in each case the goal is to achieve 8–10 kJ of energy per 10 cm^2 of treated area. It is recommended after the 6th post operative for optimal assessment of the contour deformity.
    - **Morpheus8 Body™ and Morpheus8™:** Can be repeated on the 45th postoperative day using identical parameters to those used intraoperatively.
  - **Ultrasound procedures.**
    - An ultrasound massage, in patients without excision of the skin, with parameters 1.5 W/ cm^2, frequency 3 MHz and duration of treatment of the respective area of 5 min, for a period of 10 days, starting from the second postoperative day, is recommended in each area with previous liposuction. The process accelerates the drainage of oedema and improves venous outflow, thereby accelerating the recovery period and improving the final results.

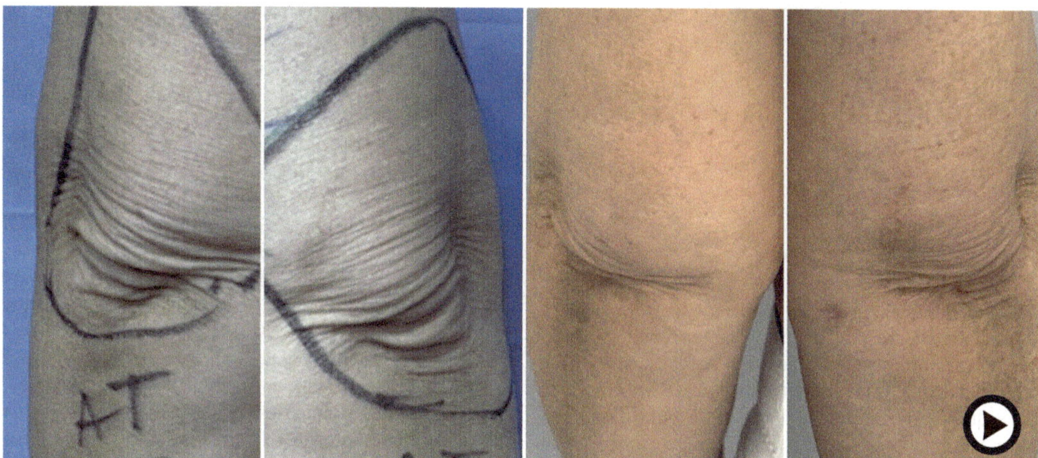

Fig. 12 6 months after Brachioplasty in combination with Vibration-Assisted Liposuction in the upper arms area; AccuTite™ in combination with Morpheus8™ (area marked with AT+M8) for tightening and improving skin quality in the elbow area. AccuTite™ followed by Morpheus8™ to improve skin elasticity and quality in the elbow area. Fourth stage in the performance of Excisional Brachioplasty in combination with Vibration-Assisted Liposuction and Radiofrequency techniques in the area of the upper arms and neighbouring areas—elbows (▶ https://doi.org/10.1007/000-b0n)

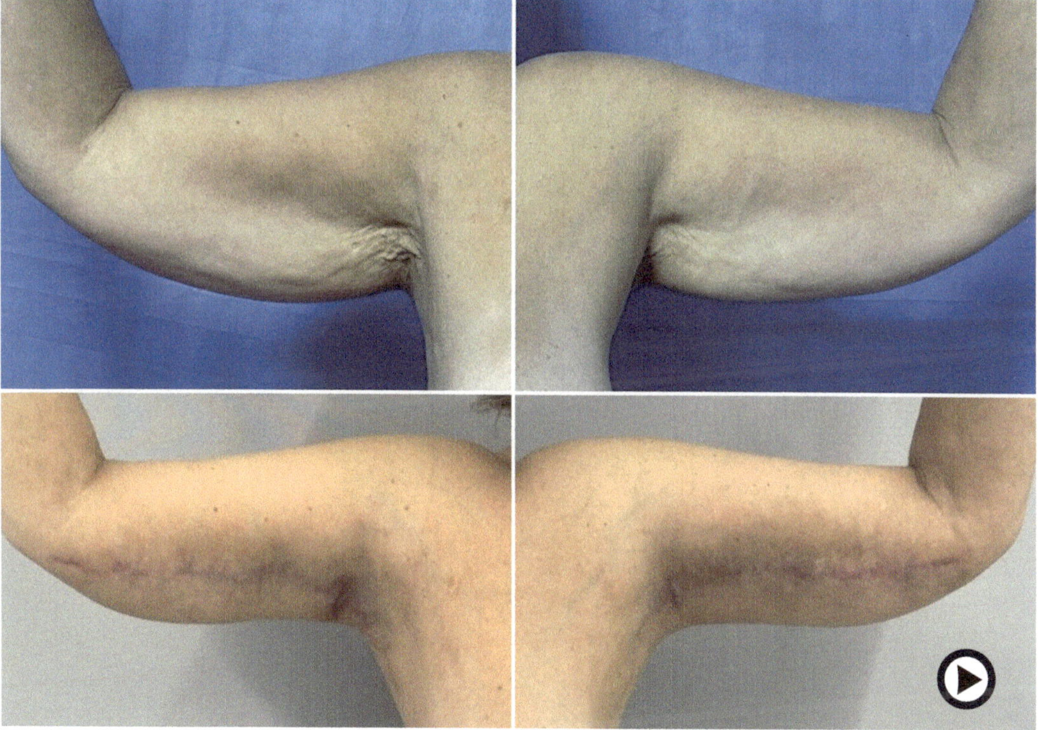

Fig. 13 6 months after Brachioplasty in combination with Vibration-Assisted Liposuction in the upper arms area; AccuTite™ in combination with Morpheus8™ for tightening and improving of skin quality in the elbow area; FaceTite™ with vibration type of liposuction and Morheus 8 Body ™ in the armpits; Morpheus 8 Body ™ in the upper arm for overall improvement in the skin elasticity. Morpheus8 Body™ on Burst Mode circularly in the area of the upper arms for the purpose of achieving an overall improvement of the skin quality in the area. Fifth, last, stage in the performance of Excisional Brachioplasty in combination with Vibration-Assisted Liposuction and Radiofrequency techniques in the area of the upper arms and neighbouring areas—armpits and elbows (▶ https://doi.org/10.1007/000-b0r)

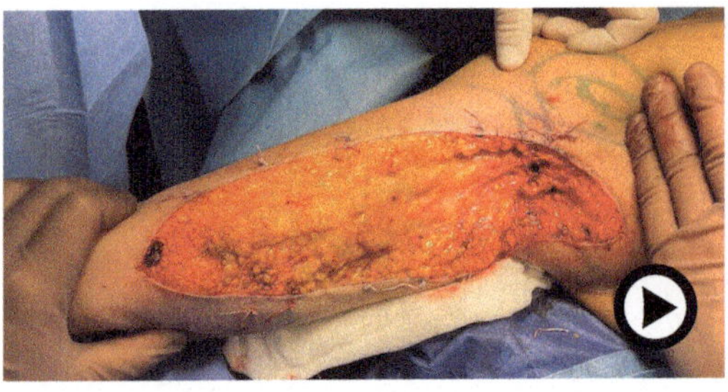

Fig. 14 Intraoperative view after the performance of Stage 1 and Stage 2 brachioplasty combined with liposuction and radiofrequency techniques. After closure of the surgical defect, it is proceeded to the next stages described as a sequence above. Brachioplasty of the type of segmental resection closure. Second stage in the performance of excisional brachioplasty in combination with vibration-assisted liposuction and radiofrequency techniques in the area of the upper arm and neighbouring areas—armpits and elbows (▶ https://doi.org/10.1007/000-b0s)

References

1. Correa-Iturraspe M, Fernandez JC. Dermolipectomia braquial. Prensa Med Argent. 1954;41:2432.
2. Pitanguy I. Correction of lipodystrophy of the lateral thoracic aspect and inner side of the arm and elbow. Clin Plast Surg. 1975;2:477–83.
3. Baroudi R. Body sculpturing. Clin Plast Surg. 1984;11(3):419–43.
4. Lockwood TE. Superficial fascial system (SFS) of the trunk and extremities: a new concept. Plast Reconstr Surg. 1991;87(6):1009–18.
5. El Khatib HA. Classification of brachial ptosis; strategy for treatment. Plast Reconstr Surg. 2007;119:1337–42.
6. Al Aly S. Body contouring after massive weight loss. Missouri: St. Louis; 2006. p. 312–7.
7. Rubin P, Jellew ML, Richter DF, Uebel CO. Body contouring and liposuction. Philadelphia: Saunders Elsevier; 2013. p. 19–24.
8. Hurwitz DJ. Comprehensive body contouring. Theory and practice. Berlin: Springer; 2016. p. 170–4.
9. Hurwitz DJ, Holland SW, The L. Brachioplasty: an innovative approach to correct excess tissue of the upper arm, axilla and lateral chest. Plast Reconstr Surg. 2006;117:403–11.
10. Mulholland RS. The BodyTite book. 2nd ed. London: IntechOpen; 2021. p. 227–39.
11. Mulholland RS. Radiofrequency energy for non-invasive and minimally invasive skin tightening. Clin Plast Surg. 2011;38:437–48.
12. Levy AS, Grant RT, Rothaus KO. Radiofrequency physics for minimally invasive aesthetic surgery. Clin Plast Surg. 2016;43:551–6.
13. Hoyos AE, Prendergast PM. High definition body sculpting. Berlin: Springer; 2014. p. 129–36.

Lateral Tension Upper Body Lift Procedures: How to Combine with Minimal and Non-invasive Techniques to Alter the Results

Introduction

It is important to discuss with the patient both the position and the length and possible hypertrophic evolution of the postoperative scar. The excision volume is determined by means of 'pinch-test', marking a wavy ellipse on the lateral surface of the chest extending from the axilla to below the level of the iliac crest. The wavy shape aims to prevent the possible hypertrophic nature of the postoperative scar. A key factor is determination of the future position of the nipple-areola complex (NAC), which is displaced laterally during the closure of the surgical defect (Figs. 1 and 2).

Technique

Lateral Tension Upper Body Lift—How to Combine with Non-invasive Techniques

In the Postoperative Period to Alter the Results

The author examines and describes the following technique (Fig. 3):

In lateral position it is proceeded to a cutaneous–subcutaneous excision following the rule of the segmental-closure resection type [1]. After thorough haemostasis, undermining both posteriorly and anteriorly is performed. Baroudi sutures with 0/0 Vicryl are placed, after which the surgical defect is closed in layers (Fig. 4; Video 1). The author uses Redon drainage, which is brought out at a declivous location. Then the patient is repositioned, and a similar approach is applied to the contralateral side.

In position of lying on one's back, a repositioning of NAC as free nipple transfer [1] (Fig. 5).

Application of Non-invasive and Minimally Invasive Techniques in Lateral Tension Body Lift Procedures

- Given the significant separation of tissues both anteriorly and posteriorly and the possible compromise of the blood supply to the available flap, the author recommends that additional minimally invasive and non-invasive procedures be part of the late postoperative period.
- In cases of intraoperative combination, the author recommends avoiding the flap areas, but with possible treatment of neighbouring areas—such is the area of the armpits—treatment is described in Section Mastopexy and Section Brachioplasty in the book.

Supplementary Information The online version contains supplementary material available at https://doi.org/10.1007/978-3-031-33350-7_14. The videos can be accessed individually by clicking the DOI link in the accompanying figure caption or by scanning this link with the SN More Media App.

E. Sharkov, *Body Contouring Surgery*, https://doi.org/10.1007/978-3-031-33350-7_14

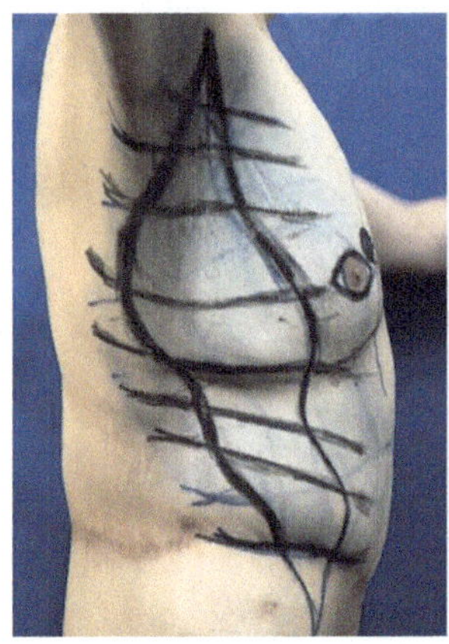
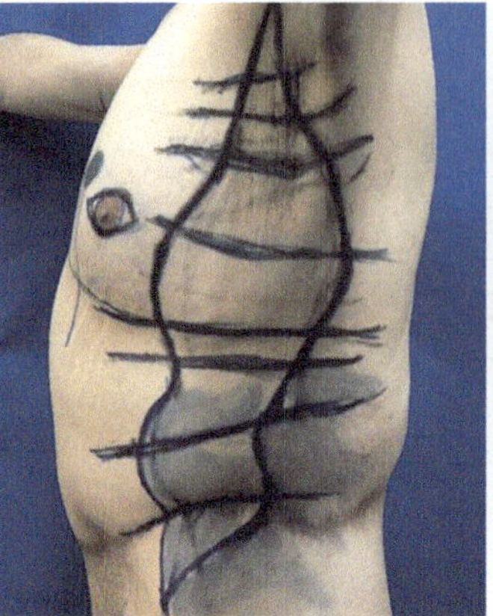
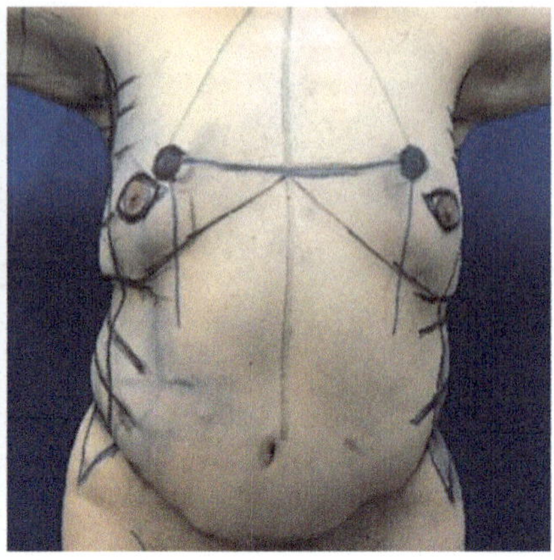

Fig. 1 A patient after massive weight loss and previous belt lipectomy. Preoperative marking of the excision area on the lateral surface of the chest and in the area of the flanks laterally. The marking is in the form of a wavy ellipse, marking the future position of the nipple-areola complex (NAC), which will be subject of free nipple transfer

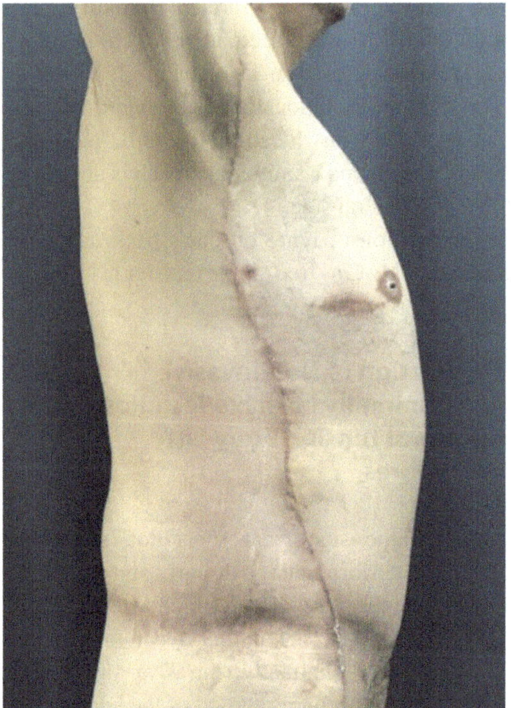

Fig. 2 Third postoperative month and view of the postoperative scar in a lateral tension upper body lift procedure performed in a patient with previous belt lipectomy intervention due to massive weight loss after bariatric intervention

A. Secondary procedures
   - **Radiofrequency procedures:**
     - **BodyTite™, FaceTite™, AccuTite™** are used to correct contour irregularities and/or additionally tighten the skin [2, 3]. In the case of significant defect—BodyTite cannula is used and in the case of smaller or minimal deformity—the FaceTite and AccuTite cannulas are used.
     - The goal is 70 °C internal probe for destruction of subcutaneous fat and 40 °C external probe for additional tightening of the skin. Usually deposit 8–10 kJ of energy per 10 cm^2. Wait 6 months to optimally assess the contour deformity.
     - **EVOLVE X™** provides improvement of the skin tone through collagen stimulation, reduction in the fat deposits and stimulation of the muscle tone. Wait for 6 months, the treatment of the areas would have an exothermic effect on the underlying fat cells from the induced myostimulation, which could

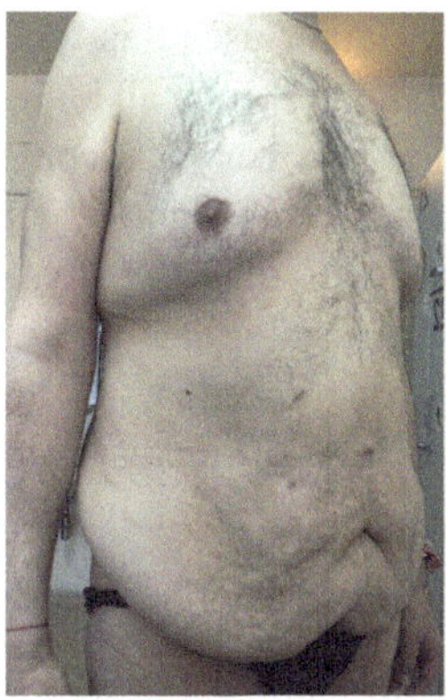
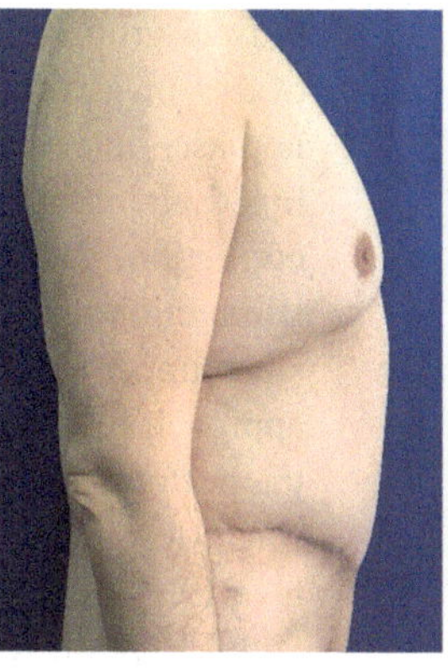
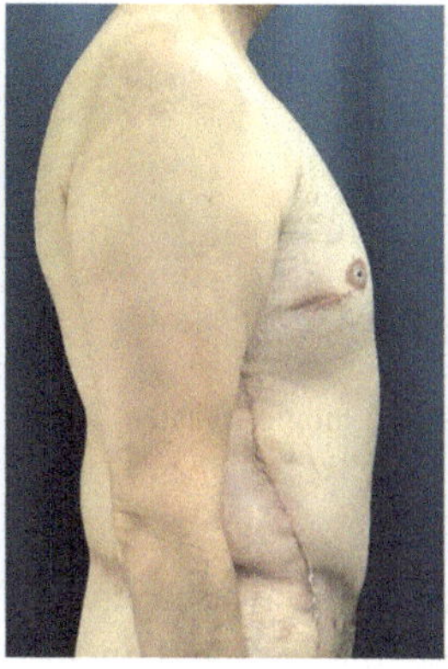
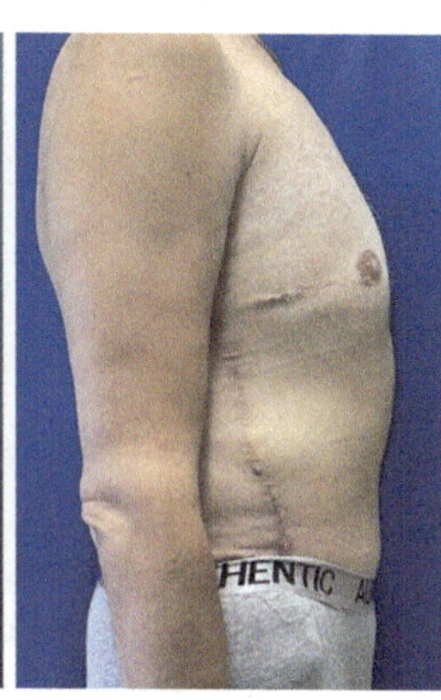

Fig. 3 The following is indicated from left to right: a patient with massive weight loss after bariatric intervention and before belt lipectomy surgical intervention; the second photo shows the result of the patient 1 year after belt lipectomy surgical intervention and before lateral tension upper body lift procedure; the third photo shows the result in the third postoperative month after the lateral tension upper body lift was performed; the 4th photo illustrates the final result in the 6th postoperative month after Lateral Tension Upper Body Lift

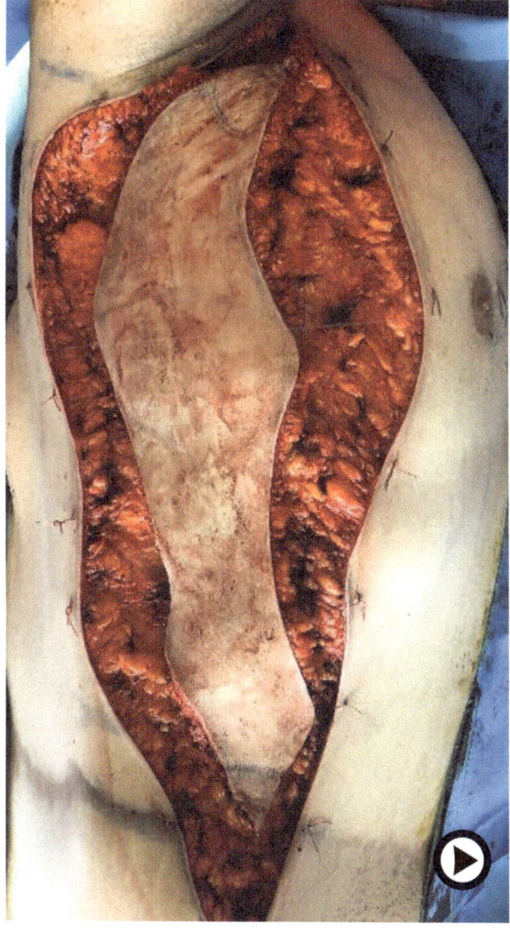

Fig. 4 View of the removed cutaneous–subcutaneous excess during a lateral tension upper body lift procedure. The resulting defect is 20 cm wide and 60 cm long (▶ https://doi.org/10.1007/000-b0t)

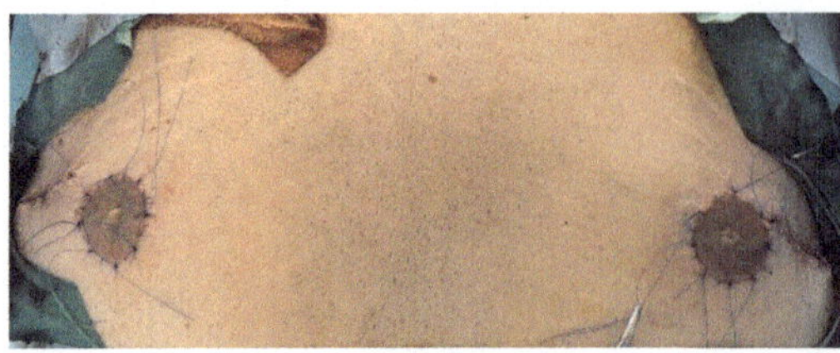

Fig. 5 Repositioned NAC as free nipple transfer—final stage of the procedure

result in prolongation of the tissue swelling and possible seromas in the respective areas.

  - The procedure could involve both the abdominal area and the chest area in male patients, as well as the flanks.
  - **Morpheus8 Body™**—The parameters are 7–5–3 mm burst mode depth with 30 kJ, at 3 stacks. The procedure is performed 45, and possibly 90 days postop. The procedure is used in the area of the abdomen, flanks, breasts and armpits and aims to improve skin elasticity and quality.

- **Electrical muscle stimulation (EMS)—truSculpt® flex**—is aimed at specific muscle groups. The author uses this type of non-invasive technique both in abdominoplasty interventions (in cases of combined abdominoplasty with hernia defect correction, the author avoids using myostimulation procedures) and in lateral tension upper body lift procedures. The approach requires at least 6 months from the performed surgical procedure, for reasons described above identical to the EVOLVE X procedures. When combined with EVOLVE X™, the approach is to finish the radiofrequency cycle of procedures and then proceed to the cycle of myostimulation procedures—2 procedures are performed weekly, and the total number of procedures is 6.

References

1. Thorek M. Possibilities in the reconstruction of the human form. NY Med J Rec. 1922;116:572.
2. Mulholland RS. The BodyTite book. 2nd ed. London: IntechOpen; 2021. p. 227–39.
3. Mulholland RS. Radiofrequency energy for non-invasive and minimally invasive skin tightening. Clin Plast Surg. 2011;38:437–48.

Facelift Procedures in Combination with Minimally Invasive Techniques

Introduction

Facelift procedures are used in

- Patients after the age of 50 due to age changes
- Patients after massive weight loss with the aim of lifting and removing excess soft tissue in the area of the face and neck
- Patients with obesity—the area of the neck and/or lower 1/3 of the face could be subjected to liposuction with/without radiofrequency treatment with/without ultrasound definition
- Patients with obesity and significant ptosis in the area of the neck and lower third of the face—the areas can be subjected to liposuction, which can be combined with excision of the soft tissue excess
- Genetic predisposition

Historically, several eminent specialists with immeasurable contribution in the field of facelift interventions can be listed, among them

- In 1901, in Berlin, Eugen Holländer performed the first procedure aimed at removing excess skin in the lower third of the face—excision of an elliptical skin area just preauricularly. Erich Lexer was the first to introduce at the same time a similar technique, but already with undermining of the cutaneous–subcutaneous flap a few centimetres distal from the site of the skin excision [1]
- In 1968, Tord Skoog was the first to publish a technique with subfacial dissection of the platysma [2]. Later, Hamra and Barten described composite flap of skin and SMAS in their deep plane facelift approach [3, 4]
- The short-scar technique was introduced for the first time by Baker and Tonnard [5]
- Feldman was the first to introduce the platysmal 'corset' technique [6], meanwhile the modern techniques of lipofilling were introduced for the first time by Coleman [7].

Knowing the anatomical structures is the basis for achieving long-lasting and maximally effective results when lifting tissues in the face and neck area:

- **Superficial muscular aponeurotic system (SMAS)**—the SMAS extends from the platysma to the galea aponeurotica and is continuous with temporoparietal fascia and galea. It connects to the dermis via vertical septa [8].
- **Facial nerve**. The facial nerve (VII) provides sensory innervation for the mimic muscles of the face, but also provides motor innervation for m. levator anguli oris, m. buccinator and m. mentalis. Distal to stylomastoid foramen,

E. Sharkov, *Body Contouring Surgery*, https://doi.org/10.1007/978-3-031-33350-7_15

the following are the nerves branch off the facial nerve:

- **Posterior auricular nerve** controls movements of some of the scalp muscles around the ear
- Branch to posterior belly of **digastric muscle**, as well as the **stylohyoid muscle**
- Five major facial branches (at parotid plexus)—from superior to inferior:
  - **Temporal branch**
  - **Zygomatic branch**
  - **Buccal branch**
  - **Marginal mandibular branch**—one of the most frequently injured nerve branches during facelift procedures
  - **Cervical branch**

Dissection in the deep plane can mostly be performed safely, because the facial nerve innervates the facial muscles on the deep surface of these muscles (except for the muscles which are lying deep to the facial nerve, the mentalis, the levator anguli oris and the buccinator) [9].

- **Erb's point (McKinney's point)** [10]—n. auricularis magnus and n. transversus colli, coming from n. accesorius, v. jugularis externa et v. jug.anterior, go on 6.5 cm caudally to meatus acusticus externus along the posterior edge of SCM in subSMAS. Especially in thin individuals, the skin in this area is tightly grown into the muscle fascia, and when separating the tissues, although being subcutaneously, the above-mentioned structures may be injured.
- **Retaining ligaments**
  The retaining ligaments in the face provide an anchorage of superficial structures to underlying bone. The platysma-cutaneous ligaments and the platysma-auricular ligament connect the platysma to the dermis. The osteocutaneous ligaments, the zygomatic ligament and the mandibular ligament attach to the skin and bone, leading to a counteraction of gravitational forces. These ligaments should be released surgically to obtain a fully mobile facelift flap [11–14].
- **Greater auricular nerve**
  Injury to the greater auricular nerve is the most seen nerve injury after rhytidectomy. Care should be taken in elevation over the sternocleidomastoid muscle.
- **Vascularization**
  The composite flap is vascularized by **facial**, **angular** and/or **inferior orbital arteries**. The facial artery supplies the platysma and goes on as the angular artery, which connects with the branches of the arteria supratrochlearis and arteria infraorbitalis.

The author recommends the following options from his practice in determining the type and combination of techniques to achieve optimal results (the degree of cutaneous–subcutaneous excess and the corresponding refinement of the need for a surgical or minimally invasive technique are considered):

(a) Patients under the age of 50 with minimal skin excess—FaceTite™ radiofrequency techniques in combination with Morpheus8™
(b) Patients under the age of 50 with moderate skin excess—FaceTite™ radiofrequency techniques in combination with Morpheus8™
(c) Patients under the age of 50 with minimal or moderate skin excess and present subcutaneous fat component—FaceTite radiofrequency techniques, followed by vibration or manual liposuction and Morpheus8™
(d) Patients under the age of 50 with minimal or moderate skin excess and present subplatysmal fat component—VASERlipo® ultrasound of subplatysmal fat, followed by lipoaspiration of the subplatysmal and subcutaneous fat and Morpheus8™
(e) Patients under the age of 50 with significant skin excess with/without present subcutaneous fat component—FaceTite radiofrequency techniques, followed by vibration or manual liposuction, in cases of present fat deposits, and Morpheus8™ (the patient should be informed about a positive influence on the aesthetic problem within 50–70%) or facelift with/without lipoaspiration techniques
(f) Patients over the age of 50 with minimal skin excess—FaceTite™ radiofrequency techniques in combination with Morpheus8™

(g) patients over the age of 50 with moderate skin excess—FaceTite radiofrequency techniques in combination with Morpheus8™ (patient should be informed—expected improvement within 50–70%) or facelift surgical intervention
(h) patients over the age of 50 with minimal or moderate skin excess and present subcutaneous fat component—FaceTite radiofrequency techniques, followed by moderate vibration or manual liposuction and Morpheus8™ (patient should be informed—expected improvement within 50–60%)
(i) patients over the age of 50 with significant skin excess with/without present subcutaneous fat component with/without subplatysmal fat component—facelift procedure. An option for patients who do not want a surgical intervention is FaceTite™ with Morpheus8™, clearly informing the patient that he or she can expect a 30–50% improvement

Surgical Techniques

Skin incision in the sideburns, which continues in the preauricular area just before or behind the tragus and subsequently passes under the lobulus auriculae and behind the pinna, **initial subcutaneous dissection** is approached, after which the following approaches are possible:

(a) **Complete subcutaneous dissection**
(b) **In case of subsequent SMAS-dissection**, it includes a transverse incision at the level below the arcus zygomaticus and interrupting the preauricular incision, continuing to the angulus mandibulae along the anterior edge of the m. sternocleidomastoideus, after which SMAS is dissected, as the end point of its dissection is the anterior edge of the gl. parotis [15]. It is possible to perform the so-called extended SMAS-dissection, which allows single-stage filling in the malar area and theoretically allows significant contouring of the jaw and the neck. In this option of SMAS-dissection, the level of the transverse incision is above the arcus zygomaticus and it continues in the preauricular area and along the course of the m. sternocleidomastoideus. The dissection is extended, lifting the SMAS-platysma flap above the anterior end of the gland; then the dissection continues superficially above the level of m. zygomaticus major to avoid unwanted denervation of the same [16].

Regardless of the preferred approach of subcutaneous facelift or 'traditional' or 'extended' SMAS-dissection, the subsequent technique in relation to SMAS could be

- **Baker SMAS-ectomy** [17]—a strip of SMAS is cut diagonally between the angulus mandibulae and the lateral canthus, then the movable SMAS is sutured to its immovable component, and the platysma is sutured to the proc. mastoideus. Options exist in the form of an excised strip of SMAS. The author's preferred approach is the inverted L type ('golf-stick')
- **SMAS-plication** [18], in which along the above-described diagonal line (or another type of variation in terms of shape), plication is performed instead of excision
- **MACS-lifting** [19] with minimal access and need for purse-string sutures in SMAS and malar fat pad with vertical anchorage; techniques with bi- and tricuspid flap. The intervention ends with tightening of the skin and removal of the excess

Tissue lifting often requires additional techniques for contouring in the neck area—a **submental incision** is required, which is followed by subcutaneous separation. The need to reduce the adipose tissue along the muscle fibres is evaluated and, if necessary, the present *subplatysmal fat tissue* is also removed. The next surgical step is to perform a *Feldman 'corset' type platysmaplasty* with duplication along the midline of the m. platysma (there are options with interruption of the platysma by means of a surgical incision). The possible additional techniques to further contour and emphasize the mandibular margin include *resection of the submandibular glands and possible partial resection of m. digastricus.*

Author's Preferred Surgical Technique

- In the presence of platysmal bridles and dehiscence of the platysma along the midline, it is initially approached with a submental incision. In the presence of fat deposits, infiltration of Klein solution is performed, followed by lipoaspiration with a 2.5 mm 'spatula' type cannula manually or by vibration liposuction using a 3 mm short angled cannula. The subplatysmal adipose tissue is separated and a gentle excision of the same is performed. Corset platysmaplasty;
- After making a skin incision in the sideburns, which continues in the preauricular area just before or behind the tragus and subsequently passes under the lobulus auriculae and behind the pinna, a complete subcutaneous dissection is approached until communication is reached with the submental access. The osteocutaneous ligaments are released, then a **SMAS-ectomy** is performed—a strip of SMAS of the inverted L ('golf-stick') type, after which the movable SMAS is sutured to its static component, and the platysma is sutured to the proc. mastoideus. Skin excision is performed, then redon-drainage is brought out, the surgical wound is closed in layers, and the contralateral side is approached in an identical manner [20].

Minimally Invasive Surgical Approach Depending on the Preoperative Assessment and Patient's Status (Author's Preferred Option)

***FaceTite*™ is a radiofrequency procedure aimed at skin tightening and fat excess 'melting' in the area of the neck and lower third of the face. The procedure is performed using a bipolar cannula, with the internal electrode providing destruction of the fat deposits by reaching a temperature of 70 °C, while the external electrode providing skin tightening by heating the surface to 40–42 °C** [21–24]**. The radiofrequency energy emitted between the two electrodes stimulates the collagen, resulting in fibres and subsequent contraction with a lifting effect on the skin. The procedure is used under local anaesthesia, which can also be combined with sedation, if the patient wishes. The optimal effect of the procedure is visible between the 6th and 12th postoperative month, and the durability of the effect is about 6 years.**

The author uses several entry points through which the procedure is performed—an entry point immediately along the submental midline; two points under the jaw, laterally to the so-called NO GO AREA and two entry points just below the mandible angle. For significant skin excess, an entry point just anterior to the anterior edge of SCM is also recommended. When treating the lower third of the face, the author uses an entry point immediately in front of the tragus of the pinna (Fig. 1**—the entry points are marked in red).**

The neck area and the area of the lower third of the face are treated with FaceTite. The plane is strictly subcutaneous, the energy is supplied linearly retrograde by means of two techniques—'lining' with the aim of tightening and lifting the skin, 'stamping' with the aim of melting the subcutaneous fatty tissue.

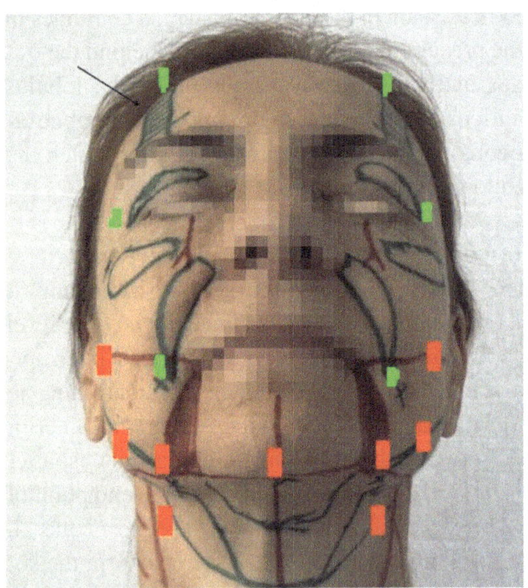

Fig. 1 Visualization of the entry points aimed at treating the neck and the lower third of the face using FaceTite™ (marked in red) and the entry points aimed at treating the areas of the nasolabial fold (NLF), malar fat pad, upper and lower eyelid, and lifting of the eyebrows using AccuTite ™ (marked in green)

The supplied energy varies from 5 to 14 kJ in the neck area and 1.0–2.0 kJ per side in the area of the lower third of the face.

The author recommends that the area of therapy should not pass over the line connecting the tragus of the ear with the corner of the mouth, because in this area the branches of the facial nerve have a more superficial course; similarly, given the innervation of the lower lip, it is recommended to avoid the area marked with a red triangle on the left and right under the corners of the mouth—NGA.

***AccuTite*™ is a radiofrequency procedure aimed at skin tightening and fat excess 'melting' in the area of the lower third of the face, nasolabial fold (NLF), malar fat pad, upper eyelids, lower eyelids, lifting of the eyebrows. The procedure is performed using a bipolar cannula, with the internal electrode providing a permanent destruction of the fat deposits by reaching a temperature of 70 °C, while the external electrode providing skin tightening by heating the surface to 40–42 °C** [21–24]**. The radiofrequency energy emitted between the two electrodes has a main effect through stimulation of collagen fibres and subsequent contraction with a lifting effect on the skin. The procedure is used under local anaesthesia, which can also be combined with sedation, if the patient wishes. The optimal effect of the procedure is visible between the 6th and 12th postoperative month, and the durability of the effect is about 6 years.**

The author uses several entry points through which the procedure is performed, depending on the treated area—the entry points are marked in green in Fig. 1**: immediately above and lateral to the corner of the mouth bilaterally—treatment of the NLF area; 1.0–1.5 cm laterally from the lateral canthus of the eye in order to reach the areas of the upper, lower eyelid and malar fat pad; immediately at the border with the hairy part of the scalp bilaterally for the purpose of lifting and access to the eyebrows.**

Depending on the treated areas, the work parameters and techniques are as follows

- **Nasolabial fold (NLF)—subcutaneously; technique of stamping in order to melt the fat excess; 0.2–0.4 kJ per side; 40 C external cut off and 70 C internal cut off**
- **Malar fat pad—subcutaneously; technique of stamping in order to melt the fat excess; 0.2–0.4 kJ per side; 40 C external cut off and 70 C internal cut off. The author recommends a combination with Morpheus8™ to optimize the results achieved**
- **Upper eyelids—subcutaneously; technique of lining in order to tighten the skin; 0.2–0.3 kJ per side; 36 C external cut off and 66 C internal cut off. The author recommends a combination with Morpheus8 Prime™ to optimize the results achieved**
- **Lower eyelids—subcutaneously; technique of lining in order to tighten the skin; 0.2–0.3 kJ per side; 37 C external cut off and 67 C internal cut off. The author recommends a combination with Morpheus8 Prime™ to optimize the results achieved;**
- **Eyebrows—supraperiosteally; it is worked in an area that is laterally limited by a vertical line located 1 cm medially from the temporal crist. Medially, this area is limited by a vertical line located 1 cm medial to the lateral border, respectively, the width of the area is 1 cm. Caudally, the area extends 1 cm above the orbital rim. The parameters are as follow - technique of lining with 40 C external and 70 C internal cut off; 0.4–0.7 kJ per side. The area is indicated by an arrow in** Fig. 1.

A. Patients under the age of 50 with minimal skin excess—FaceTite™ radiofrequency techniques in combination with Morpheus 8 (Figs. 2 and 3)

The work parameters that the author recommends are as follows

- Infiltration (Klein Solution)—60–100 mL
- Temperature parameters of the FaceTite cannula—40 °C external cut off/70 °C internal cut off
- Energy to be cumulated on the area of the neck—4.0–7.0 kJ for the neck area, depending on how big the case is/techniques—mainly of tightening (lining) to tighten and lift the skin
- Morpheus8™ at the end of the procedure with parameters as follows: whenever done in com-

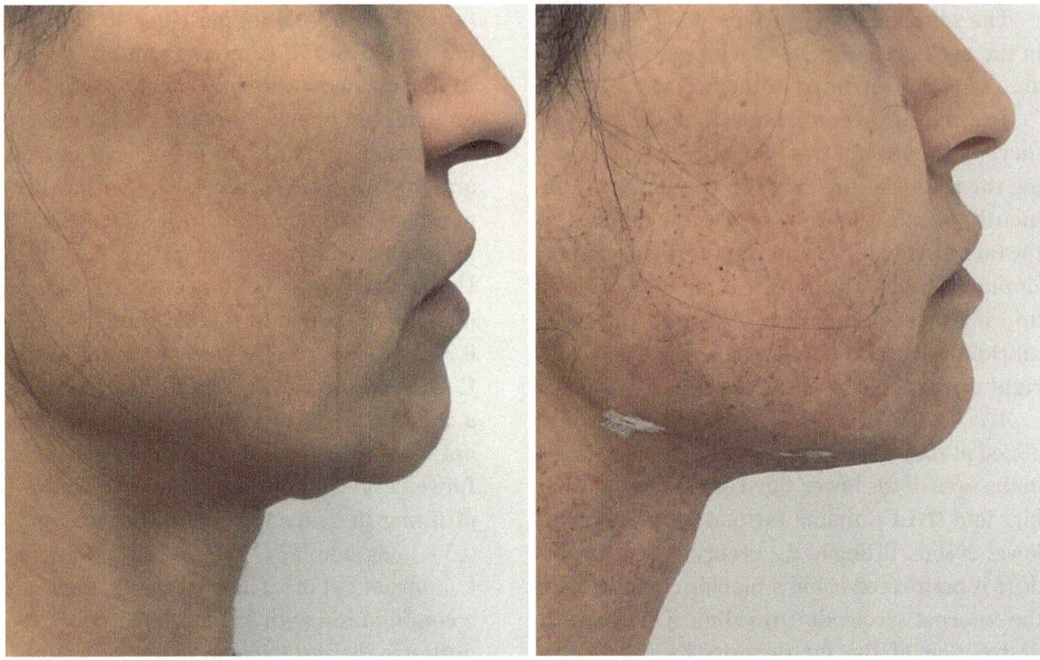

Fig. 2 3 days after FaceTite™ with Morpheus8™ in a 41-year-old female patient Treatment of slight skin excess in the area of the neck

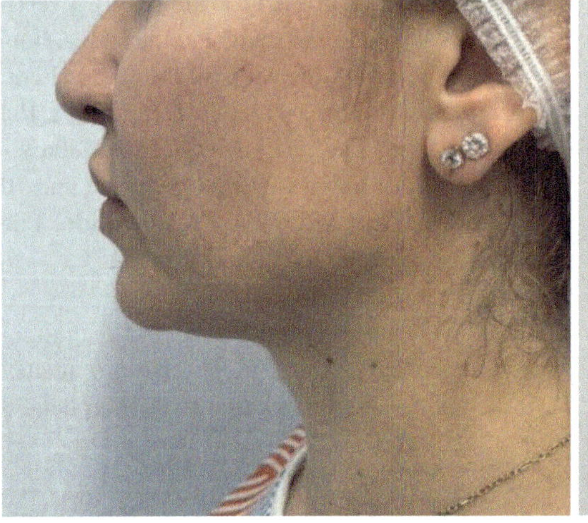

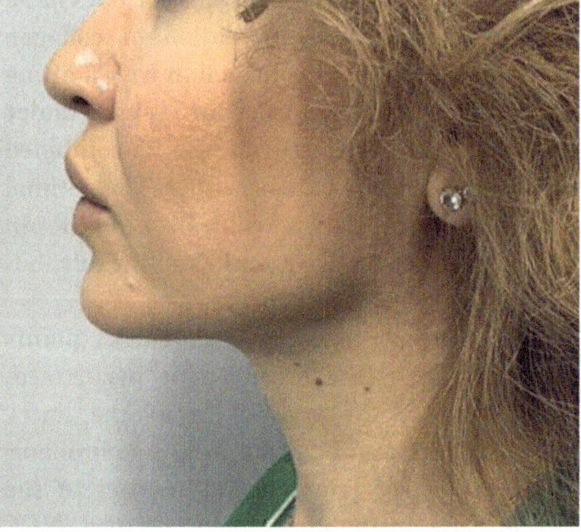

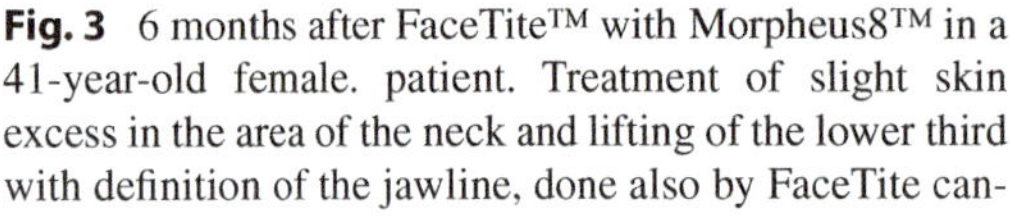

Fig. 3 6 months after FaceTite™ with Morpheus8™ in a 41-year-old female. patient. Treatment of slight skin excess in the area of the neck and lifting of the lower third with definition of the jawline, done also by FaceTite cannula in combination with Morpheus8™. In this specific case also melting ('stamping') in the area of the 'buldog' was performed

bination with FaceTite or AccuTite™, the author recommends less overlapping: 4 mm/30–35 energy/3 stacks per place/fixed mode/1 pps followed by 3 mm/30 energy/2 stacks per place/fixed mode/1 pps followed by 2 mm/15 energy/one stack per place/cycle mode

– *In cases of poor jawline definition and excess skin in the area of the marionette lines*—AccuTite™ and/or FaceTite™ could be added in order to lift the lower third of the face. The parameters to be applied in those cases are: 1.5–2.0 kJ per side, from an entry point just in front of the tragus (Fig. 12, Fig. 3). Usually 15–20 mL of infiltration solution per side is adequate as amount. Morpheus8™ could be added in the same time as a following procedure, the parameters are identical as those mentioned from above.

B. Patients under the age of 50 with moderate skin excess—FaceTite™ radiofrequency techniques in combination with Morpheus8™ (Fig. 4)

The work parameters that the author recommends are as follows

- Infiltration (Klein Solution)—60–100 mL
- Temperature parameters of the FaceTite cannula—40 °C external cut off/70 °C internal cut off.
- Energy to be cumulated on the area of the neck—7.0–8.0 kJ for the neck area, depending on how big the case is/techniques—mainly of tightening ('lining') to tighten and lift the skin
- Morpheus8™ at the end of the procedure with parameters as follows: whenever done in combination with FaceTite™ or AccuTite™, the author recommends less overlapping: 4 mm/30–35 energy/3 stacks per place/fixed mode/1 pps followed by 3 mm/30 energy/2 stacks per place/fixed mode/1 pps followed by 2 mm/15 energy/one stack per place/cycle mode
  - *In cases of poor jawline definition and excess skin in the area of the marionette lines*—AccuTite™ and/or FaceTite™ could be added in order to lift the lower third of the face. The parameters to be applied in those cases are 1.5–2.0 kJ per side, from an entry point just in front of the tragus (Fig. 12, Fig. 4). Usually 15–20 mL of infiltration solution per side is adequate as amount. Morpheus8™ could be added in the same time as a following procedure, the parameters are identical as those mentioned from above.

C. **Patients under the age of 50 with minimal or moderate skin excess and present subcutaneous fat component—FaceTite radiofrequency techniques followed by manual or vibration-based liposuction and Morpheus8™** (Figs. 5 and 6 and Fig. 7)

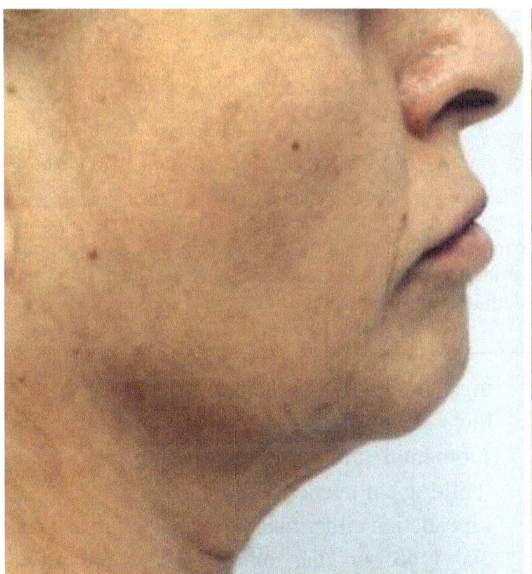
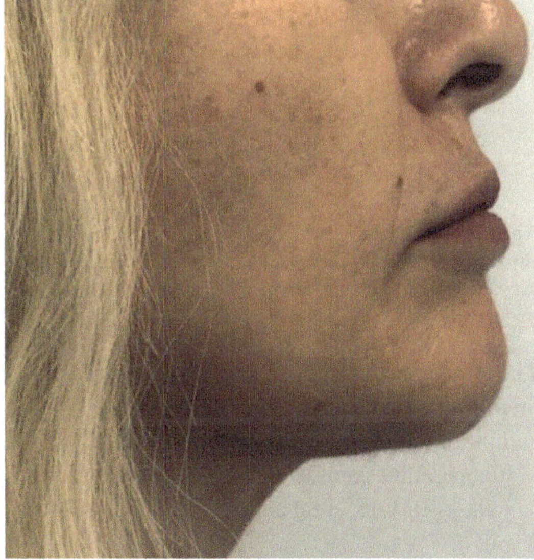

Fig. 4 1 year after FaceTite™ with Morpheus8™ in a 45-year-old female patient. Treatment of slight skin excess in the area of the neck and lifting of the lower third with definition of the jawline

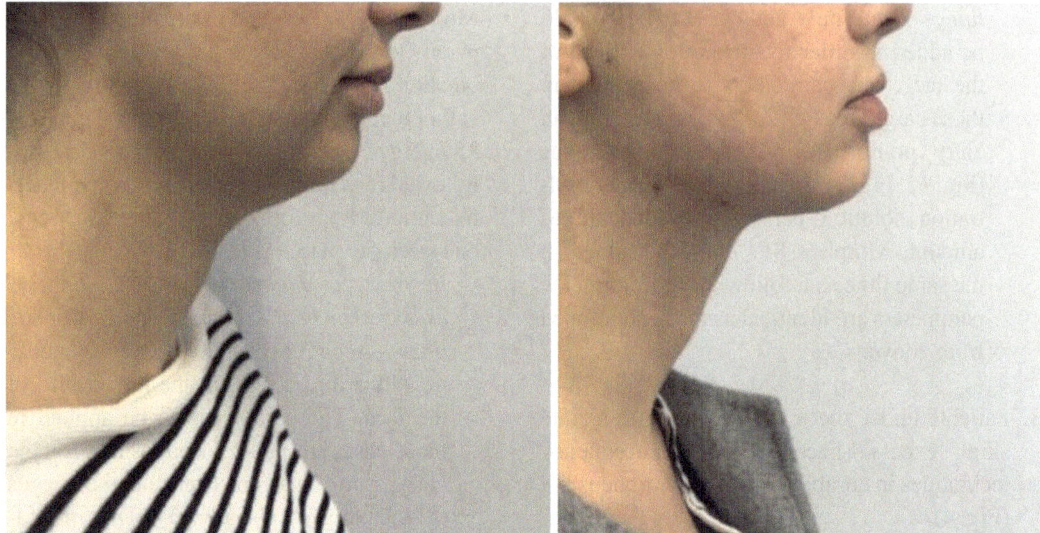

Fig. 5 1 month after FaceTite™ with liposuction, manually with 2.5 mm 'spatula' type cannula, and Morpheus8™ in a 33-year-old female patient. Treatment of slight skin excess, slight amount of submental fat and slight amount of fat in the 'bulldog' area. Lifting of the lower third with definition of the jawline

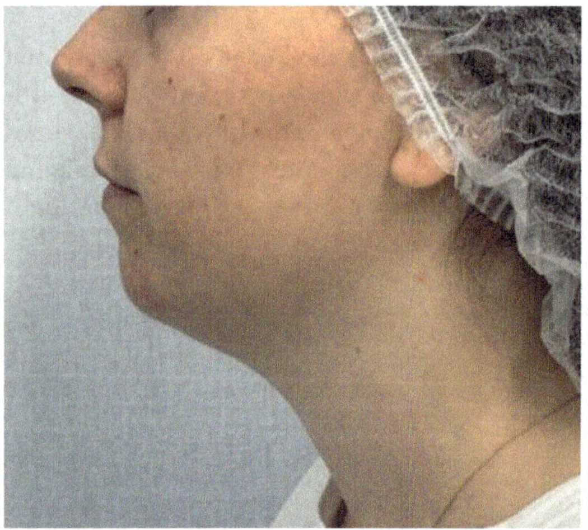

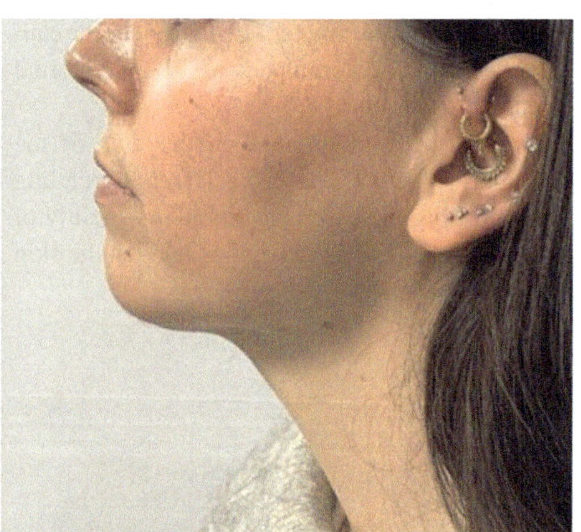

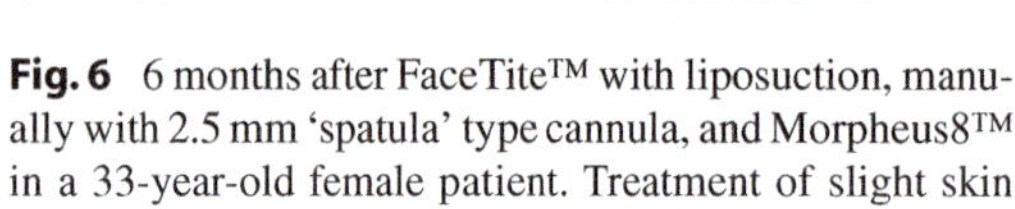

Fig. 6 6 months after FaceTite™ with liposuction, manually with 2.5 mm 'spatula' type cannula, and Morpheus8™ in a 33-year-old female patient. Treatment of slight skin excess, slight amount of submental fat and slight amount of fat in the 'bulldog' area. Lifting of the lower third with definition of the jawline

The work parameters that the author recommends are as follows

- Infiltration (Klein Solution)—60–100 mL;
- Temperature parameters of the FaceTite cannula—40 °C external cut off/70 °C internal cut off
- Energy to be cumulated on the area of the neck—6.0–9.0 kJ for the neck area, depending on how big the case is/techniques of tightening ('lining') to tighten and lift the skin, followed by 'stamping' (melting) the fat in the submental area and also in the area of the 'bulldog', if needed
- Liposuction either manually with 2.5 mm 'spatula' type cannula, either done by vibration-assisted liposuction 3 mm short angled cannula
- Morpheus8™ at the end of the procedure with parameters as follows: whenever done in com-

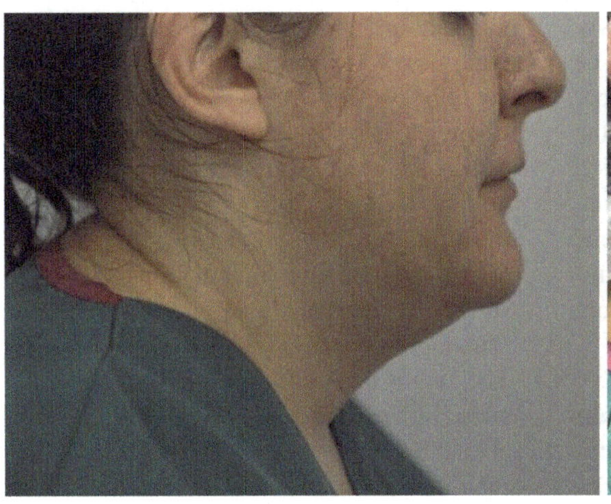
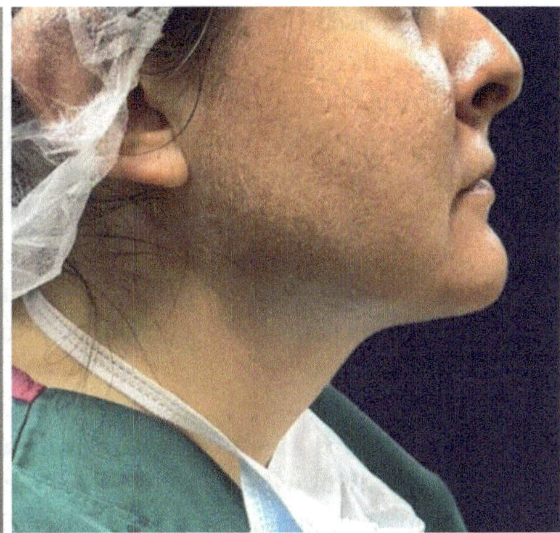

Fig. 7 6 months after VASERlipo® with liposuction done by VERTEX N3 type of cannula in a 35-year-old female patient. Treatment of skin excess and subplatysmal fat. This patient was done with cooperation with Nikolaos Sgouros MD

bination with FaceTite™ or AccuTite™, the author recommends less overlapping: 4 mm/30–35 energy/3 stacks per place/fixed mode/1 pps followed by 3 mm/30 energy/2 stacks per place/fixed mode/1 pps followed by 2 mm/15 energy/one stack per place/cycle mode

- *In cases of poor jawline definition and excess skin in the area of the marionette lines*—AccuTite™ and/or FaceTite™ could be added in order to lift the lower third of the face. The parameters to be applied in those cases are 1.5–2.0 kJ per side, from an entry point just in front of the tragus (Fig. 12, Fig. 5). Usually 15–20 mL of infiltration solution per side is adequate as amount. Morpheus8™ could be added in the same time as a following procedure, the parameters are identical as those mentioned from above.

D. **Patients under the age of 50 with minimal or moderate skin excess and present subplatysmal fat component—VASERlipo® of subplatysmal fat followed by vibration-based liposuction with/without Morpheus8™** (Fig. 7).

The work parameters that the author recommends are as follows

- Infiltration (Klein Solution)—120–150 mL
- Temperature parameters of the VASERlipo® FaceKit—50C VASER MODE—to tighten and lift the skin from overall 3 entry points—one just under the chin on the midline, and an entry point just under the angle of the mandible on the left and on the right side. With the face probe of the VASER around 40–60 s should be done in the subcutaneous layer. This should be followed by 40–60 s work on to the subplatysmal fat from the middle point, gently, in a radius of 2–3 cm, and not furthermore
- Liposuction either manually with 2.5 mm spatula type cannula or done by VERTEX N3 type of cannula. Suction should be done from all entry points, but suction of the subplatysmal fat should be done only from the midline one, following the same rules as area of treatment, mentioned from above
- Morpheus 8™ at the end of the procedure with parameters as follows: whenever done in combination with VASER, the author recommends less overlapping: 4 mm/30–35 energy/3 stacks per place/fixed mode/1 pps followed by 3 mm/30 energy/2 stacks per place/fixed mode/1 pps followed by 2 mm/15 energy/one stack per place/cycle mode
  - *In cases of poor jawline definition and excess skin in the area of the marionette lines*—AccuTite™ and/or FaceTite™

could be added in order to lift the lower third of the face. The parameters to be applied in those cases are 1.5–2.0 kJ per side, from an entry point just in front of the tragus. Usually 15–20 mL of infiltration solution per side is adequate as amount. Morpheus8™ could be added in the same time as a following procedure, the parameters are identical as those mentioned from above.

E. **Patients under the age of 50 with significant skin excess with/without present subcutaneous fat component—FaceTite™ radiofrequency techniques followed by vibration assisted liposuction, in case of available fat deposits, and Morpheus8™ (the patient should be informed about a positive influence on the aesthetic problem within 50–70%) or facelift with/without lipoaspiration techniques** (Figs. 8, 9, 10, 11 and 12).

The work parameters that the author recommends in a minimally invasive approach (Figs. 8, 9 and 10) are as follows

- Infiltration (Klein Solution)—80–120 mL
- Temperature parameters of the FaceTite cannula—40 °C external cut off/70 °C internal cut off
- Energy to be cumulated on the area of the neck—10–14 kJ for the neck area, depending on how big the case is/techniques of tightening (lining) to tighten and lift the skin, followed by stamping (melting) the fat in the submental area and also in the area of the 'bulldog', if needed
- The author recommends an entry point to be added on the front edge of SCM to cumulate a greater amount of energy
- *Liposuction either manually with 2.5 mm spatula type cannula or done by vibration-assisted liposuction with 3 mm short angled cannula. Liposuction in those cases should be carefully estimated by properly evaluating the contraction capability of the skin prior to the procedure. In those specific cases, the author addresses the fat deposits by slight manual liposuction in cases between 40 and 50 of age* (Fig. 9), *and being more aggressive in patients under 40* (Fig. 10) *with adequate contraction capability of the skin. Not being very aggressive in severe cases of skin laxity is also addi-*

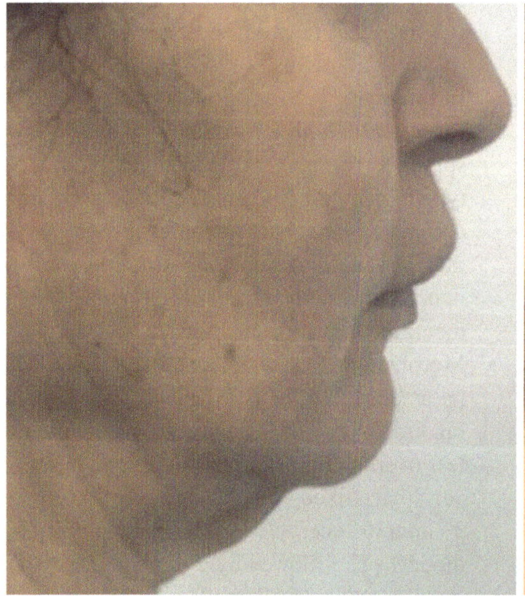

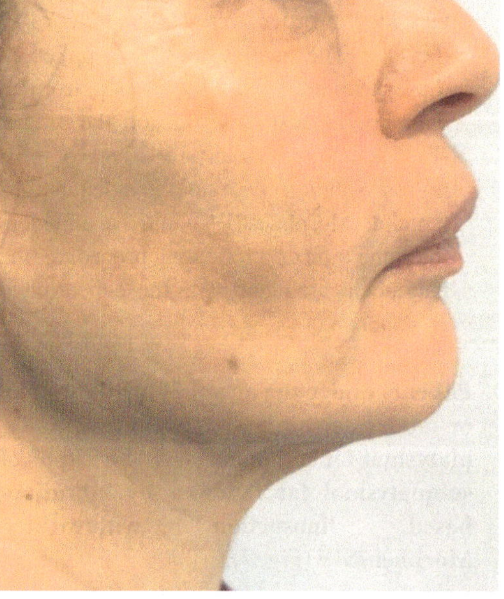

Fig. 8 A 48-year-old female patient. 1 year after FaceTite™ and Morpheus8™ without liposuction. Treatment of skin excess in the area of the neck and lower third of the face

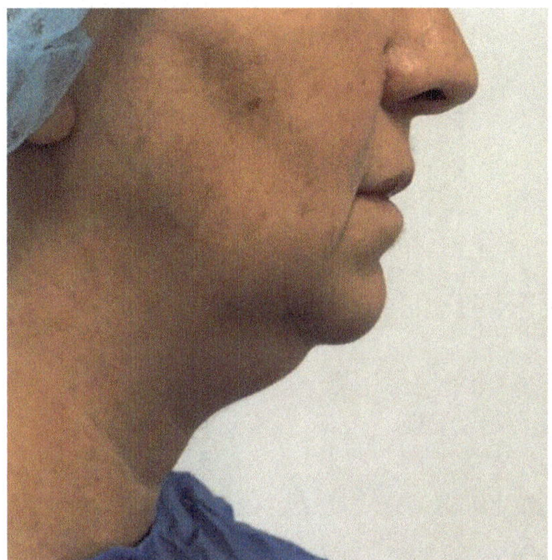

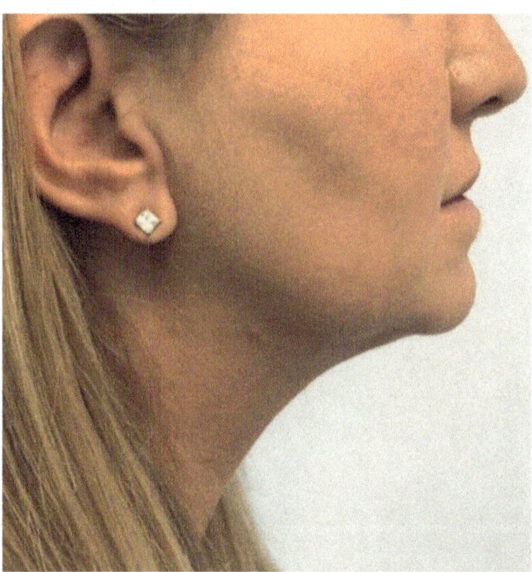

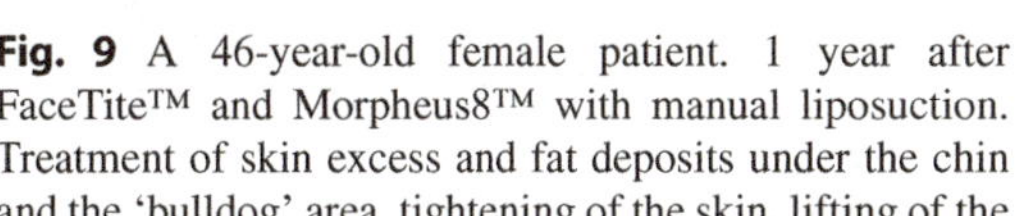

Fig. 9 A 46-year-old female patient. 1 year after FaceTite™ and Morpheus8™ with manual liposuction. Treatment of skin excess and fat deposits under the chin and the 'bulldog' area, tightening of the skin, lifting of the lower third of the face and definition of the jawline. In this specific case, 10 mL of pure fat were suctioned from the submental area, and 2 mL per side from the 'bulldog' area

tional prevention for the skin contraction in radiofrequency procedures chosen as treatment plan for those types of patients;

- Morpheus8™ at the end of the procedure with parameters as follows: whenever done in combination with FaceTite™ or AccuTite™, the author recommends less overlapping:
- 4 mm/30–35 energy/3 stacks per place/ fixed mode/1 pps followed by 3 mm/30 energy/2 stacks per place/fixed mode/1 pps followed by 2 mm/15 energy/one stack per place/cycle mode.
  - *In cases of poor jawline definition and excess skin in the area of the marionette lines*—AccuTite™ and/or FaceTite™ could be added in order to lift the lower third of the face. Parameters to be applied in those cases are 1.5–2.0 kJ per side, from an entry point just in front of the tragus (Figs. 8, 9 and 10). Usually 15–20 mL of infiltration solution per side is adequate as amount. Morpheus 8 could be added in the same time as a following procedure, the parameters are identical as those mentioned from above.

When selecting a surgical technique, the approach is described in the text of paragraph 1.6 above (Figs. 11 and 12).

F. **Patients over the age of 50 with minimal skin excess—FaceTite™ radiofrequency techniques in combination with Morpheus8™** (Fig. 13).

The work parameters that the author recommends are as follows

- Infiltration (Klein Solution)—60–100 mL
- Temperature parameters of the FaceTite cannula—40 °C external cut off/70 °C internal cut off
- Energy to be cumulated on the area of the neck—6.0–10 kJ for the neck area, depending on how big the case is/techniques—mainly of tightening (lining) to tighten and lift the skin;
- Morpheus8™ at the end of the procedure with parameters as follows: whenever done in combination with FaceTite™ or AccuTite™, the author recommends less overlapping:

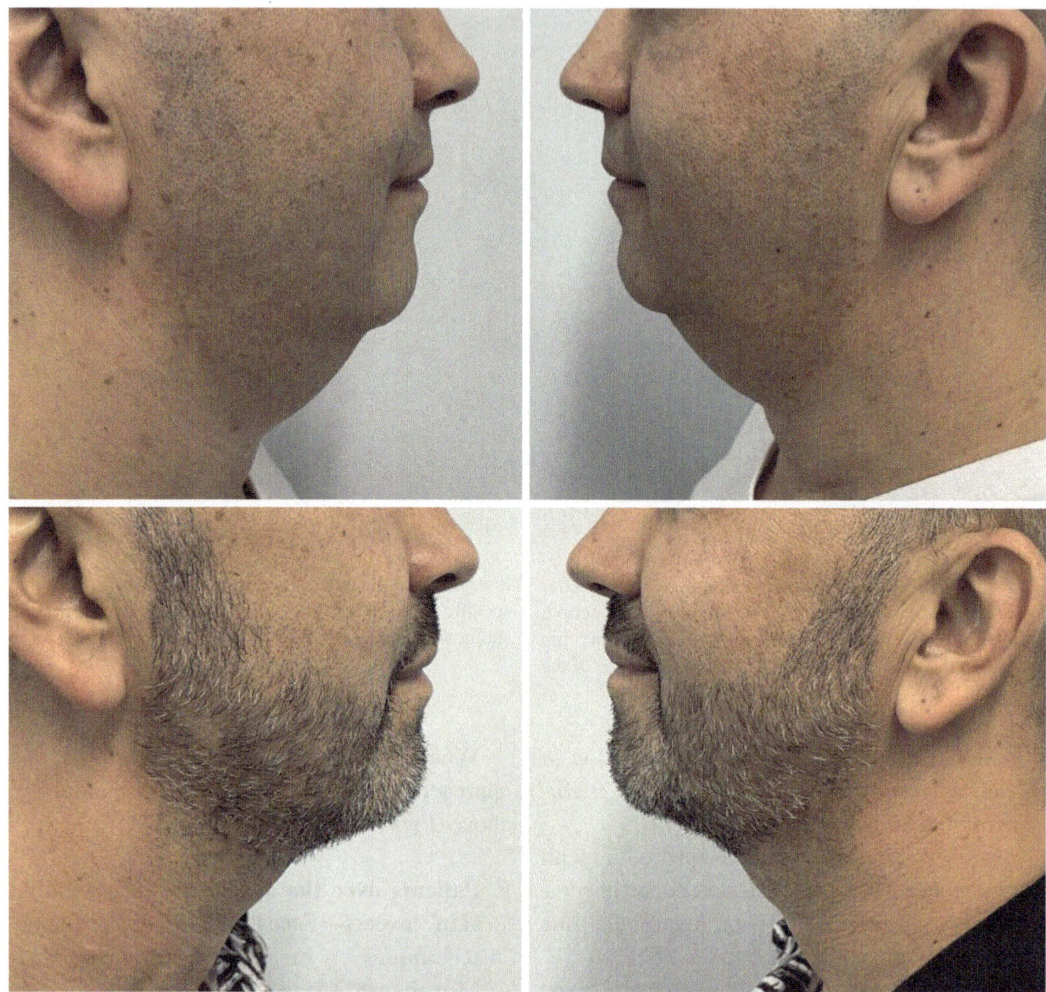

Fig. 10 A 39-year-old male patient. 6 months after FaceTite™ and Morpheus8™ with vibration-assisted liposuction. Treatment of skin excess and fat deposits under the chin and the 'bulldog' area, tightening of the skin, lifting of the lower third of the face and definition of the jawline. In this specific case, 40 mL of pure fat were suctioned from the submental area, and 2 mL per side from the 'bulldog' area

- 4 mm/30–35 energy/3 stacks per place/fixed mode/1 pps followed by 3 mm/30 energy/2 stacks per place/fixed mode/1 pps followed by 2 mm/15 energy/one stack per place/cycle mode
  – *In cases of poor jawline definition and excess skin in the area of the marionette lines*—AccuTite™ and/or FaceTite™ could be added in order to lift the lower third of the face. The parameters to be applied in those cases are 1.5–2.0 kJ per side, from an entry point just in front of the tragus (Fig. 12, Fig. 13). Usually 15–20 mL of infiltration solution per side is adequate as amount. Morpheus8™ could be added in the same time as a following procedure, the parameters are identical as those mentioned from above.

G. **Patients over the age of 50 with moderate skin excess—FaceTite™ radiofrequency techniques in combination with Morpheus8™ (the patient should be informed about a positive influence on aesthetic problem within 50–70%,** Fig. 14) **or facelift surgical intervention.**

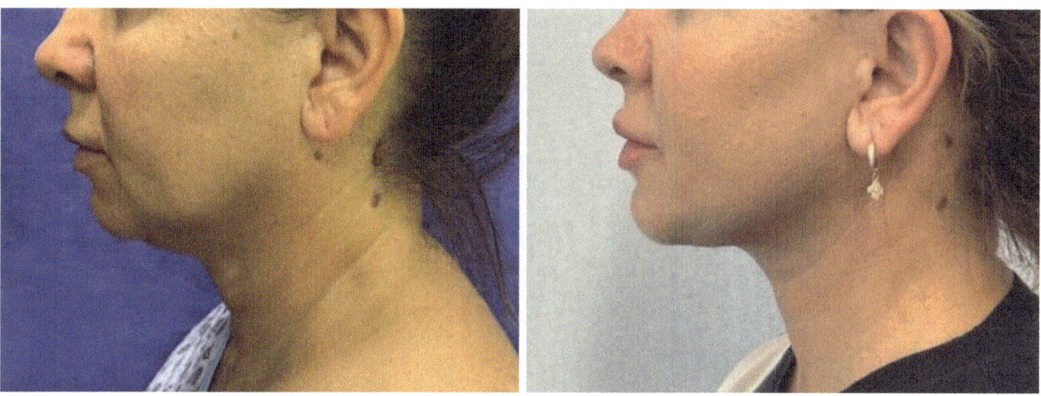

Fig. 11 A 49-year-old female patient. 6 months after facelift with liposuction and plication of the platysma. The procedure was done following the preferable protocol from behalf of the author, as described from above

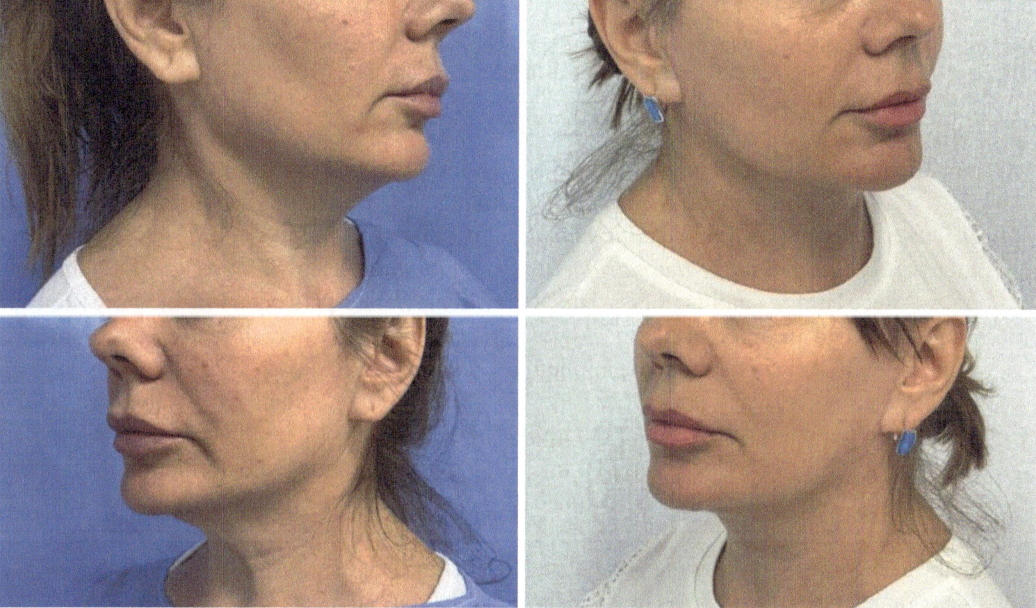

Fig. 12 A 49-year-old female patient. 1 year after facelift with plication of the platysma and without liposuction. The procedure was done following the preferable protocol from behalf of the author, as described from above

The work parameters that the author recommends when choosing a minimally invasive technique are as follows

- Infiltration (Klein Solution)—60–100 mL
- Temperature parameters of the FaceTite cannula—40 °C external cut off/70 °C internal cut off
- Energy to be cumulated on the area of the neck—8.0–10 kJ for the neck area, depending on how big the case is/techniques—mainly of tightening (lining) to tighten and lift the skin
- Morpheus 8™ at the end of the procedure with parameters as follows: whenever done in combination with FaceTite™ or AccuTite™, the author recommends less overlapping:
- 4 mm/30–35 energy/3 stacks per place/fixed mode/1 pps followed by 3 mm/30 energy/2 stacks per place/fixed mode/1 pps followed by

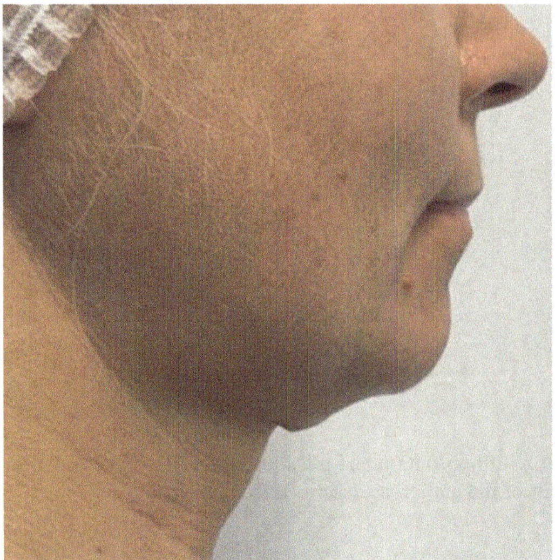
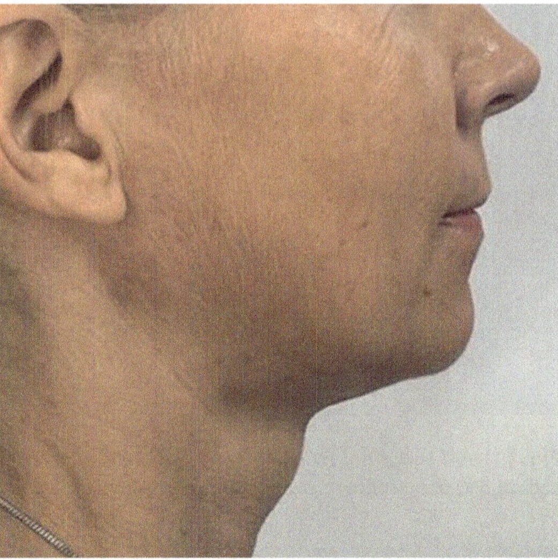

Fig. 13 1 year after FaceTite™ with Morpheus8™ in a 51-year-old female patient. Treatment of slight skin excess in the area of the neck and lifting of the lower third with definition of the jawline

2 mm/15 energy/one stack per place/cycle mode

- *In cases of poor jawline definition and excess skin in the area of the marionette lines*—AccuTite™ and/or FaceTite™ could be added in order to lift the lower third of the face. Parameters to be applied in those cases are 1.5–2.0 kJ per side, from an entry point just in front of the tragus (Fig. 12, Fig. 14). Usually 15–20 mL of infiltration solution per side is adequate as amount. Morpheus8™ could be added in the same time as a following procedure, the parameters are identical as those mentioned from above.

When choosing **a surgical technique**—(Fig. 17).

H. **Patients over the age of 50 with minimal or moderate skin excess and present subcutaneous fat component—FaceTite™ radiofrequency techniques followed by moderate vibration-based liposuction and Morpheus8™ (the patient should be informed about a positive influence on the aesthetic problem within 50–60%) or facelift**

The work parameters that the author recommends in a minimally invasive approach (Fig. 15) are as follows

- Infiltration (Klein Solution)—80–120 mL
- Temperature parameters of the FaceTite cannula—40 °C external cut off/70 °C internal cut off
- Energy to be cumulated on the area of the neck—12–13 kJ for the neck area, depending on how big the case is/techniques of tightening ('lining') to tighten and lift the skin, followed by stamping ('melting') the fat in the submental area and also in the area of the 'bulldog', if needed
- The author recommends an entry point to be added on the front edge of SCM to cumulate additional amount of energy
- *Liposuction manually with 2.5 mm spatula type cannula. Liposuction in those cases should be carefully estimated by properly evaluating the contraction capability of the skin prior to the procedure. Not being very aggressive in severe cases of skin laxity is also additional prevention for the skin contraction in radiofrequency procedures chosen as treatment plan for those types of patients*
- Morpheus8™ at the end of the procedure with parameters as follows: whenever done in com-

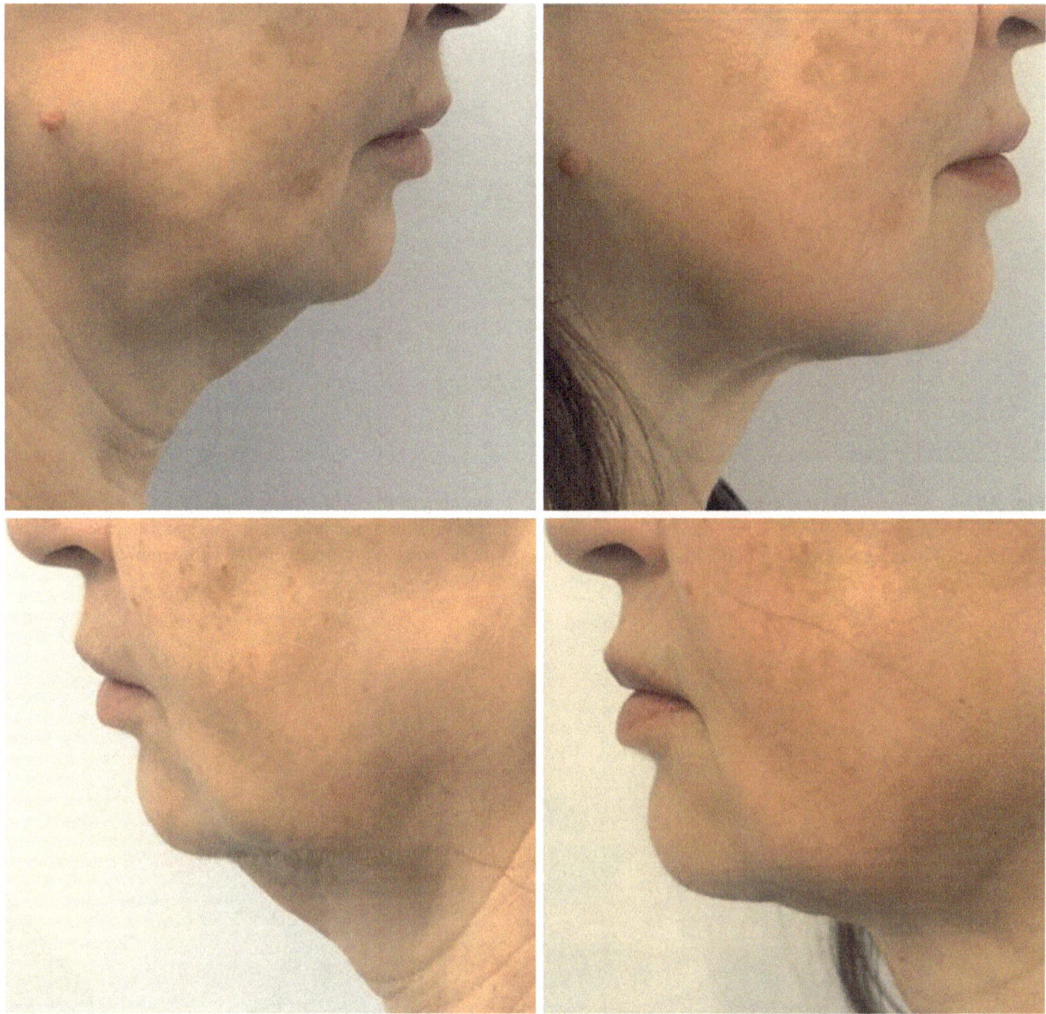

Fig. 14 1 year after FaceTite™ with Morpheus8™ in a 54-year-old female patient. Treatment of slight skin excess in the area of the neck and lifting of the lower third of the face

bination with FaceTite™ or AccuTite™, the author recommends less overlapping:

- 4 mm/30–35 energy/3 stacks per place/fixed mode/1 pps followed by 3 mm/30 energy/2 stacks per place/fixed mode/1 pps followed by 2 mm/15 energy/one stack per place/cycle mode.
  - *In cases of poor jawline definition and excess skin in the area of the marionette lines*—AccuTite™ and/or FaceTite™ (Fig. 15) could be added in order to lift the lower third of the face. The parameters to be applied in those cases are 1.5–2.0 kJ per side, from an entry point just in front of the tragus. Usually 15–20 mL of infiltration solution per side is adequate as amount. Morpheus 8 could be added in the same time as a following procedure, the parameters are identical as those mentioned from above.

When choosing a surgical technique, the approach is described in the text of paragraph 1.6 above—(Fig. 17).

I. **Patients over the age of 50 with significant skin excess with/without present subcutaneous fat component with/without subplatysmal fat component—facelift procedure. An**

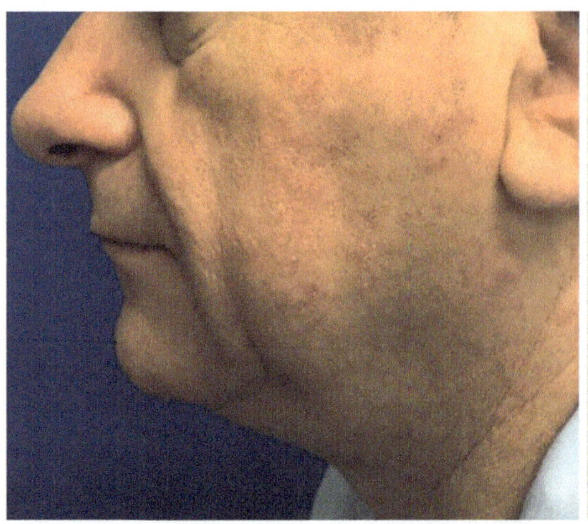
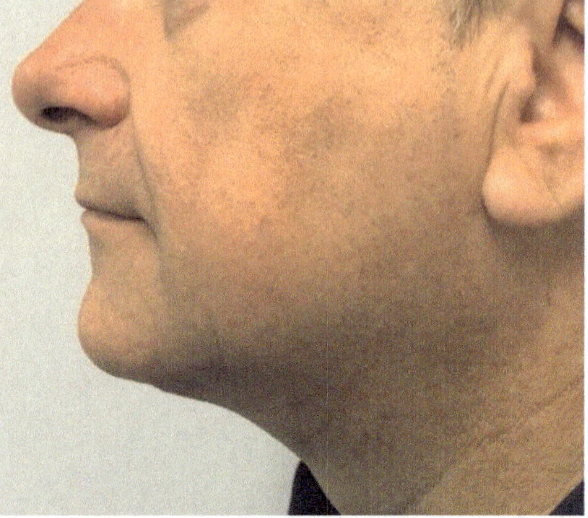

Fig. 15 A 54-year-old male patient. 6 months after FaceTite™ and Morpheus8™ with manual liposuction. Treatment of skin excess and fat deposits under the chin, tightening of the skin, lifting of the lower third of the face and definition of the jawline. In this specific case, 8 mL of pure fat were suctioned from the submental area

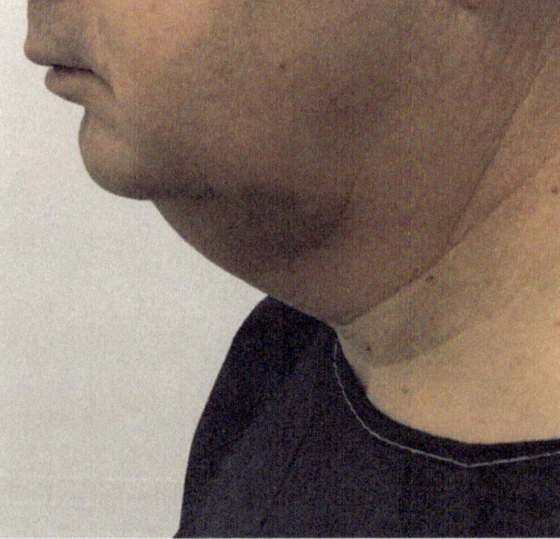
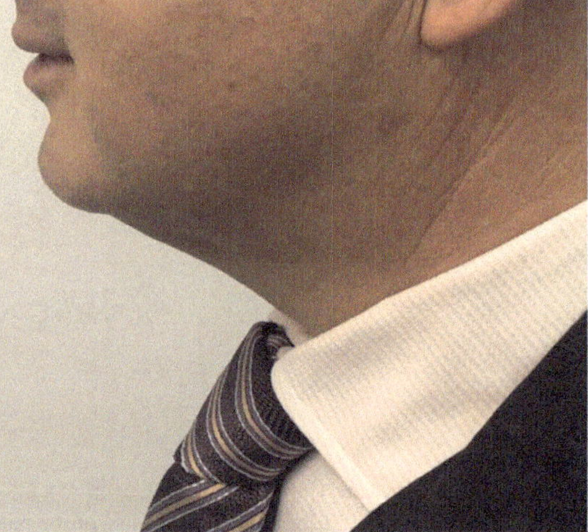

Fig. 16 A 56-year-old male patient. 1 year after FaceTite™ and Morpheus8™ for tightening of the skin of the neck and lifting of the lower third of the face without liposuction

option for patients, who do not want a surgical intervention, is FaceTite™ with Morpheus 8™, clearly informing the patient that he or she can expect a 30–50% improvement.

The work parameters that the author recommends in a minimally invasive approach (Fig. 16) are as follows

- Infiltration (Klein Solution)—80–120 mL
- Temperature parameters of the FaceTite cannula—40 °C external cut off/70 °C internal cut off
- Energy to be cumulated on the area of the neck—13–14 kJ for the neck area, depending on how big the case is/techniques of tightening (lining) to tighten and lift the skin, followed by stamping (melting) the fat in the submental area and also in the area of the 'bulldog', if needed
- The author recommends an entry point to be added on the front edge of SCM to cumulate additional amount of energy
- *Liposuction manually with 2.5 mm spatula type cannula. Liposuction in those cases should be carefully estimated by properly*

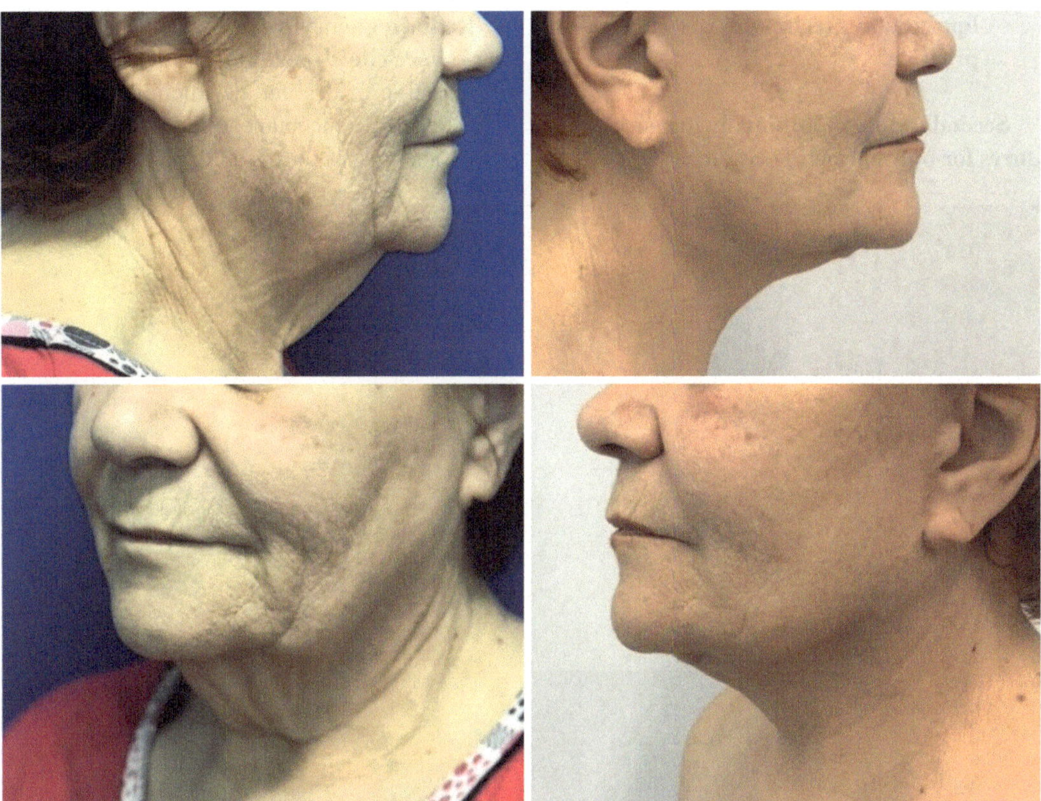

Fig. 17 1 year after extended facelift in a 64-year-old female patient, following the author preferable intraoperative protocol, described from above in this chapter

evaluating the contraction capability of the skin prior to the procedure. Not being very aggressive in severe cases of skin laxity, is also additional prevention for the skin contraction in radiofrequency procedures chosen as treatment plan for those types of patients;

- Morpheus8™ at the end of the procedure with parameters as follows: whenever done in combination with FaceTite™ or AccuTite™, the author recommends less overlapping:
- 4 mm/30–35 energy/3 stacks per place/fixed mode/1 pps followed by 3 mm/30 energy/2 stacks per place/fixed mode/1 pps followed by 2 mm/15 energy/one stack per place/cycle mode.

When choosing a surgical technique, the approach is described in the text of paragraph 1.6 above (Fig. 17).

- **Intraoperative combinations of minimally invasive surgical techniques**

- **The author DOES NOT recommend combination of surgical lifting and treatment of the elevated cutaneous–subcutaneous flap with radiofrequency energy at one stage. The author believes that, given the ablative effect of the procedures, this could compromise the blood supply to the flap and create an additional risk of possible tissue necrosis.**
- **The author considers possible the following combinations of facelift surgical procedures and radiofrequency treatment of neighbouring areas—AccuTite™ of upper and lower eyelid, malar fat pad, and eyebrow lifting, as the procedure parameters are described above in this chapter.**
- **In the presence of fat deposits in the area of the neck and the lower third of the face, the combination of facelift surgical technique and vibration assisted**

liposuction technique is a routine practice.

Secondary use of minimally invasive procedures for optimal lasting results:

- **Radiofrequency procedures:**
  - **FaceTite™**—additionally tighten the skin and provides fat destruction in case of available subcutaneous and/or skin excess. The goal is to reach 70 °C for destruction

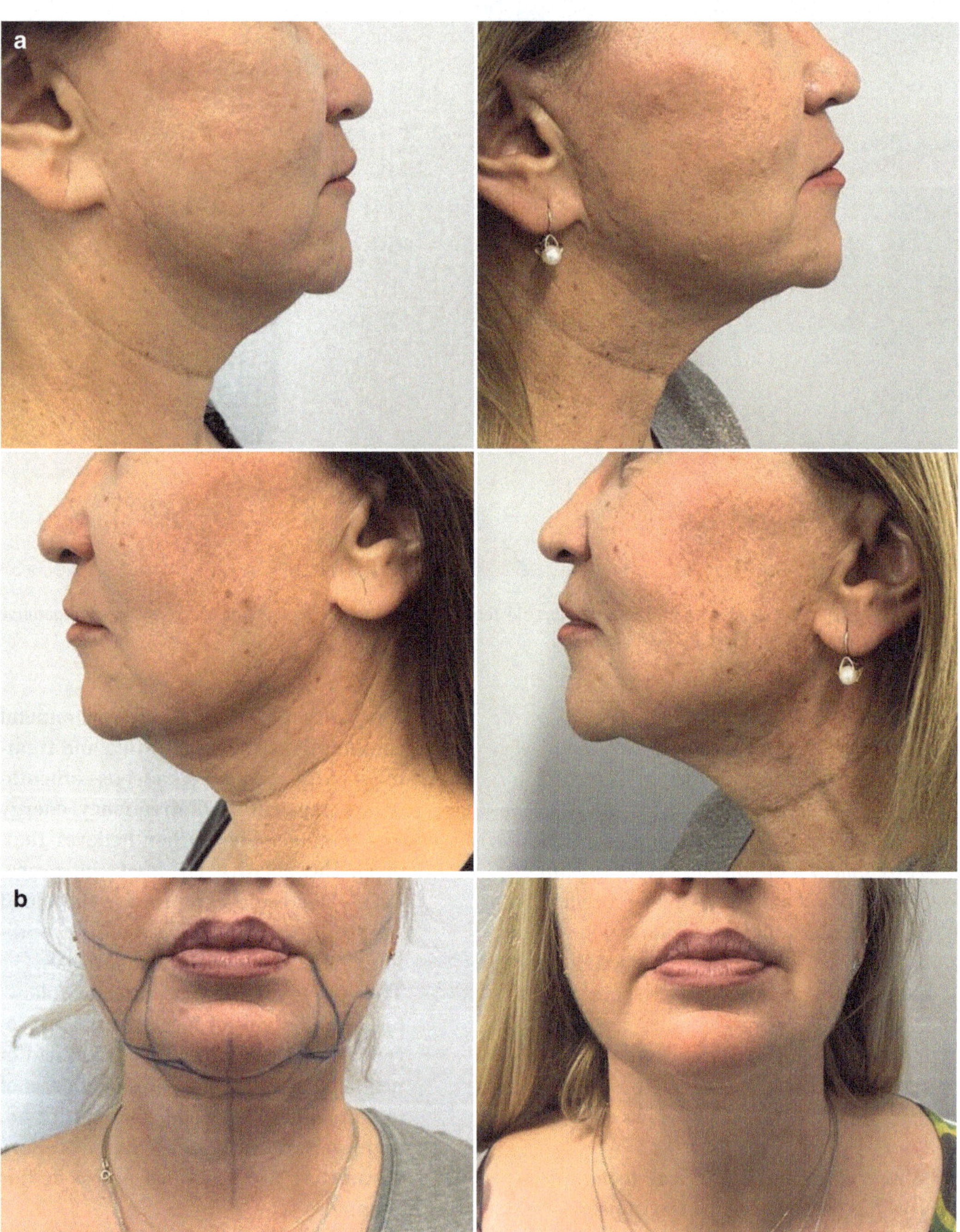

Fig. 18 (**a**) 6 months after FaceTite™ for additional tightening of the skin in a 60-year-old patient done by another surgeon 2 years ago with a facelift procedure. (**b**) 6 months after FaceTite™ for additional tightening of the skin in a 45-year-old patient done by another surgeon 1 year ago with a Facelift procedure

of subcutaneous fat accumulation and 40 °C for additional tightening of the skin. It is recommended after the 6th month in order to optimally assess the contour deformity after the surgery (Fig. 18a, b).

- **Morpheus8™**—3 procedures in between 45 days, starting on the 45th day post op. Additional beneficial impact on the tightening of the skin. Those 3 procedures could be repeated every year for longer lasting results. The parameters are as follows: 4 mm/30–35 energy/3 stacks per place/fixed mode/1 pps/50% overlapping followed by 3 mm/30 energy/2 stacks per place/fixed mode/1 pps 30% of overlapping followed by 2 mm/15 energy/one stack per place/cycle mode.
- **Ultherapy®**—Additional beneficial impact on the tightening of the skin and lasting of the results. Starting from the sixth post op month, two procedures in between 3 months per year could be done. The parameters are described in Chapter 2 'Non-invasive techniques' in this book.

References

1. Locher WG, Feinendegen DL. Aus der Frühzeit der Ästhetischen Chirurgie: Eugen Holländer (1867–1932) und Erich Lexer (1867–1937) als face-lift-Pioniere [the early days of aesthetic surgery: facelift pioneers Eugen Holländer (1867–1932) and Erich Lexer (1967–1937)]. Handchir Mikrochir Plast Chir. 2020;52(6):545–51.
2. Zimbler MS. Tord skoog: face-lift innovator. Arch Facial Plast Surg. 2001;3(1):63.
3. Hamra ST. Composite rhytidectomy. Plast Reconstr Surg. 1992;90:1–13.
4. Barton FE. The SMAS and the nasolabial fold. Plast Reconstr Surg. 1992;89:1054–9.
5. Tonnard P, Verpaele A, Monstrey S, et al. Minimal access cranial suspension lift: a modified S-lift. Plast Reconstr Surg. 2002;109(6):2074–86.
6. Feldman JJ. Corset platysmaplasty. Plast Reconstr Surg. 1990;85(3):333–43.
7. Coleman SR. Long-term survival of fat transplants: controlled demonstrations. Aesthet Plast Surg. 1995;19(5):421–5.
8. Mitz V, Peyronie M. The superficial musculo-aponeurotic system (SMAS) in the parotid and cheek area. Plast Reconstr Surg. 1976;58(1):80–8.
9. Ahmed MH, Couto RA, Duraes EFR, Çakmakoğlu Ç, Swanson M, Surek C, Zins JE. Facelift part I: history, anatomy, and clinical assessment. Aesthet Surg J. 2020;40(1):1–18.
10. McKinney P, Katrana DJ. Prevention of injury to the great auricular nerve during rhytidectomy. Plast Reconstr Surg. 1980;66(5):675–9.
11. Moss CJ, Mendelson BC, Taylor GI. Surgical anatomy of the ligamentous attachments in the temple and periorbital regions. Plast Reconstr Surg. 2000;105(4):1475–90.
12. Muzaffar AR, Mendelson BC, Adams WP Jr. Surgical anatomy of the ligamentous attachments of the lower lid and lateral canthus. Plast Reconstr Surg. 2002;110(3):873–84.
13. Furnas DW. The retaining ligaments of the cheek. Plast Reconstr Surg. 1989;83:11–6.
14. Alghoul M, Bitik O, McBride J, Zins JE. Relationship of the zygomatic facial nerve to the retaining ligaments of the face: the sub-SMAS danger zone. Plast Reconstr Surg. 2013;131(2):245e–52e.
15. Aston SJ. Platysma-SMAS cervicofacial rhytidoplasty. Clin Plast Surg. 1983;10(3):507–20.
16. Stuzin JM, Baker TJ, Gordon HL, Baker TM. Extended SMAS dissection as an approach to midface rejuvenation. Clin Plast Surg. 1995;22(2):295–311.
17. Baker DC. Lateral SMASectomy. Plast Reconstr Surg. 1997;100(2):509–13.
18. Berry MG, Davies D. Platysma-SMAS plication facelift. J Plast Reconstr Aesthet Surg. 2010;63(5):793–800.
19. Patrick T, Alexis V. The MACS-lift short scar rhytidectomy. Aesthet Surg J. 2007;27(2):188–98.
20. Niamtu J III. The art and science of facelift surgery. Philadelphia: Saunders Elsevier; 2019. p. 62–183.
21. Mulholland RS. The BodyTite book. 2nd ed. London: IntechOpen; 2021. p. 227–39.
22. Mulholland RS. Radiofrequency energy for non-invasive and minimally invasive skin tightening. Clin Plast Surg. 2011;38:437–48.
23. Theodorou SJ, Del Vecchio D, Chia CT. Soft tissue contraction in body contouring with radiofrequency-assisted liposuction: a treatment gap solution. Aesthet Surg J. 2018;38:S74–83.
24. Levy AS, Grant RT, Rothaus KO. Radiofrequency physics for minimally invasive aesthetic surgery. Clin Plast Surg. 2016;43:55.

Back Bra Lift with Minimally Invasive Procedures of Neighbouring Areas. Minimally Invasive Procedures of the Back as Isolated Treatment in the Area

Introduction

In the properly selected patient, lipoplasty provides nice improvement in contour, with a relatively low risk of overlying residual skin deformity. Skin in the upper back is robust, with thicker epidermis and dermis to aid in retraction following liposuction. With this, however, fat in the upper back, being thicker and fibrous, can make it relatively more resistant to traditional methods of liposuction. Because of this, many may be candidates for direct excision of this tissue.

The intervention is used to remove cutaneous–subcutaneous excess and lift soft tissues in the back area in the following cases

- In patients after massive weight loss
- In obese patients, in whom the area could be subjected to ultrasound definition with vibration-based liposuction
- In patients with reduced skin elasticity and predominant skin excess as a result of natural processes of ageing
- In patients with previous liposuction

Surgical Techniques/Methods

A. Bra Line Back Lift

Markings are made in the standing position. We utilize a standard six position photographic technique to record the entire lateral and upper back condition. Boundaries of the patient's ideal scar position are confirmed by marking the borders of a bra of the patient's choice. When the final incision line has been determined, bimanual palpation is used to strongly gather the redundant skin and excess adiposity such that this redundancy centres the final incision line. This gathering of tissue is performed at multiple spots across the entire line of resection and marked. These points are then connected as a continuum identifying the final area for resection. Note that the resection is the least in the midline because of the strong zone of adherence there. It is this strong adherence along the spine that permits forces from lower body lifting from having any dramatic effect on the upper back. The resection is strongly tapered into the inframammary fold at the level of the anterior axillary line to avoid a dog ear. Realignment marks are then made across the area for resection to allow for precise realignment intraoperatively. The markings are made with the arms at the patient's side, allowing for the maximum amount of tissue to be gathered to achieve an optimal result [1, 2] (Fig. 1).

An incision is made, and skin and subcutaneous tissue are dissected straight down to the loose areolar plane above the muscle fascia without any undermining. Cutaneous–subcutaneous excesses with elliptical shape are excised. Dissection is performed 3 cm in the

E. Sharkov, *Body Contouring Surgery*, https://doi.org/10.1007/978-3-031-33350-7_16

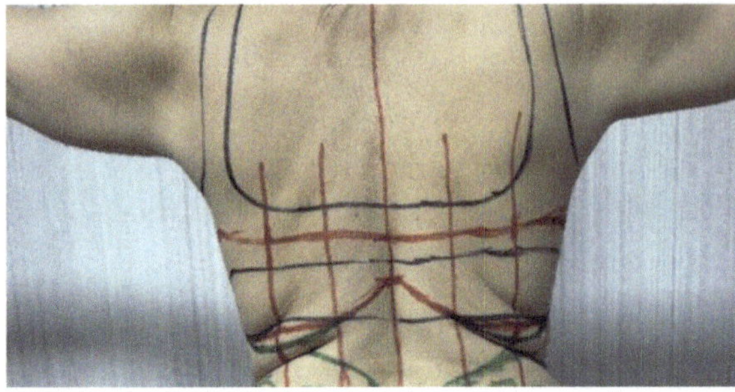

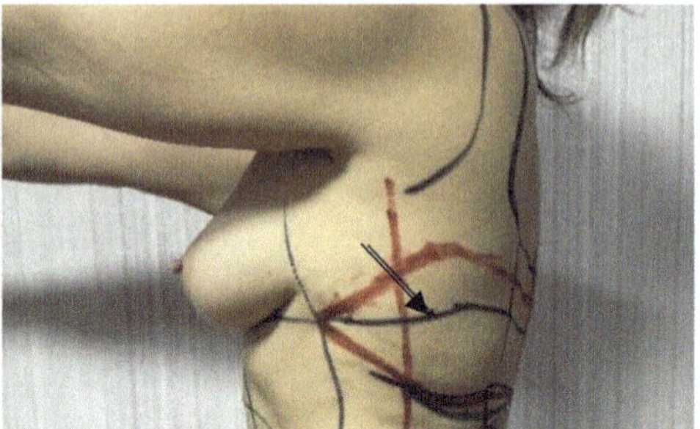

Fig. 1 Preoperative drawing—the black arrow shows the future position of the final scar—it is projected along the course of the inframammary fold. The scar remains hidden in the bra. In anterior aspect, the excision may reach the anterior axillary line

caudal direction, and cranially 1 cm, for the purpose of easier adaptation and lowering the risk of stretching the postoperative cicatrix.

The resection is completed, and skin edges are temporarily aligned with penetrating towel clamps using the realignment marks as reference points. A three-layer closure is then performed starting laterally and progressing towards the spine. This closure is done by taking bites of the superficial fascial system, then underlying muscular fascia, and then the opposite side of the superficial fascia (SFS) [3, 4]. Subcutaneous suture with Vicryl 0, Vicryl 2/0, Vicryl 3/0. Skin suture with Prolene 3/0 (Fig. 2).

B. **VASERlipo® + vibration-assisted liposuction**—The author recommends this type of combination of minimally invasive procedures in cases of a present subcutaneous fat component and preserved skin elastics (Fig. 3). Under general anaesthesia, after infiltration of Klein solution, the tissues are treated with ultrasound energy—80% V mode, superficially, 80% C mode deep with 2 ring probe, after which vibration-assisted liposuction is performed with 3 mm and 4 mm long curved and long bent Mercedes type of cannulas [5].

C. **Bra Line Back Lift in combination with minimally invasive treatment of neighbouring area (ultrasound treatment, followed by vibration assisted liposuction in the area of the flanks)** (Figs. 4, 5 and 6).

The advantages of this approach are as follows

- **Complete contouring in the torso area dorsally (upper back and flanks)**
- **The ultrasound treatment and subsequent lipoaspiration in the area of the flanks provide an additional opportunity to optimally pull the cutaneous–subcutaneous flap in the cranial direction in relation to the Bra Line Back Lift procedure: optimal results in terms of skin excess in the area of the back + reduced tension during the wound closure—reduced risk of dehiscence and reduced risk of dilatation and caudal dislocation of the postoperative scar**
- **The excisional technique in the area of the back leads to additional lifting in the area of the flanks, which reduces the risk of contour irregularities and optimizes the results of the lipoaspiration procedure in this area**
- **Lifting in the area of the back with lipoaspiration procedure in the area of the flanks could limit the length of the postoperative scar in a single-stage or subsequent abdominoplasty**

D. **BodyTite™ radiofrequency treatment of the tissues to tighten the skin and lift the tissues in the area of the back**

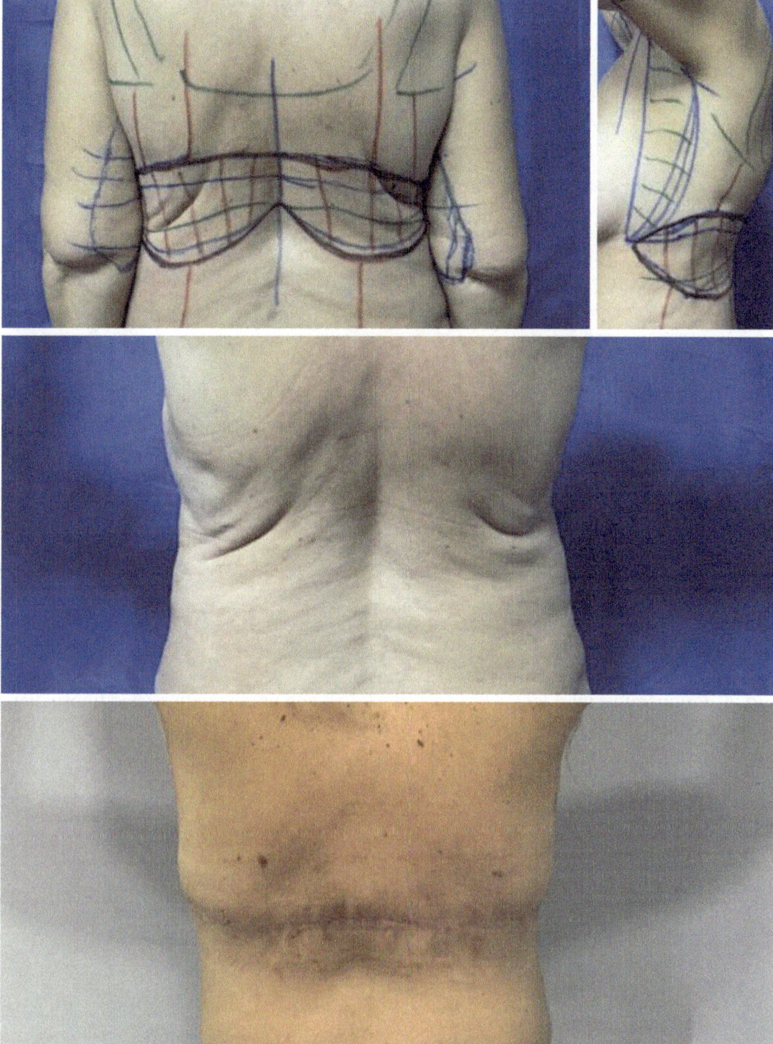

Fig. 2 Bra Line Back Lift in combination with L-type brachioplasty in a 54-year-old female patient with previous liposuction in the area of the back performed in another clinic more than 5 years ago. Demonstration of preoperative drawing with the existing preoperative status and early postoperative outcome with the corresponding position of the postoperative scar—30th postoperative day—early results

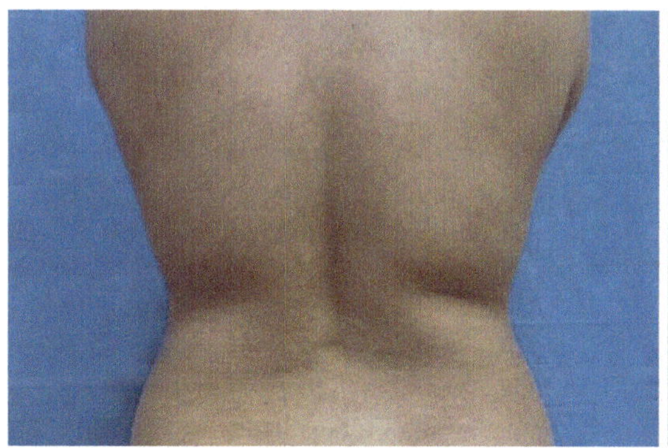

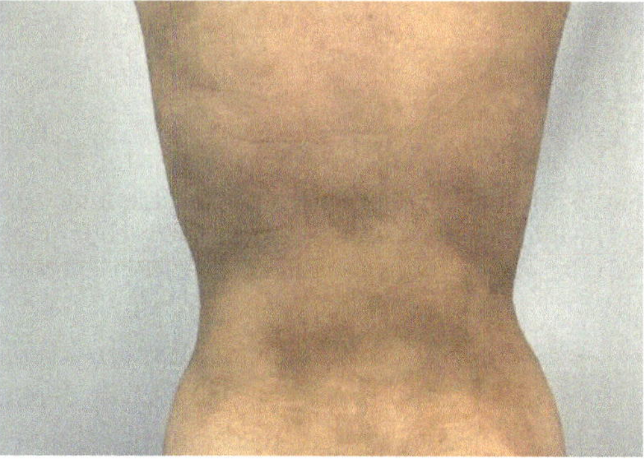

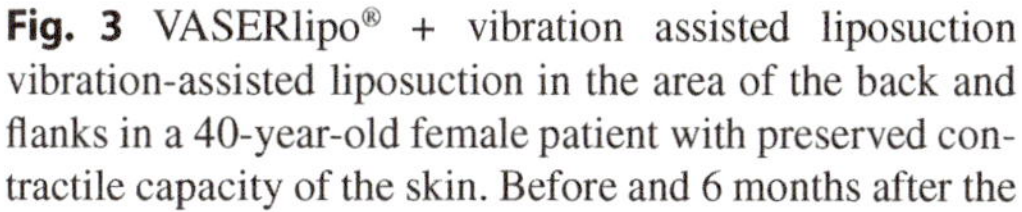

Fig. 3 VASERlipo® + vibration assisted liposuction vibration-assisted liposuction in the area of the back and flanks in a 40-year-old female patient with preserved contractile capacity of the skin. Before and 6 months after the procedure, during which lipoaspiration was performed, respectively, 400 mL of lipoaspirate per side from the area of the flanks and 250 mL per side from the area of the back

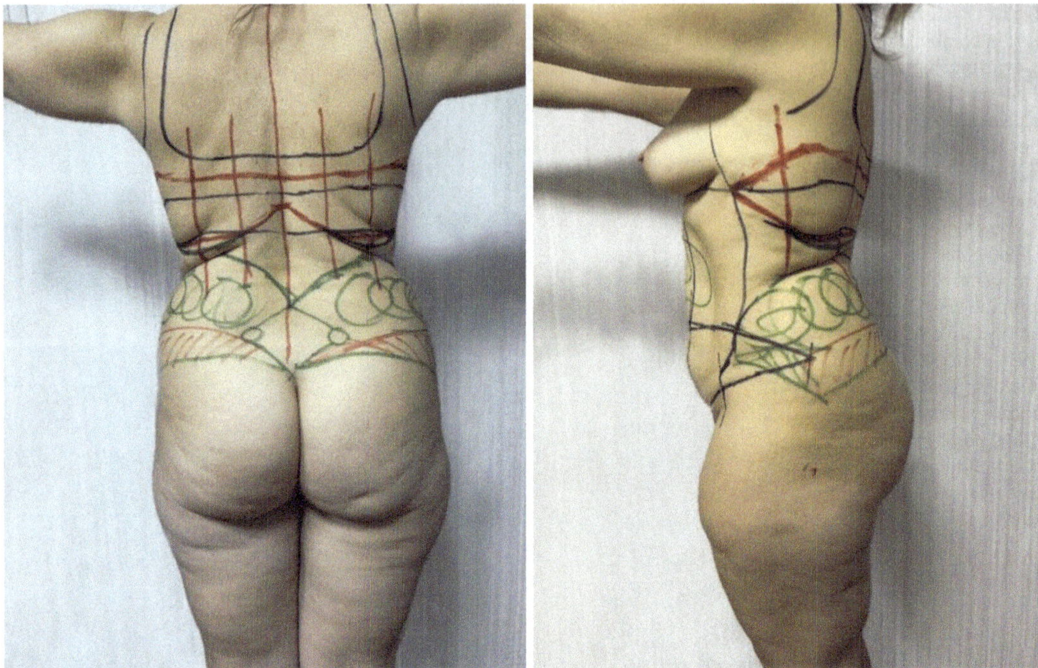

Fig. 4 Preoperative markings—Bra Line Back Lift and ultrasound-assisted liposuction of the flanks. Abdominoplasty was performed in the same stage

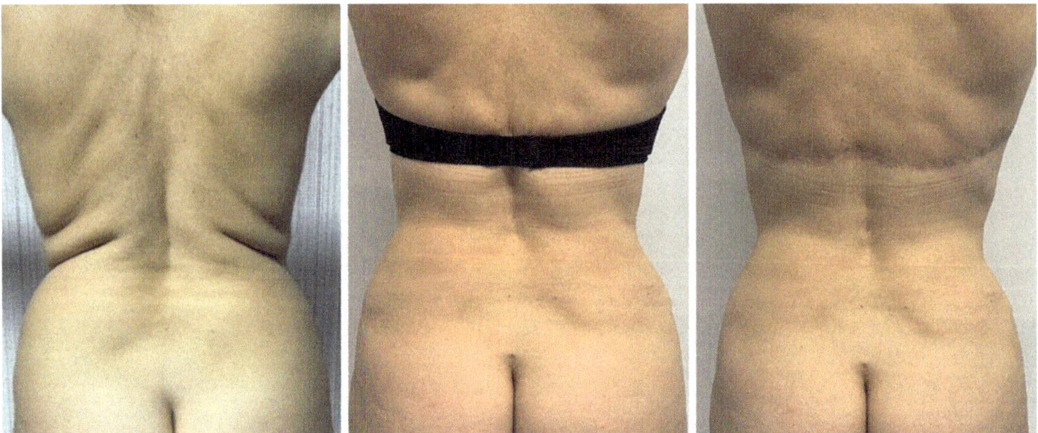

Fig. 5 40-year-old female patient—1 year after surgery—Bra Line Back Lift excisional intervention using the technique described above in the Chapter in combination with VASERlipo® + vibration-assisted liposuction vibration based liposuction of the flanks—450 mL per side. Abdominoplasty was performed in the same stage

- BodyTite—20 W cannula/40 power/40 ext. cut/15–20 kJ energy per side, 2 cm depth. The technique is, respectively, 'lining' (tightening the skin by reaching 40 °C ext. cut off) [6–9]
- The advantage of the procedure is the lifting of the tissue (with a sufficiently good aesthetic outcome in young patients and preserved skin elasticity) without the presence of a large postoperative scar (Fig. 7)
- The procedure could be repeated to optimize the result after the sixth month

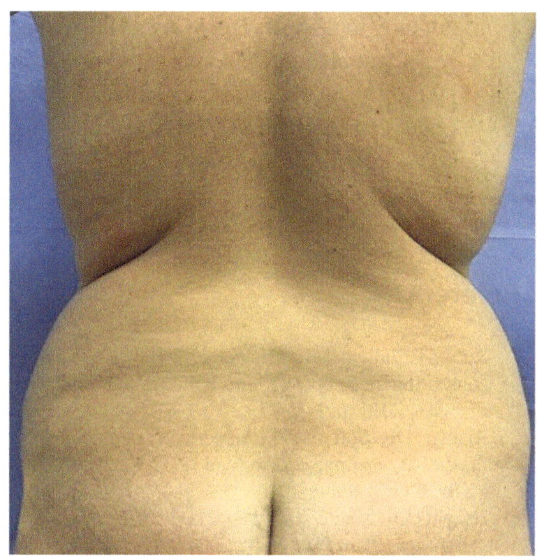
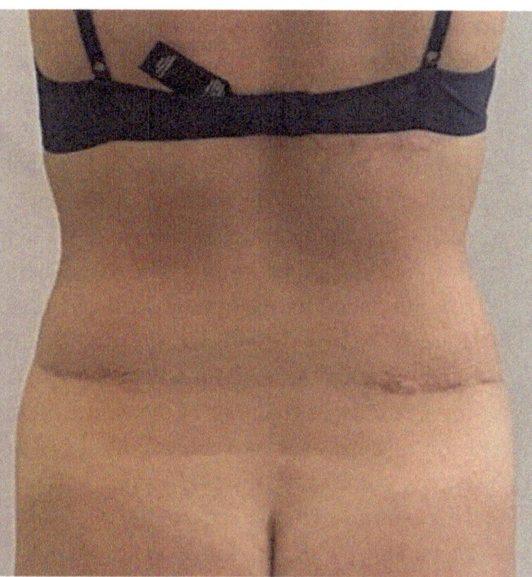

Fig. 6 Preoperative view of a 37-year-old woman with massive weight loss 1 year after surgery—when the preoperative markings have been done properly, there is NO VISIBLE SCAR. Bra Line Back Lift excisional intervention using the technique described above in the Chapter in combination with VASERlipo® + vibration-assisted liposuction vibration-based liposuction of the flanks—500 mL per side. Extended abdominoplasty was performed in the same stage

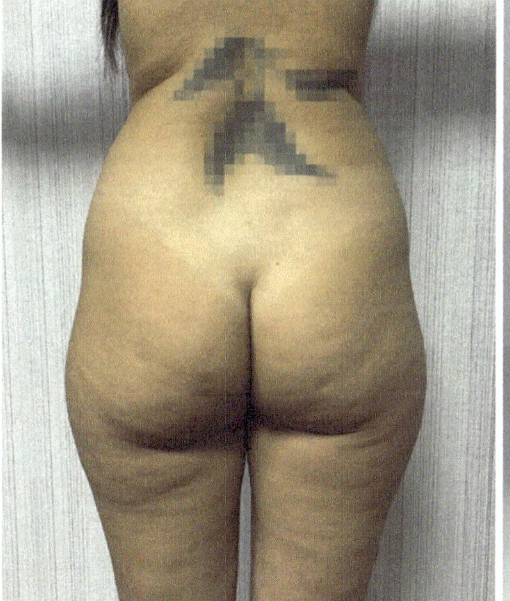
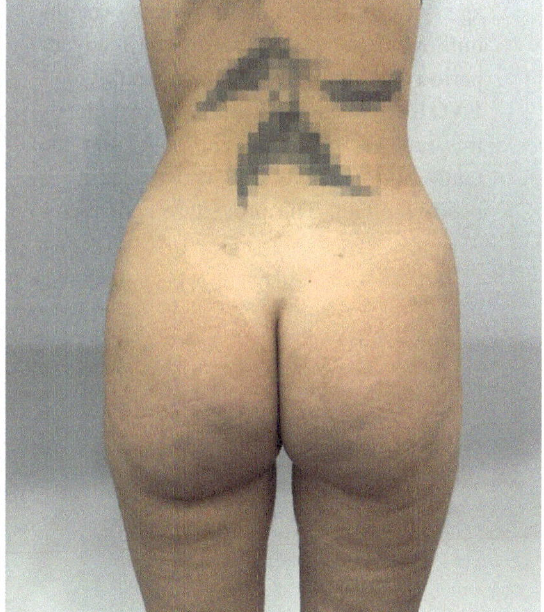

Fig. 7 Sixth postoperative month in a 32-year-old patient after BodyTite™ of the back in combination with BodyTite™ and vibration assisted liposuction in the area of the flanks, outer and inner thighs

- **Secondary procedures:**
  - **BodyTite™** is used to correct contour irregularities and/or additionally tighten the skin in case of available subcutaneous and/or skin excess. In the case of additional need of tightening in the area of the back, such a procedure shouldn't be done sooner than the 6th post op month. The parameters recommended by the author in those cases are as follow—70 °C for destruction of subcutaneous fat accumulation and 40 °C for additional tightening of the skin, and in each case the goal is to achieve 15–20 kJ of energy per 10 cm^2 of treated area.
  - **Ultrasound procedures**
  - In patients without skin excision—in the area of the flanks during combined treatment of the back and flanks—an ultrasound massage with parameters 1.5 W/cm^2, frequency 3 MHz and duration of treatment of the respective area of 5 min, for a period of 10 days, starting from the tenth postoperative day. The process accelerates the drainage of oedema and improves venous outflow, thereby accelerating the recovery period and improving the final results.
  - **EVOLVE X™**—The author recommends this type of intervention to start after the tenth postoperative day when seeking a positive effect. The procedure contributes not only to the faster recovery of the treated areas, but also to achieving optimal results by tightening the underlying muscles, additional fat resorption and tightening the skin.

References

1. Rubin P, Jellew ML, Richter DF, Uebel CO. Body contouring and liposuction. Philadelphia: Saunders Elsevier; 2013. p. 149–77.
2. Richter DF, Soft A. The upper lateral thoracic lift. Plastic surgery pulse news, vol. 2. St Louis: Quality Medical Publishing; 2010.
3. Hurwitz DJ. Single-staged total body lift after massive weight loss. Ann Plast Surg. 2004;52(5):435–41.
4. Aly AS. Body contouring after massive weight loss. St Louis: Quality Medical Publishing; 2006.
5. Hoyos AE, Prendergast PM. High definition body sculpting, vol. 129. Berlin: Springer; 2014. p. 147–55.
6. Mulholland RS. The BodyTite book. 2nd ed. London: IntechOpen; 2021. p. 227–39.
7. Mulholland RS. Radiofrequency energy for non-invasive and minimally invasive skin tightening. Clin Plast Surg. 2011;38:437–48.
8. Theodorou SJ, Del Vecchio D, Chia CT. Soft tissue contraction in body contouring with radiofrequency-assisted liposuction: a treatment gap solution. Aesthet Surg J. 2018;38:S74–83.
9. Levy AS, Grant RT, Rothaus KO. Radiofrequency physics for minimally invasive aesthetic surgery. Clin Plast Surg. 2016;43:55.

Complications of Minimally Invasive Procedures

Complications

Thermal Injury [1]

The above-mentioned radiofrequency procedures for tissue treatment may have an undesirable effect in the form of thermal injury, if an incorrect approach is used by the surgeon.

If a thermal effect is present, it can be *in the area distal from the entry point, in the area of the entry point, proximal to the entry point, in the area of the postoperative cicatrix in combined procedures*.

In the Area Distal from the Entry Point

Cause—Too superficial treatment of the tissues; supply of radiofrequency energy during antegrade movement of the cannula; non-compliance with the parameters reached and the signal sent by the equipment, which has safety features and provides adequate visual and auditory signal when the set temperature is reached; 'unstretched' skin in the area of treatment; insufficient ultrasound gel on the skin surface during tissue treatment.

Prophylaxis and prevention—When treating tissues, the surgeon should work at an adequate depth subcutaneously—the tip of the internal probe should not be visible and seen through the skin; the energy should be supplied by means of 'lining or stamping' technique only retrograde; compliance by the operator with the auditory and visual signals from the equipment when the preset parameters are reached, and the tissues can be further evaluated regarding their heating and warming by palpation and/or by means of an additional thermal camera; during the procedure the skin surface should be stretched and smooth, which can be done both by the operator with his non-dominant hand and by the assistant, and the treated area should be well covered with ultrasound gel.

Therapy—In most of the cases, applying dressings with local treatment and secondary healing process provides satisfactory results. In cases where the skin layers are affected in depth, excision and secondary suture with/without local or other type of plastic surgery procedure is required, as the author does not report such cases in his practice and considers their probability as casuistry and poor knowledge of the technique by the operator.

In the Area of the Entry Point

Cause, prophylaxis and prevention—inaccurate supply of energy and heating in the area of the entry point. The prevention of this type of injury consists in the use of an adequate technique by the operator, in which, supplying the energy slowly retrograde, the application is stopped 0.5 cm before the entry point.

Therapy—In most of the cases, applying dressings with local treatment and secondary healing process provides satisfactory results. In cases where the skin layers are affected in depth, excision and secondary suture with/without local

E. Sharkov, *Body Contouring Surgery*, https://doi.org/10.1007/978-3-031-33350-7_17

or other type of plastic surgery procedure is required, as the author does not report such cases in his practice and considers their probability as casuistry and poor knowledge of the technique by the operator.

Proximal to the Entry Point

Cause, prophylaxis and prevention—The cause of this type of injury can be associated with the inaccurate supply of energy and heating in the area proximal to the entry point. The prevention consists in the use of an adequate type of handpiece—new generation handpieces for BodyTite™, FaceTite™, and AccuTite™ have a coated internal probe.

In the Area of the Postoperative Scar in Combined Procedures

Cause—The ablative effect of radiofrequency energy and an aggressive approach by the operator around thinned soft tissue flap (Fig. 1).

Prophylaxis and prevention—To supply energy at least 2–3 cm distal from the postoperative scar in cases of combined excisional-radiofrequency procedures. For optimal prevention and prophylaxis at this stage, the author recommends, when combining an excisional procedure and a radiofrequency procedure, the latter to be applied with Morpheus8™ or Morpheus8 Body™, and in second stage, after minimum 6 months to approach with BodyTite™, FaceTite™, AccuTite™, if necessary.

Therapy—Excision and secondary suture with/without local or other type of plastic is required.

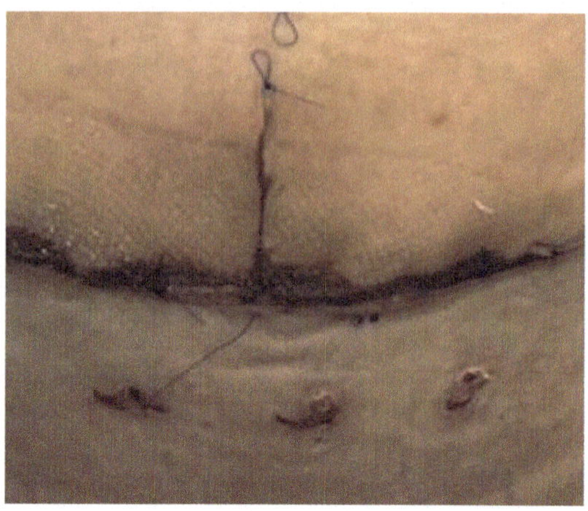

Fig. 1 Scar necrosis in a female patient with abdominoplasty in combination with BodyTite™. On the 45th postoperative day, an excision was performed with refreshing the edges of the defect and secondary suture

Fibrotic Nodules

Cause—When the energy is applied through one or a small number of entry points, the treated area will receive the necessary amount of energy, but all this amount will also accumulate at the respective entry point, which will lead to fibrous compaction of the same [1].

Prophylaxis and prevention—supply energy through several entry points.

Therapy—corticosteroid injection procedure.

Postoperative Oedema and Swelling

Cause—Inflammatory tissue induration and/or residual subcutaneous fat.

Prevention and prophylaxis—The author recommends for prevention purposes: lipoaspiration after radiofrequency melting of subcutaneous fat, when this is indicated for the specific patient; elastic compression in the area—5 days in the neck area and 14 days in the body area, 24 h a day; after the fifth day in the neck area—massages for lymphatic drainage 2 times a day for 5 min per side/ultrasound massage with parameters 1.5 W/cm^2, frequency 3 MHz and duration of 5 min, for a period of 10 days, starting from the 1st postoperative day—body areas. The process accelerates the drainage of oedema and improves venous outflow, thereby accelerating the recovery period and improving the final results.

Therapy—Electromyostimulation and massages for lymphatic drainage; ultrasound procedures; in case of inflammatory process—incision, drainage, local anti-inflammatory therapy and systematic antibiotic therapy, if necessary.

Neurapraxia

Cause—in most cases it is a temporary effect of the applied local infiltration anaesthesia and/or thermal and/or radiofrequency 'irritation' of the respective nerve branches [1]. In all cases it is completely temporary.

Prevention and prophylaxis—To avoid the so-called NGA in the areas of the face, which are described in Chapter Facelift of the textbook.

Therapy—In his practice, the author reports two cases of disturbances in the motility and sensitivity of the corner of the mouth, as in both cases the disturbances disappeared in 14 days and 30 days, respectively. The applied therapy is only Milgamma N (vitB12 complex) tablets, one tablet 3 times a day for 14 days. The author believes that any disturbance in the sensory and/or motor innervation of treated areas is entirely temporary and reversible due to the nature of the procedure.

Insufficiently Satisfactory Result

The procedure can be applied again 6 months after the first intervention to optimize the results.

Inflammations and Infections

The author follows a work protocol with intra- and postoperative antibiotic prophylaxis Ciprofloxacin 2 × 500 mg daily for 7 days.

Hematomas

Cause—A possible complication when the procedure is combined with lipoaspiration techniques and/or excisional procedures.

Prophylaxis and prevention—Awareness regarding the medications routinely taken by the patient; intraoperative haemostasis; use of **tranexamic acid** in the infiltration solution when performing procedures in the body area; postoperative compression; drainage in combination with excisional procedure.

Therapy—In most cases, no additional therapy is required, except in cases of significant collections, which would require puncture of liquefied hematoma in the late postoperative period.

Seromas

Cause, prophylaxis and prevention, therapy—When treating large areas, seromas can be observed in combination with excisional and/or lipoaspiration technique. Adequate postoperative compression in the treated area for the indicated period of time is essential. Significant amounts as a collection may require single or repeated puncture and evacuation of the collection.

Morpheus8™, Morpheus8 Body™, Morpheus prime™

Thermal Injury

Cause—Thermal injury is possible in case of dried blood on the tip; moist skin surface; use of chlorhexidine to clean the skin surface; poor contact between the tip and the skin surface.

Prophylaxis and prevention—The skin of the treated area is cleaned with an alcohol-containing disinfectant and chlorhexidine is not used; the skin surface is dry; periodic cleaning of the tip surface during the procedure; good contact between the tip and the skin surface.

Therapy—applying epithelializing agents in combination with antibiotic and corticosteroid therapy topical—Fusicort, Epithelial Duo Cream, Cicatridina cream.

Fibrous Nodules

Cause—The author considers the treatment of highly thinned skin with high energy surface parameters (depth of 1 mm and energy over 25 kJ) as a possible cause of this type of complication.

Prophylaxis and prevention—To treat such type of skin at a depth of 2 mm with parameters of the set energy up to 15 kJ and operation in cycle mode. In a subsequent procedure and adequate recovery with no side effects, the parameters can be increased to 20 kJ.

Therapy—Corticosteroid injection procedures.

Pigmentations

Cause—Non-observance of post-procedural instructions and exposure to sun in the early period after the procedure.

Prophylaxis and prevention—To use of 50+ sun protection factor and non-exposure to direct sunlight in the next 14 days.

Therapy—Laser procedures aimed at erasing pigmentations—picosecond laser.

VASERlipo® Ultrasound Procedures

Thermal Injury

If a thermal effect is present, it could be *in the area distal from the entry point, in the area of the entry point, proximal to the entry point, in the area of the postoperative cicatrix in combined procedures* [2].

In the Area Distal from the Entry Point

Cause—superficial treatment of the tissues; excessive accumulation of energy along the same subcutaneous 'tunnel' of treatment; exceeding the duration of treatment of the area and not complying with the amount of infiltrated solution.

Prophylaxis and prevention—the tip of the cannula should not be visible and seen through the skin; the energy should be supplied by means of 'fanning' technique; 1 min treatment of the tissues per 100 mL infiltrated solution.

Therapy—in most of the cases, applying dressings with local treatment and secondary healing process provides satisfactory results. In cases where the skin layers are affected in depth, excision and secondary suture with/without local or other type of plastic surgery procedure is required.

In the Area of the Entry Point

Cause, prophylaxis and prevention—The cause of this type of injury can be associated with the inaccurate supply of energy and heating in the area of the entry point. The prevention consists in the use of adequate technique and local protection by cooling with a gauze compress irrigated with saline in the area between the cannula and the skin.

Therapy—In most of the cases, applying dressings with local treatment and secondary healing process provides satisfactory results. In cases where the skin layers are affected in depth, excision and secondary suture with/without local or other type of plastic surgery procedure is required, as the author does not report such cases in his practice and considers their probability as casuistry and poor knowledge of the technique by the operator.

Proximal to the Entry Point

Cause, prophylaxis and prevention—inaccurate supply of energy and heating in the area proximal to the entry point. The prevention consists in the use of adequate technique and local protection by cooling with a gauze compress irrigated with saline in the area between the cannula and the skin.

Therapy—In most of the cases, applying dressings with local treatment and secondary healing process provides satisfactory results. In cases where the skin layers are affected in depth, excision and secondary suture with/without local or other type of plastic surgery procedure is required, as the author does not report such cases in his practice and considers their probability as casuistry and poor knowledge of the technique by the operator.

In the Area of the Postoperative Scar in Combined Procedures

Cause—An aggressive approach by the operator in the area of a thinned cutaneous–subcutaneous flap.

Prophylaxis and prevention—To supply energy at least 1.0 cm distal from the postoperative scar in cases of combined excisional-ultrasound procedures.

Therapy—Excision and secondary suture with/without local or other type of plastic is required. Hyperbaric therapy can also be used for hard-to-heal wounds (Figs. 2 and 3).

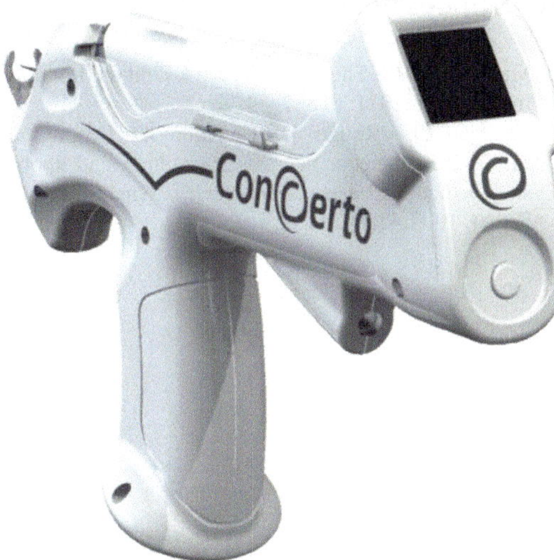

Fig. 2 CONCERTO®—The author uses the protocol described above for therapy of fibrous adhesions by means of carboxytherapy

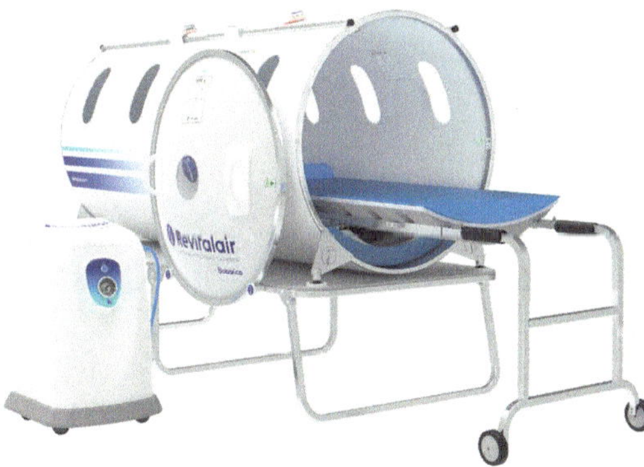

Fig. 3 Revitalair® hyperbaric therapy is the author's hyperbaric therapy for hard-to-heal wounds

Adhesions

Cause—Exceeding the necessary amount of ultrasound energy in the treated area.

Prophylaxis and prevention—The supplied ultrasound energy should provide an optimal effect, and at the end of treatment of the area there should be no resistance to the movement of the cannula in the subcutaneous tissue. This will provide an optimal effect regarding the desired result, but the duration of treatment should not drastically exceed the above-mentioned 1 min per 100 mL of infiltrated solution.

Therapy—The author uses carboxytherapy (Fig. 2). The protocol is as follows:

- Injections at around 3–5 mm depth (according to the volume)
- Point of injection 2 cc (you can increase to point 5 cc, if the patient well accepts it)
- Sessions per week
- From 6 to 12 sessions according to the need

Vibration-Based Liposuction

Contour Irregularities

Cause—Insufficient experience of the surgeon.

Prophylaxis and prevention—The author uses 3 mm and 4 mm curved and bent Mercedes type cannulas; the areas are treated by means of 'criss-cross' for smoother results; the areas are treated by means of ultrasound, which liquefies the fat and helps to achieve an optimal result by minimizing the likelihood of postoperative contour irregularities; precise sparing approach to the superficial fat component.

Therapy

A. **in case of 'bulging'—BodyTite™, FaceTite™, AccuTite™** are used to correct contour irregularities It is recommended to use the specified tip depending on the area of the surgical defect, as in the case of a significant defect—the BodyTite cannula is used and in the case of a smaller or minimal deformity—the FaceTite and AccuTite cannulas are, respectively, used. The goal is to reach the following parameters: 70 °C for destruction of subcutaneous fat deposits and 40 °C for additional tightening of the skin, and in each case the goal is to achieve 8–10 kJ of energy per 10 cm^2 of treated area. It is recommended after the sixth month to optimally assess the contour deformity.

B. **In Case of Sagging—Lipofilling**
The author uses the **LipoCube™** (Fig. 4) technology for maximum purification of the extracted fat.

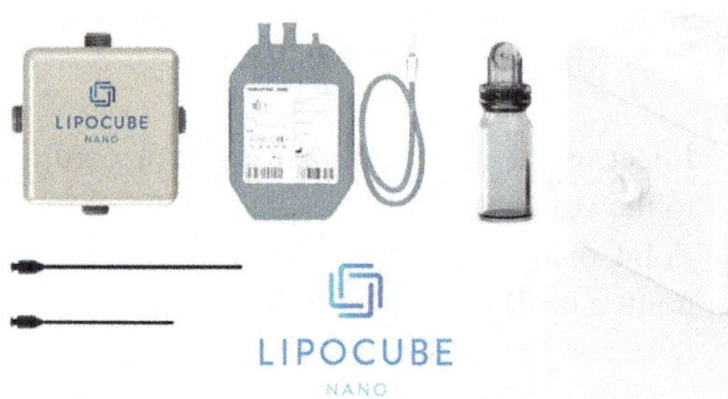

Fig. 4 LipoCube™ technology for purification of extracted fat

References

1. Mulholland RS. The BodyTite book. 2nd ed. London: IntechOpen; 2021. p. 857–74.
2. Grolleau JL, Rouge D, Chavoin JP, Costagliola M. Severe cutaneous necrosis after ultrasound lipolysis. Medicolegal aspects and review. Ann Chir Plast Esthet. 1997;42(1):31–6.

Algorithm in Times of COVID for Adequate Approach in the Preoperative Evaluation Before Body Contouring Surgery

Algorithm

The Author Used Cluster Analysis Using the K-Means Cluster Method

Two variables were selected to be used for this analysis which have no relationship between each other—they are the body mass index (BMI) and the age of the respondents.

In this approach, the number of clusters to be obtained is predetermined. After several attempts, the optimal number of groups was reached, namely five in total:

Initial cluster centres					
	Cluster				
	Cluster 1	Cluster 2	Cluster 3	Cluster 4	Cluster 5
BMI	35.25	25.70	60.00	28.30	33.50
Age	41.00	29.00	42.00	67.00	16.00

Final cluster centres					
	Cluster				
	Cluster 1	Cluster 2	Cluster 3	Cluster 4	Cluster 5
BMI	26.44	23.72	54.95	26.93	25.59
Age	50.19	33.68	40.00	52.46	27.59

Number of cases in each cluster		
Cluster	Cluster 1	69.000
	Cluster 2	85.000
	Cluster 3	2.000
	Cluster 4	24.000
	Cluster 5	54.000
Valid		234.000
Missing		0.000

As can be seen from the analysis, the five clusters obtained of these two variables can be characterized as follows:

Cluster 1: This group includes 69 individuals. They have average BMI values of around 26, but are at a relatively high average age—50 years.

Cluster 2: This is the group with the highest relative share of all groups—it includes 85 individuals, which is more than a third of the studied population. This group includes individuals at an average age of 33–34 years, who have the lowest BMI compared to all other groups—23.7.

Cluster 3: Only 2 cases are included here, which can be considered as exceptions because of the extremely high BMI values. In general, this cluster will not be studied in the further analysis due to the small number of cases in it.

Cluster 4: This group includes 24 individuals of the studied population. The average age is high—52.5 years, and BMI is higher than the average for the population and higher than all other clusters (except for the extreme Cluster 3).

Cluster 5: This group includes 54 individuals. The BMI value is close to the average, but this is the group with the lowest average age—27–28 years.

E. Sharkov, *Body Contouring Surgery*, https://doi.org/10.1007/978-3-031-33350-7_18

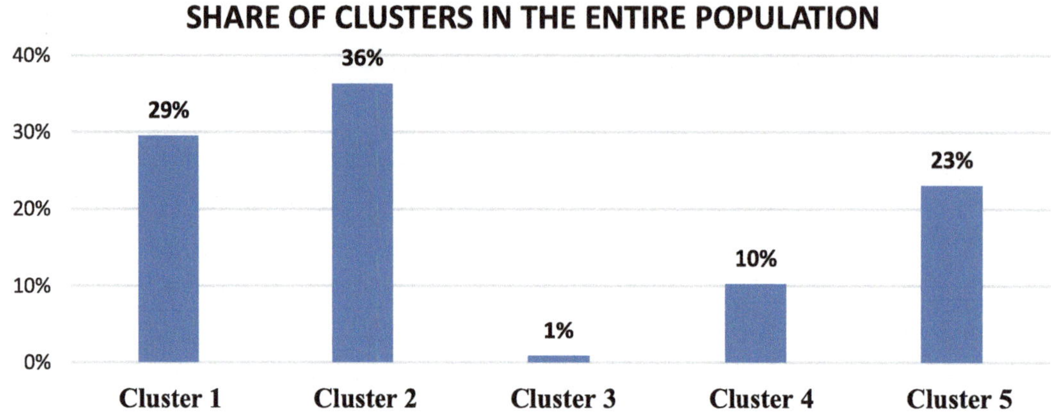

Table 1 Previous interventions by clusters

%	Cluster 1	Cluster 2	Cluster 4	Cluster 5	Totally
Previous plastic surgery intervention	30%	26%	21%	20%	25%
	21	22	5	11	59
					–
Bariatric surgery	1%	1%	33%	0%	4%
	1	1	8	0	10
			A B E		–
Surgical intervention other than plastic surgery	22%	35%	13%	4%	22%
	15	30	3	2	51
	e	E			–
No previous surgical intervention	46%	38%	33%	76%	49%
	32	32	8	41	114
				a B d	–
Column name	**A**	**B**	**D**	**E**	**F**

The author checks how these groups behave according to all the variables in the database used (previous interventions; method of losing weight; preoperative local status; diagnosis, surgical protocol—respectively Tables 1, 2, 3, 4 and 5). The idea is to construct a model that can be used to predict the expected diagnosis and surgical protocol based only on different demographic and preoperative criteria.

Only those variables are presented by the author below, in which we observe significant statistical differences, excluding Cluster 3:

Result—Comparing with all other clusters, Cluster 4, consisting of 24 individuals with an average BMI value of 26.9 and an average age of 52.46, has undergone predominantly bariatric procedures. The conclusion that can be drawn is that patients with previous bariatric intervention are mostly patients around 50 years of age and with a prevailing BMI of 26.9, which is classified as overweight, but not obesity.

Result—Cluster 1 are patients who lost weight only by dietary regimen. Those patients are more than all other clusters regarding the choice of this type of weight loss in terms of statistical significance. The conclusion is that the dietary regimen is main choice as a weight loss method for patients around 50 years and with BMI value of 26.44.

Result—Bariatric interventions are statistically the main choice as a weight loss method in Cluster 4, with an average age of 52.46 and a BMI value of 26.93, compared to all other clusters. The conclusion can be drawn that Cluster 1 and Cluster 4, which include patients around 50 years of age and BMI values around 26/over-

Table 2 Weight loss method by clusters

%	Cluster 1	Cluster 2	Cluster 4	Cluster 5	Totally
Dietary regimen	44%	20%	0%	24%	27%
	30	17	0	13	62
	b D e	d		d	–
Physical regimen	0%	1%	0%	0%	0%
	0	1	0	0	1
					–
Dietary and physical regimen	0%	76%	67%	0%	35%
	0	65	16	0	81
		A E	A E		–
Bariatric intervention	0%	2%	33%	0%	4%
	0	2	8	0	10
			A B E		–
No weight reduction	56%	0%	0%	76%	34%
	38	0	0	41	79
	B D			a B D	–
Column name	**A**	**B**	**D**	**E**	**F**

Table 3 Preoperative local status by clusters

%	Cluster 1	Cluster 2	Cluster 4	Cluster 5	Totally
Soft-tissue ptosis	44%	98%	71%	24%	62%
	30	83	17	13	145
	e	A D E	a E		–
Soft-tissue ptosis with a predominant skin component	0%	2%	29%	0%	4%
	0	2	7	0	9
			A B E		–
Fat deposits	56%	0%	0%	76%	34%
	38	0	0	41	79
	B D			a B D	–
Column name	**A**	**B**	**D**	**E**	**F**

weight/ achieve weight loss by dietary regimen and/or bariatric intervention.

Result—Patients without weight reduction are predominantly present in Cluster 5 in terms of statistical significance. The conclusion is that patients at a young age (27.59) approach surgical interventions for the purpose of contouring the body without weight reduction.

The table thus presented shows the following results and conclusions

- Patients with 'soft tissue ptosis' from Cluster 2 are higher number in terms of statistical significance comparing with other clusters. The conclusion that can be drawn is that these are patients of active age, around 33 years, who have normal BMI values (23.72) through a dietary and physical regimen, as in cases where surgical correction is performed, it is due to 'soft tissue ptosis'.
- In Cluster 4, at an average age of 52.46 years, the soft-tissue ptosis with a prevailing skin component is more in terms of statistical significance compared to the same preoperative finding in representatives of the other clusters. In Cluster 1, at an average age of 50 years, the fat deposits are more in terms of statistical significance compared to the same finding in representatives of Cluster 4. The conclusion is that in patients at an average age of 50 years (Cluster 1 and Cluster 4), the dietary regimen (without accompanying physical regimen) and/or bariatric intervention are the main choice of body weight reduction, as in the second case the soft-

Table 4 Diagnosis by clusters

%	Cluster 1	Cluster 2	Cluster 4	Cluster 5	Totally
Cutis laxa. St.p. MWL	0%	7%	17%	0%	4%
	0	6	4	0	10
			a e		–
Venter propendens	22%	48%	54%	4%	31%
	15	41	13	2	73
	e	A E	a E		–
Ptosis gl.m.bill	16%	26%	13%	13%	18%
	11	22	3	7	43
					–
Lipomatosis	48%	4%	0%	61%	29%
	33	3	0	33	69
	B D			B D	–
Gynecomastia	3%	1%	0%	19%	6%
	2	1	0	10	13
				a b	–
Other	12%	14%	17%	4%	11%
	8	12	4	2	26
					–
Column name	**A**	**B**	**D**	**E**	**F**

Table 5 Surgical protocol by clusters

%	Cluster 1	Cluster 2	Cluster 4	Cluster 5	Totally
Abdominoplasty	25%	54%	63%	4%	35%
	17	46	15	2	82
	e	A E	a E		–
Mastopexy	16%	25%	8%	13%	18%
	11	21	2	7	41
					–
Breast contouring in men	4%	4%	4%	19%	7%
	3	3	1	10	17
				b	–
Liposuction	45%	1%	0%	61%	28%
	31	1	0	33	65
	B D			B D	–
Other	10%	16%	25%	4%	12%
	7	14	6	2	29
			e		–
Column name	**A**	**B**	**D**	**E**	**F**

tissue ptosis, with a predominant skin component, is a mandatory finding. Patients who rely only on a diet will have fat deposits, and as a consequence, not so satisfactory results in terms of aesthetics from the applied surgical interventions for contouring the body.

Based on the presented data, we can make the following model:

Cluster 1: This group includes individuals with average BMI values of around 26, at a relatively high average age—50 years, without weight reduction or with weight loss only with a dietary regimen, with preoperative local status—fat deposits or soft-tissue ptosis

Cluster 2: This group includes mainly individuals at the age of about 33–34 years, with low BMI, who may have undergone a surgical intervention other than plastic surgery; they have lost weight mainly with a dietary and physical regimen, and are present with soft-tissue ptosis

Cluster 3: A very rare group of patients—their main characteristic is an extremely high BMI

Cluster 4: A relatively high average age—52.5 years, high BMI; they have undergone a previous bariatric surgery or they have lost weight through a dietary and physical regimen; they have either soft-tissue ptosis (similar to Cluster 2) or, when bariatric procedure has been done, soft-tissue ptosis with a prevailing skin component

Cluster 5: This group includes mainly young people under 30 years, with BMI around 25.59, almost certainly with no previous surgical intervention or only a previous plastic surgical intervention, with no weight reduction or weight loss only with a dietary regimen and almost necessarily with fat accumulations

Thus, it is possible to predict a probable diag nosis and surgical protocol based only on the described preoperative indicators:

The following results can be derived from the table thus presented and the logical sequence of the above-described cluster dependencies

- Cluster 2, active young people at an average age of 33, who most often choose a combined dietary and physical regimen for weight reduction, as a result of which, in cases where they seek a plastic intervention for body contouring, it is in order to remove the excess skin and subcutaneous tissue as a preoperative finding, respectively, the cases with 'Venter propendens' are more compared to the other Clusters 1 and 5 in terms of statistical significance.
- Cluster 1 includes patients at an average age of about 50, who choose, statistically significantly more than any other weight loss option, a dietary regimen as an isolated option without combination with a physical regimen. This leads to a preoperative finding of fat deposits; therefore, the patients with a preoperative finding of 'lipomatosis' are more compared to Clusters 2 and 4 in terms of statistical significance.
- Cluster 4 again includes patients at an average age of about 50, which makes them a group similar to that of Cluster 1, but in this case, these are patients who choose a bariatric intervention for weight reduction, which is most often due to the impossibility of choosing another option associated with previous overweight. Logically, the preoperative finding is associated with cutaneous–subcutaneous excess with a predominant skin component; therefore, patients with 'Venter propendens' are more than Cluster 5 in terms of statistical significance.
- Cluster 5 includes patients at a young age of about 28 years, most often without or with an insignificant weight reduction; therefore, the preoperative finding is associated with more patients with 'lipomatosis' compared to Clusters 2 and 4 in terms of statistical significance.

Based on the results, the following conclusions can be made

- 'Venter propendens' predominates as a diagnosis in patients (Cluster 2) at an average age of 33 years, who have reached an average BMI value of 23.72 through dietary and physical regimen, compared to patients aged around 50 years (Cluster 1), who have reached a BMI value of 26.44 through dietary regimen, as well as compared to young patients (Cluster 5) without reduction in weight. While in the second case, this is explainable (due to the younger age and preserved skin elasticity in Cluster 5, lipomatosis is the leading finding), the statistically significant difference of the finding in Cluster 2 and Cluster 1 can be explained as insufficient weight reduction when choosing only a dietary regimen, which leads to insufficient soft-tissue ptosis and, accordingly, the leading preoperative finding—lipomatosis.

- In Cluster 4, which, despite its similarity with Cluster 1 in terms of age characteristics and average BMI values, patients are again with the leading diagnosis of 'venter propendens', which can be explained by the fact that the choice of surgical intervention—'bariatric intervention' has resulted in massive weight loss, in contrast with Cluster 1.
- Cluster 5 includes young people, and Cluster 1—people at an average age of 50 years, and despite the different choice of weight reduction, they have the leading diagnosis of 'lipomatosis' in statistically significant cases both as number and as percentage ratio.

Derivation of an algorithm of behaviour in surgical and organizational aspect based on anamnestic and physical data.

Based on the last table and all the results and conclusions made above, the following indicative model can be summarized to guide the expectations of the medical team for a possible probable diagnosis and surgical protocol—an immediate benefit in times of online consultations and pandemic conditions:

- Cluster 2 consists of active young people, who have chosen a dietary and physical regimen leading to cutaneous–subcutaneous excess in different parts of the body (statistically significant mostly in the abdominal area), and who are presented with the predominant diagnosis of venter propendens; due to this, the 'abdominoplasty' intervention is statistically significant compared to Cluster 1 and Cluster 5. Therefore, representatives of Cluster 2 are most likely to undergo liposuction, which is directly related to their age, BMI, and weight loss method.
- Cluster 1 consists of patients at an average age of 50 years, who have chosen an isolated dietary regimen as a weight loss method, which in most cases leads to an unsatisfactory results; and, therefore, this type of patients have a finding of fat deposits, respectively, 'lipomatosis', and are more likely to undergo liposuction for contouring compared to Cluster 2 and Cluster 4 in terms of statistical significance. Cluster 1 is most likely to undergo an abdominoplasty surgical correction, which is directly related to their age, BMI, and weight loss method.
- Cluster 4 consists of patients with a similar BMI value and age, compared to Cluster 1. The difference here is the higher percentage of patients who have chosen bariatric procedure as weight loss method. This choice results in massive weight loss, dominant skin excess in all areas of the body and most often the first choice of surgical intervention—abdominoplasty (similar to Cluster 2).
- Cluster 5 consists of young patients under the age of 30, in whom there is no reduction in weight, and due to obesity their leading diagnosis is lipomatosis and, accordingly, their leading choice of surgical technique is liposuction (Fig. 1).

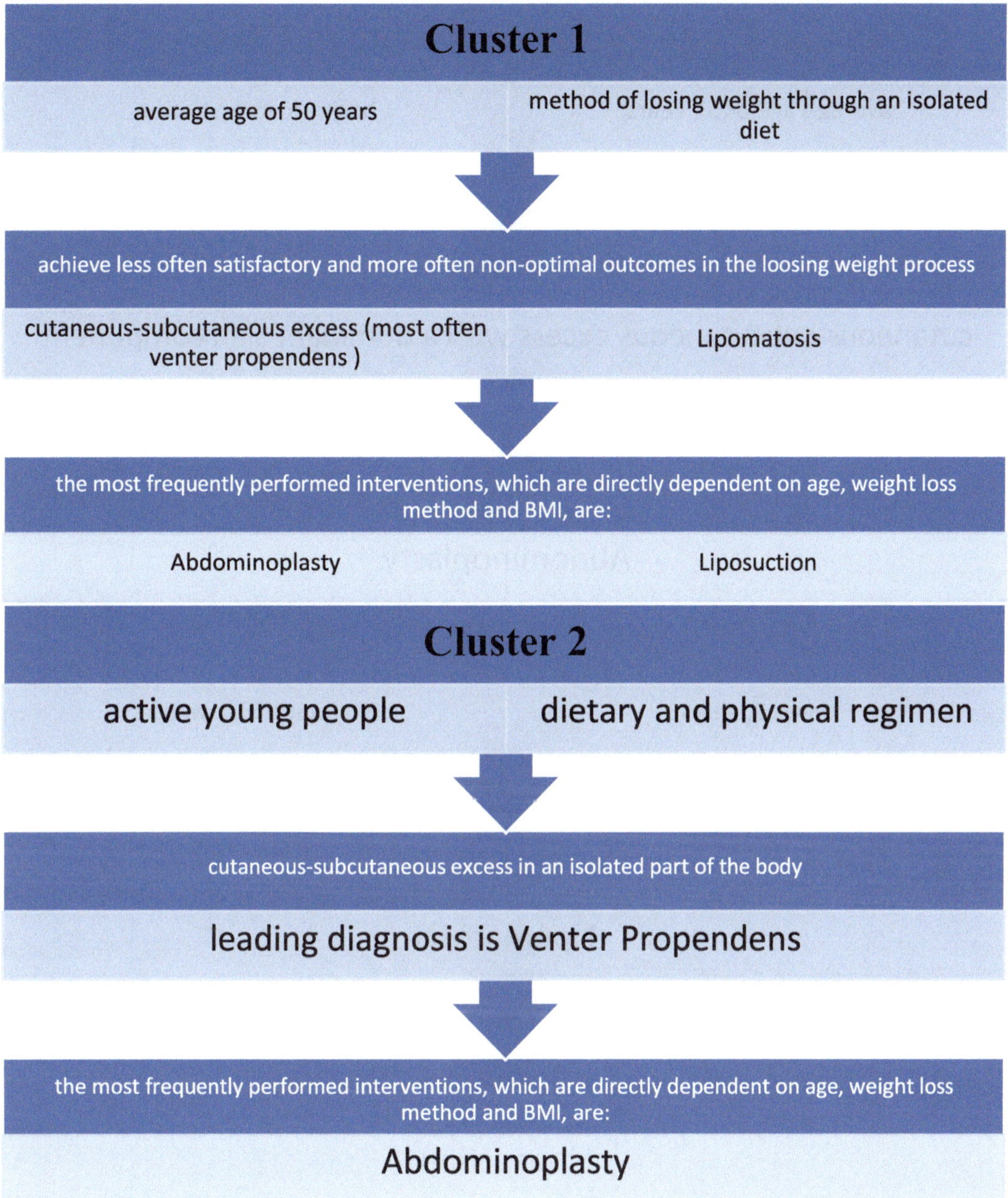

Fig. 1 Algorithm for predicting surgical interventions

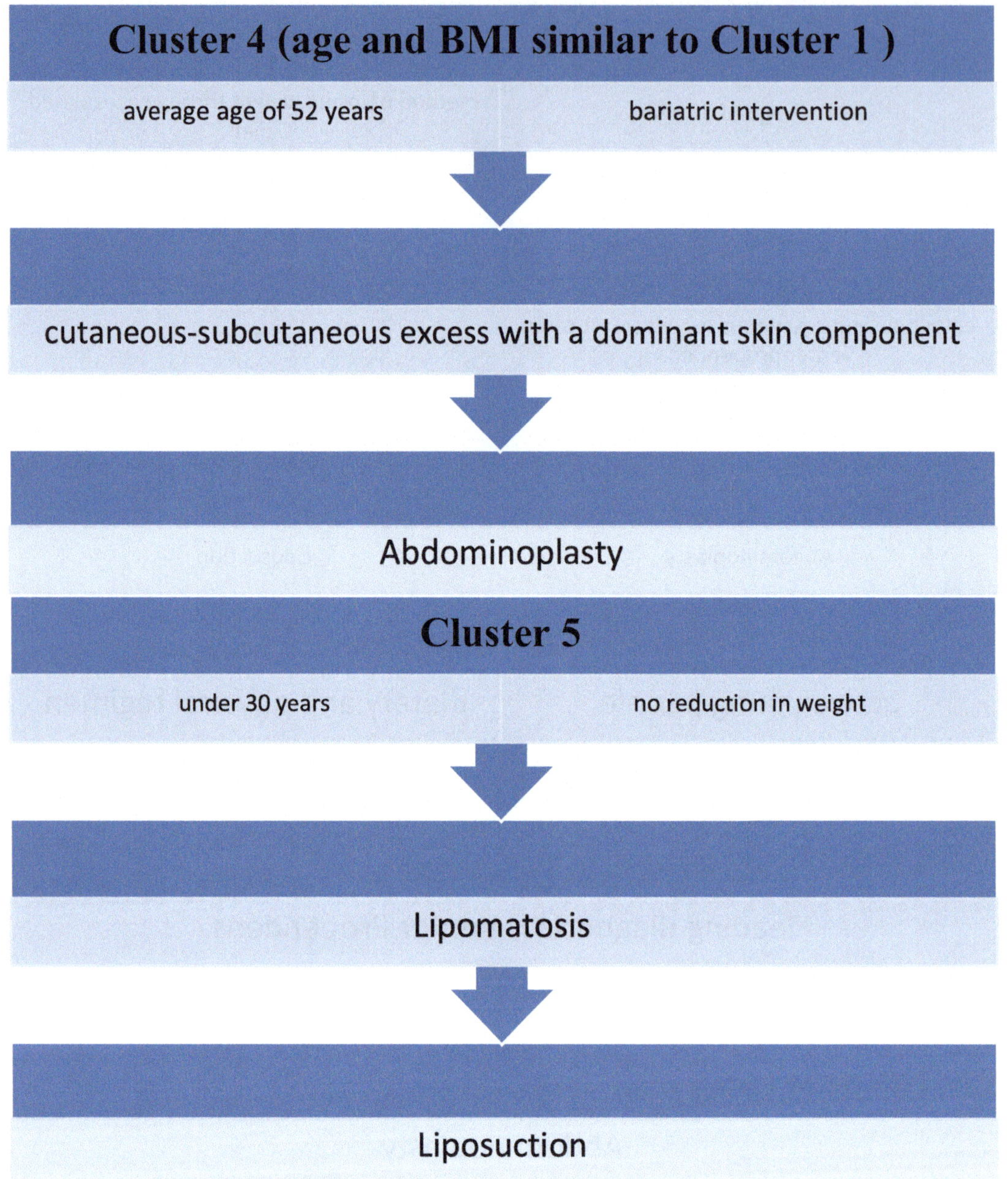

Fig. 1 (continued)

Body Contouring Surgery: Summary

The procedures aimed at contouring the body involve an extremely diverse group of interventions both in terms of invasiveness and in terms of technology used—ultrasound, radiofrequency, vibration-based. The author describes the possible combinations preferred in his practice in order to achieve optimal results and at the same time a low risk of possible side effects.

The described procedures vary from non-invasive through minimally invasive to excisional surgical interventions.

The author demonstrates the use of non-invasive procedures—EVOLVE X™ radiofrequency stimulation; TrueSculptFlex myostimulation; ultherapy ultrasound technology, which he applies to optimize the final results in the postoperative period, and in certain cases also to treat an undesirable reaction.

Use of minimally invasive techniques according to the type of radiofrequency interventions: BodyTite™, FaceTite™, AccuTite™, Morpheus8™, Morpheus8 body™ are widely used in the author's practice, emphasizing both their isolated application and their combination with other minimally invasive and/or surgical procedures. Their use in the postoperative period is also demonstrated in order to optimize the results and correct unsatisfactory results. Special attention is paid to the type and method of application of the radiofrequency intervention, which the author prefers and considers to be the safest one when combined with an excisional technique. The author's preferred combinations with ultrasound procedures and vibration-based liposuction are described.

The author uses u VASERlipo® ultrasound technology in his practice in order to achieve smoother results when contouring the body and/or defining specific muscle groups. Combinations with radiofrequency interventions are indicated—the combination with Morpheus8 Body™ is preferred by the author in most cases for additional tightening of the skin. Combinations with excisional procedures are described, which the author successfully applies, given the vessel-sparing effect of ultrasound energy.

MicroAire® vibration liposuction is a preferred option of the lipoaspiration technique, which the author considers to be sparing in terms of the operator's workload and, even more importantly, extremely contributory in terms of definition in body contouring procedures.

The author describes excisional surgical techniques used by him in different parts of the body. The results of both isolated excisional procedures and a combination with minimally invasive techniques are presented. Combinations in the treatment of neighboring areas of the body to optimize the final result are described.

The author adjusts the choice of his approach both to the preoperative status of the patient and to the set goal as a final result, and last but not least to minimize the likelihood of side effects.

E. Sharkov, *Body Contouring Surgery*, https://doi.org/10.1007/978-3-031-33350-7_19

In conclusion, we can say that the possible variations in the combinations of procedures with different degree of invasiveness and different type of technology are endless. Based on his own clinical experience and the available scientific literature, the author attempts to summarize the combinations of techniques in the treatment of different areas of the body, which are preferred by him, optimal in terms of aesthetics and minimal in terms of risk.

GPSR Compliance

The European Union's (EU) General Product Safety Regulation (GPSR) is a set of rules that requires consumer products to be safe and our obligations to ensure this.

If you have any concerns about our products, you can contact us on ProductSafety@springernature.com

In case Publisher is established outside the EU, the EU authorized representative is:

Springer Nature Customer Service Center GmbH
Europaplatz 3
69115 Heidelberg, Germany

Batch number: 10406427

Printed by Printforce, the Netherlands